BMTCN® Certification Review Manual

Edited by
Beth Faiman, PhD, MSN, APRN-BC, AOCN®

Oncology Nursing Society
Pittsburgh, Pennsylvania

ONS Publications Department

Publisher and Director of Publications: William A. Tony, BA, CQIA
Managing Editor: Lisa M. George, BA
Assistant Managing Editor: Amy Nicoletti, BA, JD
Acquisitions Editor: John Zaphyr, BA, MEd
Copy Editors: Vanessa Kattouf, BA, Andrew Petyak, BA
Graphic Designer: Dany Sjoen
Editorial Assistant: Judy Holmes

Library of Congress Cataloging-in-Publication Data

Names: Faiman, Beth, editor. | Oncology Nursing Society, issuing body.
Title: BMTCN certification review manual / edited by Beth Faiman.
Other titles: Blood & marrow transplant certified nurse certification review
  manual
Description: Pittsburgh, Pennsylvania : Oncology Nursing Society, [2016] |
  Includes bibliographical references and index.
Identifiers: LCCN 2016025545 | ISBN 9781935864882
Subjects: | MESH: Bone Marrow Transplantation--nursing | Hematopoietic Stem
  Cell Transplantation--nursing | Oncology Nursing | Certification | United
  States | Examination Questions
Classification: LCC RD123.5 | NLM WY 18.2 | DDC 617.4/410592--dc23 LC record available at https://lccn.loc
  .gov/2016025545

Publisher's Note

This book is published by the Oncology Nursing Society (ONS). ONS neither represents nor guarantees that the practices described herein will, if followed, ensure safe and effective patient care. The recommendations contained in this book reflect ONS's judgment regarding the state of general knowledge and practice in the field as of the date of publication. The recommendations may not be appropriate for use in all circumstances. Those who use this book should make their own determinations regarding specific safe and appropriate patient care practices, taking into account the personnel, equipment, and practices available at the hospital or other facility at which they are located. The editor and publisher cannot be held responsible for any liability incurred as a consequence from the use or application of any of the contents of this book. Figures and tables are used as examples only. They are not meant to be all-inclusive, nor do they represent endorsement of any particular institution by ONS. Mention of specific products and opinions related to those products do not indicate or imply endorsement by ONS. Websites mentioned are provided for information only; the hosts are responsible for their own content and availability. Unless otherwise indicated, dollar amounts reflect U.S. dollars.

ONS publications are originally published in English. Publishers wishing to translate ONS publications must contact ONS about licensing arrangements. ONS publications cannot be translated without obtaining written permission from ONS. (Individual tables and figures that are reprinted or adapted require additional permission from the original source.) Because translations from English may not always be accurate or precise, ONS disclaims any responsibility for inaccuracies in words or meaning that may occur as a result of the translation. Readers relying on precise information should check the original English version.

Printed in the United States of America

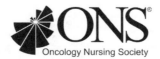

Innovation • Excellence • Advocacy

To my husband Matthew, son Max,
and family and friends.
I am thankful to have you all in my life and truly
appreciate all of your support.

Contributors

Editor

Beth Faiman, PhD, MSN, APRN-BC, AOCN®
Nurse Practitioner, Multiple Myeloma Program
Cleveland Clinic
Cleveland, Ohio

Authors

Daniela J. Casbourne, MSN, APRN, FNP-BC, AOCNP®
Lead Advanced Practice Provider, Inpatient Service
Bone Marrow and Stem Cell Transplantation Department
Winship Cancer Institute of Emory University
Atlanta, Georgia
Chapter 2. Types of Transplants and Sources of Stem Cells

Christina Ferraro, MSN, RN, NP-C, OCN®, BMTCN®
Blood and Marrow Transplant Nurse Coordinator
Cleveland Clinic, Taussig Cancer Institute
Cleveland, Ohio
Chapter 4. Transplant Preparative Regimens, Cellular Infusion, Acute Complications, and Engraftment

Ima N. Garcia, RN, MSN, ACNP-BC, AOCNP®
Nurse Practitioner, Community Hematology Liaison
The Medical Affairs Company
Chicago, Illinois
Chapter 6. Post-Transplant Issues

Rita M. Jakubowski, MSN, RN, OCN®, ANP-BC, BMTCN®
Senior Oncology Nurse Practitioner
Clinical Program Manager, Bone Marrow Transplant Program
Mount Sinai Hospital
New York, New York
Chapter 5. Graft-Versus-Host Disease

Heather Koniarczyk, MSN, NP-C, AOCNP®
Blood and Marrow Transplant Nurse Practitioner
Cleveland Clinic, Taussig Cancer Institute
Cleveland, Ohio
Chapter 4. Transplant Preparative Regimens, Cellular Infusion, Acute Complications, and Engraftment

Martha Lassiter, RN, MSN, AOCNS®, BMTCN®
Clinical Nurse Specialist
Adult Blood and Marrow Transplant Program
Duke University Health System
Durham, North Carolina
Chapter 1. Basic Concepts and Indications for Transplantation

Kimberly Noonan, RN, ANP, AOCN®
Nurse Practitioner, Multiple Myeloma
Dana-Farber Cancer Institute
Boston, Massachusetts
Chapter 6. Post-Transplant Issues

Rebecca Norton, MSN, RN, CCRN
SICU/CTICU Clinical Nurse Educator
North Florida/South Georgia Veterans Health System
University of Florida College of Nursing
Adjunct Clinical Assistant Professor
Oncology
University of Florida Health Shands Hospital
Gainesville, Florida
Chapter 6. Post-Transplant Issues

Lisa A. Pinner, RN, MSN, CPON®, BMTCN®
Nurse Educator
Lucile Packard Children's Hospital Stanford
Palo Alto, California
Chapter 7. Survivorship Issues

**Renee Spinks, MSN, APRN, ACNS-BC,
  AOCNS®**
Clinical Nurse Specialist—Oncology Services
Emory University Hospital
Atlanta, Georgia
Chapter 3. Pretransplant Issues

**Kelli Thoele, MSN, RN, ACNS-BC, BMTCN®,
  OCN®**
Clinical Nurse Specialist
Indiana University Health
Indianapolis, Indiana
Chapter 8. Professional Practice

D. Kathryn Tierney, RN, PhD, BMTCN®
Clinical Assistant Professor
School of Medicine
Stanford University
Oncology Clinical Nurse Specialist
Stanford Health Care
Palo Alto, California
Chapter 7. Survivorship Issues

Disclosure

Editors and authors of books and guidelines provided by the Oncology Nursing Society are expected to disclose to the readers any significant financial interest or other relationships with the manufacturer(s) of any commercial products.

A vested interest may be considered to exist if a contributor is affiliated with or has a financial interest in commercial organizations that may have a direct or indirect interest in the subject matter. A "financial interest" may include, but is not limited to, being a shareholder in the organization; being an employee of the commercial organization; serving on an organization's speakers bureau; or receiving research funding from the organization. An "affiliation" may be holding a position on an advisory board or some other role of benefit to the commercial organization. Vested interest statements appear in the front matter for each publication.

Contributors are expected to disclose any unlabeled or investigational use of products discussed in their content. This information is acknowledged solely for the information of the readers.

The contributors provided the following disclosure and vested interest information:

Christina Ferraro, MSN, RN, NP-C, OCN®, BMTCN®: Sanofi, Spectrum, consultant or advisory role and honoraria

D. Kathryn Tierney, RN, PhD, BMTCN®: American Society for Blood and Marrow Transplantation, Oncology Nursing Society, honoraria; Stanford Cancer Institute, research funding

Contents

Preface

For nearly 75 years, researchers have been determined to find a cure for blood and marrow cancers, solid tumors, and other genetic or immune disorders. Hematopoietic stem cell transplantation (HSCT) is a critical maneuver for many, with origins that date back to the 1940s. It wasn't until the mid-20th century that the first successful transplants were performed in humans. In the 1970s, the first indications for transplantation were identified. Subsequent investigations into the safety and efficacy of HSCT in special populations—such as in older individuals and those with organ dysfunction—and solid tumor malignancies transpired.

As of 2016, the HSCT strategy has never been safer due to ongoing advancements and improvements in the science behind transplant. Better therapies exist to treat and support a variety of hematologic cancers and blood disorders. These therapies have been shown to minimize side effects such as nausea, neutropenia, and graft-versus-host disease. Innovative procedures have been shown to improve transplant-related outcomes. Nurses have been integral to the advancement of transplant science throughout the years, especially in their knowledge of supportive care, side effect management, and patient support and education. Bone marrow transplant (BMT) nurses can now be recognized for their skills, knowledge, and dedication to patients.

The Oncology Nursing Certification Corporation and the Oncology Nursing Society (ONS) recognize the crucial role of oncology nurses and support validation of nurses' knowledge through specialty blood and marrow transplant certified nurse (BMTCN®) certification.

This study manual follows the BMTCN® Test Content Outline (Test Blueprint). Each chapter contains carefully written study questions to prepare specialty BMT nurses for the certification examination. Whether the reader is a nurse on the front line, a nurse scientist, or a nurse manager, this study manual will be an important resource for the examination for years to come.

Acknowledgments

This study manual has been in development for more than two years. I would like to gratefully acknowledge Charise Gleason for her numerous contributions to the development of this manual. Charise is an adult practitioner in the bone marrow transplant program at the Winship Cancer Institute of Emory University in Atlanta, Georgia. She started as a hematology/oncology nurse at Emory in 1998 and joined the Bone Marrow and Stem Cell Transplant Center as a nurse practitioner in 2003. Charise specializes in multiple myeloma, as well as post-transplant complications. She helped to develop the design and content, recruited authors, and provided critical review of this study manual.

I also would like to acknowledge all of the patients, nurses, and colleagues who inspire me to continue learning every day. Without their presence, encouragement, and unwavering support, this study manual would not have been possible.

Abbreviations

AACN—American Association of Critical-Care Nurses
ACP—advance care planning
ADH—antidiuretic hormone
ADL—activities of daily living
AHSCT—autologous hematopoietic stem cell transplantation
ALC—absolute lymphocyte count
allo-HSCT—allogeneic hematopoietic stem cell transplantation
AML—acute myeloid leukemia
AMS—altered mental status
ANA—American Nurses Association
ANC—absolute neutrophil count
APC—antigen-presenting cell
APRN—advanced practice registered nurse
aPTT—activated partial thromboplastin time
ASBMT—American Society for Blood and Marrow Transplantation
ATG—antithymocyte globulin
ATP—adenosine triphosphate
AV—atrioventricular
AVN—avascular necrosis
BCNU—carmustine (bis-chloroethylnitrosourea)
BEAM—carmustine, etoposide, cytarabine, melphalan
BID—twice a day
BMT—bone marrow transplant
BMTCN—blood and marrow transplant certified nurse
BMT CTN—Blood and Marrow Transplant Clinical Trials Network
BSA—body surface area
BUN—blood urea nitrogen
Ca—calcium
CBC—complete blood count
CD—cluster designation
cGy—centigray
CINV—chemotherapy-induced nausea and vomiting
CIVI—continuous intravenous infusion
CML—chronic myeloid leukemia
CMV—cytomegalovirus
CNI—calcineurin inhibitor

CNS—central nervous system
CSC—corrected serum calcium
CT—computed tomography
CTCAE—Common Terminology Criteria for Adverse Events
CTEP—Cancer Therapy Evaluation Program (National Cancer Institute)
DEXA—dual-energy x-ray absorptiometry
DHHS—U.S. Department of Health and Human Services
DIC—disseminated intravascular coagulation
DLI—donor lymphocyte infusion
DMSO—dimethyl sulfoxide
DNA—deoxyribonucleic acid
EBMT—European Society for Blood and Marrow Transplantation
EBP—evidence-based practice
EBV—Epstein-Barr virus
ECG—electrocardiogram
ECP—extracorporeal photopheresis
ELISA—enzyme-linked immunosorbent assay
EOL—end of life
EPO—erythropoietin
FA—Fanconi anemia
FACT—Foundation for the Accreditation of Cellular Therapy
FDA—U.S. Food and Drug Administration
FDP—fibrin degradation product
FEV$_1$—forced expiratory volume in one second
5-HT$_3$—5-hydroxytryptamine-3
FSH—follicle-stimulating hormone
FVC—forced vital capacity
G-CSF—granulocyte–colony-stimulating factor
GI—gastrointestinal
GM-CSF—granulocyte macrophage–colony-stimulating factor
GVD—graft-versus-disease
GVHD—graft-versus-host disease
GVT—graft-versus-tumor
Gy—gray
HbA—hemoglobin A
HBV—hepatitis B virus
HCM—hypercalcemia of malignancy
HEPA—high-efficiency particulate air

Hgb—hemoglobin
HHM—humoral hypercalcemia of malignancy
HHV—human herpesvirus
HIV—human immunodeficiency virus
HL—Hodgkin lymphoma
HLA—human leukocyte antigen
HPV—human papillomavirus
HRT—hormone replacement therapy
HSCT—hematopoietic stem cell transplantation
HSV—herpes simplex virus
HUS—hemolytic uremic syndrome
ICN—International Council of Nurses
ICU—intensive care unit
IgG—immunoglobulin G
IL—interleukin
IM—intramuscular
IOM—Institute of Medicine
IRB—institutional review board
ISCT—International Society for Cellular Therapy
ITP—idiopathic thrombocytopenic purpura
IU—international unit(s)
IV—intravenous
IVIG—intravenous immunoglobulin
JACIE—Joint Accreditation Committee of ISCT and EBMT
LDH—lactate dehydrogenase
LFT—liver function test
LH—luteinizing hormone
LLN—lower limit of normal
mAb—monoclonal antibody
MAHA—microangiopathic hemolytic anemia
MDS—myelodysplastic syndrome
MM—multiple myeloma
MMR—measles, mumps, and rubella
M-PTLD—monomorphic post-transplant lympho-proliferative disorder
MRD—matched related donor
MRI—magnetic resonance imaging
MTX—methotrexate
MUD—matched unrelated donor
Na—sodium
NCCN—National Comprehensive Cancer Network
NCI—National Cancer Institute
NCSBN—National Council of State Boards of Nursing
NIH—National Institutes of Health
NK—natural killer
NMDP—National Marrow Donor Program
ONS—Oncology Nursing Society
PBSC—peripheral blood stem cell
PCP—*Pneumocystis jiroveci* pneumonia (formerly *Pneumocystis carinii* pneumonia)

PCR—polymerase chain reaction
PFT—pulmonary function test
pH—hydrogen ion concentration
PO—oral (*per os*)
POF—premature ovarian failure
P-PTLD—polymorphic post-transplant lymphopro-liferative disorder
PRN—as needed
PT—prothrombin time
PTG—post-traumatic growth
PTH—parathyroid hormone
PTLD—post-transplant lymphoproliferative disor-der
PTSD—post-traumatic stress disorder
QOL—quality of life
RBC—red blood cell
Rh—rhesus
RIC—reduced-intensity conditioning
RNA—ribonucleic acid
SAA—severe aplastic anemia
SC—subcutaneous
SCID—severe combined immunodeficiency
SD—standard deviation
SIADH—syndrome of inappropriate antidiuretic hormone secretion
SOB—shortness of breath
SOS—sinusoidal obstruction syndrome
t-AML—therapy-related acute myeloid leukemia
TA-TMA—transplant-associated thrombotic micro-angiopathy
TB—*Mycobacterium tuberculosis*
TBI—total body irradiation
TBW—total body water
Th 1—helper T cell type 1 subset
TID—three times a day
TJC—Joint Commission
TLS—tumor lysis syndrome
t-MDS—therapy-related myelodysplastic syndrome
TMP-SMX—trimethoprim-sulfamethoxazole
TNF—tumor necrosis factor
TNF-α—tumor necrosis factor-alpha
TPN—total parenteral nutrition
TRT—testosterone replacement therapy
TTP—thrombotic thrombocytopenic purpura
UCB—umbilical cord blood
VOD—veno-occlusive disease
VRE—vancomycin-resistant *Enterococcus*
VREB—VRE bacteremia
VZV—varicella-zoster virus
WBC—white blood cell
WHO—World Health Organization

CHAPTER 1

Basic Concepts and Indications for Transplantation

Martha Lassiter, RN, MSN, AOCNS®, BMTCN®

I. Introduction
  A. The immune system comprises various components that work in tandem to provide immunity and maintain homeostasis. The use of hematopoietic stem cell transplantation (HSCT) to treat various malignant and nonmalignant diseases in the last 30 years has become an increased standard treatment for many conditions. Knowledge of basic concepts of HSCT provides a foundation for understanding the intricacies of transplantation to provide quality care and better support to patients and their families.
    1. Basic concepts of transplantation (Devine, 2013)
       a) Hematopoiesis and immunology provide the scientific basis for HSCT. Two types of bone marrow exist: red bone marrow and yellow bone marrow. Red bone marrow produces hematopoietic stem cells that create red blood cells, white blood cells, and platelets and is found in the long and flat bones. Yellow bone marrow and fat cells produce stromal stem cells that produce fat, cartilage, and bone and are found in the long bones.
       b) Components of hematopoiesis
          (1) Hematopoietic stem cells develop prior to birth and are produced in the long bones during childhood and then the axial skeleton in adulthood.
          (2) Bone marrow microenvironment: The bone marrow stroma is the housing unit and hub of cellular activity.
          (3) Cellular adhesion molecules
          (4) Chemokines, cytokines
       c) The main objective of hematopoiesis is to maintain the peripheral blood with the proper level of blood components. The pluripotent stem cells mature and differentiate into the myeloid or lymphoid progenitor cells within the bone marrow (see Figure 1-1).
          (1) Myeloid progenitor cells mature into the following:
             (a) Megakaryocytes (produce platelets)
             (b) Erythrocytes
             (c) Mast cells
             (d) Myeloblasts

Figure 1-1. Hematopoiesis

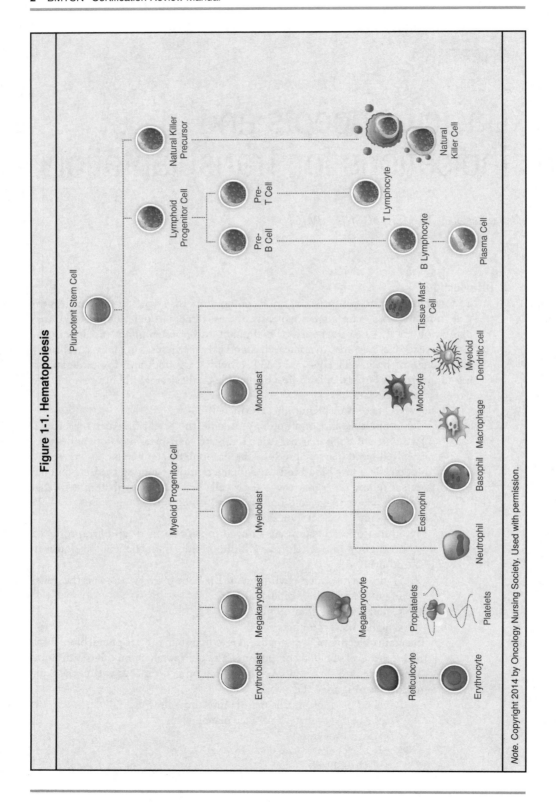

        (2) Lymphoid progenitor cells mature into the following:

            (a) Small lymphocytes, which differentiate into bone marrow–derived cells (B cells) and thymus-derived cells (T cells)

            (b) Natural killer (NK) cells

  d) Immune function is dependent on hematopoiesis.

  e) Primary organs of the immune system are involved in production, maturation, and immune activity.

        (1) Bone marrow

        (2) Thymus gland: Located in the anterior mediastinum and forms T cells

        (3) Lymph nodes: Bean-shaped glands that cluster throughout the body in the neck, chest, axillae, abdomen, and inguinal region and function as an immunologic filter

        (4) Spleen: Organ responsible for filtering white cells, platelets, and other substances

  f) The immune system consists of innate immunity and acquired immunity.

        (1) Innate immunity occurs naturally and uses phagocytes that release inflammatory mediators and NK cells.

        (2) Acquired immunity is the response of either B cells or T cells to antigens.

        (3) B-cell activation can be T-cell dependent or independent.

  g) Hematopoiesis is affected by senescence (loss of the cell's power to divide and grow) (Allsopp & Weissman, 2002; Nuss, Barnes, Fisher, Olson, & Skeens, 2011; Shao et al., 2013).

        (1) Hematopoietic stem cell senescence naturally occurs with age but also is affected by cancer treatment and transplantation.

        (2) Reduction in size of thymus and function of immune cells (not necessarily a reduction in number) is called *immunosenescence.*

        (3) Reduced size and function of thymus after puberty

        (4) Decreased cell-producing marrow with age

  h) Immune function

        (1) Myeloid cells are the first responders to injury and are not pathogen specific.

        (2) Lymphoid cells respond later and are pathogen specific.

2. Donor identification (allogeneic only) and types of transplantation (Bray et al., 2008). Types of transplant include autologous and allogeneic (see Table 1-1).

  a) Human leukocyte antigen high-resolution typing provides the degree of genetic match between a matched unrelated donor and a recipient in preparation for allogeneic transplantation.

  b) A better match is preferred because

        (1) Potential for improved overall survival with a matched donor and recipient

        (2) Reduced incidence of graft-versus-host disease (GVHD)

        (3) Improved engraftment rates

3. Role of the caregiver

  a) Provide physical and emotional support.

  b) Assist with physical recovery following HSCT.

  c) Assist with take-home medication administration.

Table 1-1. Types of Allogeneic Hematopoietic Stem Cell Transplantation

Type of Transplant	Cell Source	Advantages	Disadvantages
Syngeneic	Identical twin	No need for immuno-suppression	No graft-versus-tumor effect
Matched sibling/related	Human leukocyte antigen (HLA)-identical relative	No potential stem cell contamination Access to cells because donor is related	Only 25% of population has a sibling match Risk of graft-versus-host disease (GVHD)
Mismatched related	HLA-nonidentical relative	No potential stem cell contamination Increased number of potential donors	Increased risk of GVHD Increased risk of graft failure related to HLA disparity
Matched unrelated	HLA-identical unrelated donor	No potential stem cell contamination	Increased risk of GVHD Limited numbers of non-Caucasian donors Waiting period to identify donor
Mismatched unrelated	HLA-nonidentical unrelated donor	No potential stem cell contamination	Increased risk of GVHD High treatment-related mortality
Umbilical cord blood	Umbilical cord unit	Easy access to cell source	Limited number of cells Delayed time to engraftment Increased infection rates

Note. From "Basic Concepts of Transplantation" (p. 15), by D. Niess in S.A. Ezzone (Ed.), *Hematopoietic Stem Cell Transplantation: A Manual for Nursing Practice* (2nd ed.), 2013, Pittsburgh, PA: Oncology Nursing Society. Copyright 2013 by Oncology Nursing Society. Reprinted with permission.

      d) Perform care of central venous catheter (e.g., flushing and dressing changes).
      e) Assess for signs of infection (e.g., fevers).
      f) Monitor temperature.
      g) Perform food preparation.
      h) Provide transportation to and from the hospital or office.
      i) Aid in symptom identification.
      j) Communicate with healthcare team.
   4. Informal/family caregiver self-care
      a) Rest
      b) Balanced diet
      c) Exercise/stress reduction
      d) Management of personal health needs (e.g., medications) and personal support
   5. Goals of therapy
      a) Nonmalignant diseases: Cell line replacement (e.g., chronic granulomatous disease, sickle-cell disease, aplastic anemia)
      b) Malignant diseases: Tumor ablation

      6. Graft-versus-tumor effect
         a) Promoted by withdrawal of immunosuppressant therapy
         b) Promoted by donor lymphocyte infusions
         c) Decreased in the absence of acute GVHD
         d) Associated with higher rates of cancer relapse
      7. Immune reconstitution (Storek & Witherspoon, 2004)
         a) Dependent on patient's hematologic response to preparative regimen
         b) Dependent on rate of engraftment
         c) Dependent on survival and longevity of mature lymphocytes present at the time of transplant
         d) Delayed in patients with chronic GVHD
         e) Quantitative recovery of immune function does not always correlate with qualitative recovery.
         f) Immune reconstitution may take months to years.
      8. Phases of immune reconstitution
         a) Numeric recovery of bone marrow elements
         b) Functional recovery of cellular interactions
   B. Indications for transplantation (Pasquini & Zhu, 2016)
      1. Common malignant and nonmalignant diseases treated with HSCT (see Table 1-2)
      2. Autoimmune diseases treated under a clinical trial (Sullivan, Parkman, & Walters, 2000)
         a) Scleroderma
         b) Multiple sclerosis
         c) Systemic lupus erythematosus
         d) Rheumatoid arthritis
         e) Crohn disease

Table 1-2. Common Diseases Treated With Hematopoietic Stem Cell Transplant		
Type of Disease	**Autologous Transplant**	**Allogeneic Transplant**
Malignant		
Hematologic malignancies	Hodgkin disease Non-Hodgkin lymphoma Multiple myeloma	Acute lymphocytic leukemia Acute myeloid leukemia Chronic myeloid leukemia Myelodysplastic syndromes Non-Hodgkin lymphoma Juvenile myelomonocytic leukemia
Solid tumors	Neuroblastoma Sarcoma Germ cell tumors Brain tumors Breast cancer Ovarian cancer Melanoma Lung cancer	–

(Continued on next page)

Table 1-2. Common Diseases Treated With Hematopoietic Stem Cell Transplant *(Continued)*		
Type of Disease	**Autologous Transplant**	**Allogeneic Transplant**
Nonmalignant		
Hematologic	–	Severe aplastic anemia Fanconi anemia Thalassemia Sickle-cell disease Diamond-Blackfan anemia Chédiak-Higashi syndrome Chronic granulomatous disease Congenital neutropenia
Immunodeficiency	–	Severe combined immunodeficiency disease Wiskott-Aldrich syndrome Functional T-cell deficiency
Genetic	–	Adrenoleukodystrophy Metachromatic leukodystrophy Hurler syndrome Hunter disease Gaucher syndrome
Miscellaneous	–	Osteopetrosis Langerhans cell histiocytosis Glycogen storage diseases

Note. Based on information from Ezzone, 2009; Nuss et al., 2011; Pasquini & Wang, 2011.

From "Basic Concepts of Transplantation" (p. 14), by D. Niess in S.A. Ezzone (Ed.), *Hematopoietic Stem Cell Transplantation: A Manual for Nursing Practice* (2nd ed.), 2013, Pittsburgh, PA: Oncology Nursing Society. Copyright 2013 by Oncology Nursing Society. Reprinted with permission.

Key Points

- Nursing care of patients undergoing hematopoietic stem cell transplantation (HSCT) requires an understanding of basic hematopoiesis and immunology principles.

- As knowledge of the immune system has expanded, the patient population that might benefit from HSCT also has expanded beyond hematologic malignancies.

- Whether patients have a diagnosis of cancer or other illness, informal/family caregivers require rigorous education and support to assist with the necessary care throughout the transplant process and beyond into recovery and survivorship.

References

Allsopp, R.C., & Weissman, I.L. (2002). Replicative senescence of hematopoietic stem cells during serial transplantation: Does telomere shortening play a role? *Oncogene, 21,* 3270–3273. doi:10.1038/sj.onc.1205314

Bray, R.A., Hurley, C.K., Kamani, N.R., Woolfrey, A., Müller, C., Spellman, S., ... Confer, D.L. (2008). National Marrow Donor Program HLA matching guidelines for unrelated adult donor hematopoietic cell transplants. *Biology of Blood and Marrow Transplantation, 14*(Suppl. 9), 45–53. doi:10.1016/j.bbmt.2008.06.014

Devine, H. (2013). Overview of hematopoiesis and immunology: Implications for hematopoietic stem cell transplantation. In S.A. Ezzone (Ed.), *Hematopoietic stem cell transplantation: A manual for clinical practice* (2nd ed., pp. 1–12). Pittsburgh, PA: Oncology Nursing Society.

Ezzone, S.A. (2009). Blood and marrow transplantation. In B.H. Gobel, S. Triest-Robertson, & W.H. Vogel (Eds.), *Advanced oncology nursing certification review and resource manual* (pp. 261–303). Pittsburgh, PA: Oncology Nursing Society.

Niess, D. (2013). Basic concepts of transplantation. In S.A. Ezzone (Ed.), *Hematopoietic stem cell transplantation: A manual for nursing practice* (2nd ed., pp. 13–22). Pittsburgh, PA: Oncology Nursing Society.

Nuss, S., Barnes, Y., Fisher, V., Olson, E., & Skeens, M. (2011). Hematopoietic cell transplantation. In C. Baggott, D. Fochtman, G.V. Foley, & K.P. Kelly (Eds.), *Nursing care of children and adolescents with cancer and blood disorders* (4th ed., pp. 405–466). Glenview, IL: Association of Pediatric Hematology/Oncology Nurses.

Pasquini, M.C., & Wang, Z. (2011). Current use and outcome of hematopoietic stem cell transplantation: CIBMTR summary slides, 2011. Retrieved from http://www.cibmtr.org

Pasquini, M.C., & Zhu, X. (2016). Current uses and outcomes of hematopoietic stem cell transplantation: 2014 CIBMTR summary slides. Retrieved from http://www.cibmtr.org/referencecenter/slidesreports/summaryslides/Pages/index.aspx

Shao, L., Wang, Y., Chang, J., Luo, Y., Meng, A., & Zhou, D. (2013). Hematopoietic stem cell senescence and cancer therapy-induced long-term bone marrow injury. *Translational Cancer Research, 2,* 397–411. doi:10.3978/j.issn.2218-676X.2013.07.03

Storek, J., & Witherspoon, R.P. (2004). Immunological reconstitution after hemopoietic stem cell transplantation. In K. Atkinson, R. Champlin, J. Ritz, W.E. Fibbe, P. Ljungman, & M.K. Brenner (Eds.), *Clinical bone marrow and blood stem cell transplantation* (3rd ed., pp. 194–226). New York, NY: Cambridge University Press.

Sullivan, K.M., Parkman, R., & Walters, M.C. (2000). Bone marrow transplantation for non-malignant disease. *American Society of Hematology Education Book, 2000,* 319–338. doi:10.1182/asheducation-2000.1.319

Study Questions

1. Which of the following is an example of a myeloid cell?
   A. Thymus-derived cells (T cells)
   B. Bone marrow–derived cells (B cells)
   C. Monocytes
   D. Natural killer cells

2. Several factors affect immune reconstitution following hematopoietic stem cell transplantation (HSCT). These include all of the following EXCEPT:
   A. Recipient's response to conditioning regimen
   B. Viral infections
   C. Chronic graft-versus-host disease
   D. Longevity of mature lymphocytes present at the time of transplant

3. Hematopoiesis occurs primarily in which area?
   A. Bone marrow
   B. Spleen
   C. Thymus gland
   D. Lymph nodes

4. Which of the following statements is true about innate immunity?
   A. It occurs in response to T-cell activation.
   B. It occurs in response to B-cell activation.
   C. It is a natural process that uses phagocytes that release inflammatory mediators in response to infections or illness.
   D. It is a natural process that occurs primarily in the spleen.

5. Which is NOT a common indication for allogeneic transplantation?
   A. Acute myeloid leukemia
   B. Myelodysplastic syndrome
   C. Chronic myeloid leukemia
   D. Breast cancer

6. Graft-versus-tumor effect is promoted by which of the following?
   A. Withdrawal of immunosuppressive therapy
   B. Administration of donor lymphocyte infusion
   C. A and B
   D. Increased dose of immunosuppressive therapy

7. Which of the following is NOT a role of a caregiver?
   A. Provide physical and emotional support.
   B. Assist with recovery following HSCT.
   C. Assist with medication administration.
   D. Recommend over-the-counter medications for management of post-HSCT symptoms.

CHAPTER 2

Types of Transplants and Sources of Stem Cells

Daniela J. Casbourne, MSN, APRN, FNP-BC, AOCNP®

I. Introduction

    A. Hematopoietic stem cell transplantation (HSCT) involves the infusion of stem cells from a donor to a recipient. Three general types of transplants exist—autologous, allogeneic, and syngeneic—as well as three sources of stem cells: peripheral blood, bone marrow, and umbilical cord blood (UCB). The type of transplant needed and the source of stem cells used are based on many factors, including the type of disease being treated, the age and condition of the patient, and the current disease state. Depending on the type of disease being treated, HSCT can be used as part of the initial disease management or may be reserved for relapse. HSCT can be used with the intent to cure or with the intent to consolidate initial treatments and achieve the greatest level of disease eradication prior to beginning maintenance therapies.

    B. The handling of stem cells is an important factor in providing quality patient care. If possible, stem cells should be collected and kept in a facility that is accredited by the Foundation for the Accreditation of Cellular Therapy (FACT). A FACT-accredited facility undergoes rigorous investigation and ongoing quality development that ensures appropriate handling and storage of stem cells. FACT uses evidence-based standards to ensure high-quality patient care and facilitate positive patient outcomes (FACT, 2012).

II. Types of transplants (Ezzone, 2009; Harris, 2010; Johns Hopkins Medicine, n.d.; National Marrow Donor Program, n.d.; Niess, 2013)

    A. Autologous: An autologous transplant is the process of removing stem cells from the patient with the intent to reinfuse the cells at a later date. Before they are able to have their stem cells collected, patients undergo testing to ensure that they are disease free or, in some cases, have only minimal residual disease.

        1. The stem cells are collected and then cryopreserved until they are needed. Stem cells can be stored indefinitely if they are kept in a very controlled environment. Prior to infusion, the stem cells are checked for viability. Adequate viability of cells is essential for the reconstitution of hematopoietic function of the bone marrow. A lethal dose of chemotherapy or radiation is given to the patient prior to stem cell infusion as well. This maneuver is called the *prepara-*

tive regimen, or conditioning regimen, and is the treatment portion of the autologous transplant. The conditioning regimen used is determined by the patient's disease and overall physical status. The stem cells then are reinfused or transplanted to rescue the hematopoietic function of the bone marrow after it has been destroyed by the lethal doses of conditioning agents. Preparative regimens will be discussed in Chapter 4.

2. Advantages of autologous transplant
   a) Easily available source of stem cells
   b) Decreased risk of side effects
   c) Early engraftment
   d) Low risk of graft-versus-host disease (GVHD)
3. Disadvantages of autologous transplant
   a) Contamination of stem cells by undetectable disease cells
   b) No chance of immunologic effect of graft-versus-tumor (GVT) to assist with control of relapse

B. Allogeneic: An allogeneic transplant is the process of infusing donor stem cells into a recipient. The main types of allogeneic transplants are matched related and matched unrelated.
1. Matched related donors are of genetic relation to the patient, most often a sibling.
2. Matched unrelated donors are found through a national database of volunteer donors; the largest registry is the National Marrow Donor Program. The database comprises more than 22.5 million potential adult donors and more than 600,000 cord blood units from around the world. Testing is done to determine the strength of match through human leukocyte antigen (HLA) typing.
   a) The degree of match is very important in relation to morbidity and mortality. The higher the degree of mismatch, the greater the likelihood that the recipient will develop life-threatening complications, such as GVHD. For this reason, donors are selected who have the best match possible for the patient. If an appropriate donor is not available, other treatment options may be chosen, as the risk of death outweighs the potential benefit.
   b) Haploidentical (or half-matched related)
   c) UCB
3. As with autologous transplants, patients who undergo an allogeneic transplant receive a conditioning regimen and then stem cell infusion of donor cells. The conditioning therapies of allogeneic transplants vary not only by disease, but also by the level of myeloablation. Intensity of conditioning regimens can be reduced, therefore allowing older or less robust patients to receive transplants.
4. Advantages of allogeneic transplant
   a) Disease-free stem cell source
   b) Potential for GVT effect
5. Disadvantages of allogeneic transplant
   a) Increased risk of side effects related to polypharmacy required post-transplant
   b) Medications needed that are related to transplant (i.e., immunosuppressive drugs)
   c) GVHD, both acute and chronic (see Chapter 5)
   d) Lifestyle changes related to ongoing risks of side effects (e.g., avoiding sun exposure)

C. Syngeneic: Syngeneic HSCT uses the stem cells of an identical twin.

1. The disease-free twin donates stem cells in the same way that the allogeneic donor does. The cells then are transplanted into the identical twin.
2. This type of transplant allows for a disease-free stem cell source to be used but does not carry any GVT effect. The donor does not require the use of immuno-suppression because identical twins have the same HLA typing.

D. Other cellular therapies: Other stem cell therapies can be used in the post-transplant setting, such as donor lymphocyte infusion (DLI).

1. DLI is an infusion of lymphocytes from the original stem cell donor given in the setting of relapsed disease after allogeneic transplant. This maneuver attempts to use the immune system to fight the tumor by inducing a GVT effect.
2. Although DLI can be very effective, it also carries an increased risk of inducing GVHD. It is important that the risk-benefit ratio is weighed carefully and that the patient is thoroughly educated on the possible outcomes of this treatment.
3. Can be used with relapsed disease
4. Toxicity can be significant if either severe GVHD or bone marrow toxicity from the DLI occurs. This treatment may be done without the use of further conditioning if the tumor burden is not progressing rapidly.
5. Patients with rapidly progressing tumors will need to receive chemotherapy prior to DLI to debulk the tumor burden.
6. Research is currently looking at the use of DLI in the post-allogeneic setting as prophylaxis in patient populations with high risk of relapse post-transplant.

III. Sources of stem cells (AABB, 2013; Ezzone, 2009; Holtick, 2014; Mohty et al., 2003; Niess, 2013; Nuss, Barnes, Fisher, Olson, & Skeens, 2011)

A. Peripheral blood: Peripheral blood stem cells (PBSCs) have become the most used source of stem cells in both autologous and allogeneic transplantation. The use of granulocyte–colony-stimulating factor (G-CSF) and plerixafor increases the production of stem cells. Stem cells are mobilized out of the marrow space and into the peripheral circulation and collected through apheresis.

1. Advantages of PBSCs
   a) Engraftment of neutrophils and platelets is typically faster.
   b) Procedure can be done in the outpatient setting.
   c) Collection is well tolerated by various age groups.
   d) Early regimen-related toxicity in the allogeneic setting is decreased.
   e) Hospitalization for recipient is shorter because of earlier engraftment.
   f) An increased immunologic function is evident compared to bone marrow.
   g) No anesthesia is necessary for donor.
2. Disadvantages of PBSCs
   a) Procedure may require a central line for collection.
   b) Collection may take several days to get an adequate number of cells (possibly due to age, prior therapy, and diagnosis).
   c) Apheresis process has many possible side effects (e.g., electrolyte imbalances, thrombocytopenia).
   d) Source contains more CD34+ cells than bone marrow (related to GVHD in the allogeneic setting).
   e) An increased risk of chronic GVHD exists in the allogeneic setting.

B. Bone marrow: Prior to the discovery of G-CSF or granulocyte macrophage–colony-stimulating factor, bone marrow was the only source of stem cells. Stem cells are collected from the bone marrow by multiple needle aspirations of the marrow from the posterior or anterior iliac crests. This procedure requires that the donor undergo general anesthesia in the operating department. The marrow is mixed with an anticoagulant, and unwanted cells are filtered out. If the donor and recipient have different blood types, the product can be washed and the red cells removed.

   1. Advantages of bone marrow
      a) Harvest can be completed in a few hours.
      b) Generally well tolerated and is an outpatient procedure
      c) Decreased risk of GVHD in the allogeneic setting
   2. Disadvantages of bone marrow
      a) Requires general or epidural anesthesia
      b) Standard surgical risks of infection, bleeding, and pain at surgical site and bone damage
      c) Longer time to engraftment of cell lines
C. UCB: UCB is a rich source of stem cells. The cells are taken directly from the umbilical cords and placentas of newborn infants directly after birth. The collection of these stem cells causes no harm to the infant or mother. The cells are processed and stored in registries for later use. The cells in UCB are used when a true HLA match cannot be found in the unrelated donor registry. The stem cells in UCB have not reached immunologic maturity, allowing for a less stringent match with the potential recipient. Use of UCB in adults is limited by the size of the recipient. At times, more than one UCB unit can be used to increase the number of stem cells in the transplant. The number of stem cells, rather than identical HLA match, in a UCB transplant is a primary factor in determining outcomes and survival.

   1. Advantages of UCB
      a) Ease of access to cord blood units
      b) Short time from selection of cord blood unit until available for use
      c) Simple collection process with no harm to infant or mother
      d) Lower risk of GVHD
      e) Decreased risk of viral disease transmission
   2. Disadvantages of UCB
      a) Increased risk for passage of genetic abnormalities
      b) Limited use because of the number of stem cells in any given unit
      c) Slower engraftment than bone marrow or PBSCs
      d) Delayed post-transplant immune reconstitution
      e) Decreased GVT effect
      f) Increased risk of graft failure
      g) Impossible to get more donor cells if needed
      h) Cost

IV. Conclusion
   A. The process of stem cell transplantation has changed drastically since the first stem cell transplant was performed. Three main types of transplantations exist: autologous, syngeneic, and allogeneic. Three options for stem cell sources are used: PBSCs, bone marrow, and UCB.
   B. Strides have been made in the field of transplantation, but further research is needed to better understand the ongoing side effects that continue to cause morbidity and mortality in the peri- and post-transplant settings.

Key Points

- An autologous transplant is the process of removing stem cells from the patient with the intent to reinfuse the cells at a later date.

- An allogeneic transplant is the process of infusing donor stem cells into a recipient. Two types of allogeneic transplants exist: matched related donor and matched unrelated donor.

- The type of transplant needed and the source of stem cells used are based on many factors. Some of these factors include the type of disease being treated, the age and condition of the patient, and the current disease state.

- Three different stem cell sources are available: peripheral blood stem cells, bone marrow, and umbilical cord blood.

References

AABB. (2013). *Circular of information for the use of cellular therapy products.* Retrieved from http://www.aabb.org/aabbcct/coi/Pages/default.aspx

Ezzone, S.A. (2009). Blood and marrow transplantation. In B.H. Gobel, S. Triest-Robertson, & W.H. Vogel (Eds.), *Advanced oncology nursing certification review and resource manual* (pp. 261–303). Pittsburgh, PA: Oncology Nursing Society.

Foundation for the Accreditation of Cellular Therapy. (2012). *FACT-JACIE international standards for cellular therapy product collection, processing, and administration* [Version 5.3]. Omaha, NE: Author.

Harris, D.J. (2010). Transplantation. In J. Eggert (Ed.), *Cancer basics* (pp. 317–342). Pittsburgh, PA: Oncology Nursing Society.

Holtick, U., Albrecht, M., Chemnitz, J.M., Theurich, S., Skoetz, N., Scheid, C., & von Bergwelt-Baildon, M. (2014). Bone marrow versus peripheral blood allogeneic haematopoietic stem cell transplantation for haematological malignancies in adults. *Cochrane Database of Systematic Reviews, 2014*(4). doi:10.1002/14651858.CD010189.pub2

Johns Hopkins Medicine. (n.d.). Immunologic manipulations to treat blood and bone marrow cancers. Retrieved from http://www.hopkinsmedicine.org/kimmel_cancer_center/centers/bone_marrow_transplant/donor_lymphocyte_infusions.html

Mohty, M., Bilger, K., Jourdan, E., Kuentz, M., Michallet, M., Bourhis, J.H., … Blaise, D. (2003). Higher doses of CD34+ peripheral blood stem cells are associated with increased mortality from chronic graft-versus-host disease after allogeneic HLA-identical sibling transplantation. *Leukemia, 17,* 869–875. doi:10.1038/sj.leu.2402909

National Marrow Donor Program. (n.d.). Transplant basics. Retrieved from http://marrow.org/Transplant-Basics

Niess, D. (2013). Basic concepts of transplantation. In S.A. Ezzone (Ed.), *Hematopoietic stem cell transplantation: A manual for nursing practice* (2nd ed., pp. 13–21). Pittsburgh, PA: Oncology Nursing Society.

Nuss, S., Barnes, Y., Fisher, V., Olson, E., & Skeens, M. (2011). Hematopoietic cell transplantation. In C. Baggott, D. Fochtman, G.V. Foley, & K.P. Kelly (Eds.), *Nursing care of children and adolescents with cancer and blood disorders* (4th ed., pp. 405–466). Glenview, IL: Association of Pediatric Hematology/Oncology Nurses.

Study Questions

1. M.J. is to undergo an autologous transplant. From whom will he receive his stem cells?
   A. A matched related donor
   B. A matched unrelated donor
   C. An umbilical cord blood donor
   D. Himself

2. P.F. has undergone an allogeneic transplant using umbilical cord blood as the stem cell source. This makes her at higher risk for which of the following post-transplant complications?
   A. Graft failure
   B. Graft-versus-host disease
   C. Nausea and vomiting
   D. Complications of surgery

3. E.N. is worried about the post-transplant complication of graft-versus-host disease. Which stem cell sources have recently been shown to have decreased incidence of this serious and often debilitating problem?
   A. Umbilical cord blood and bone marrow
   B. Peripheral blood stem cells and umbilical cord blood
   C. Bone marrow and peripheral blood stem cells
   D. None of the above

CHAPTER 3

Pretransplant Issues

Renee Spinks, MSN, APRN, ACNS-BC, AOCNS®

I. Introduction
   A. The field of hematopoietic stem cell transplantation (HSCT) has evolved tremendously since the first successful allogeneic transplant for leukemia in the late 1960s (Niess, 2013). Advances in hematopoietic stem cell collection techniques, management of side effects, and the development of reduced-intensity preparative regimens have improved morbidity and mortality rates associated with stem cell transplants (Harris, 2010). However, HSCTs still carry many risks, including infection, chemotherapy toxicities, and, in the case of allogeneic transplants, graft-versus-host disease (GVHD) (Mitchell, 2009). The success of HSCT depends on matching recipients with optimal donors, collecting an adequate number of stem cells, and preparing patients and families for the challenges involved. All of these factors must be addressed well in advance of the transplant.
   B. Depending on the diagnosis, patients may undergo either an allogeneic or autologous transplant (Niess, 2013). An allogeneic transplant involves receiving cells from a related or unrelated donor with a goal of obtaining cells from an individual who is human leukocyte antigen (HLA) identical (Niess, 2013). In syngeneic transplants, the donor and recipient are identical twins, thus ensuring an exact HLA match. If a precise match is not possible, a transplant with a partial HLA match may be considered (Schmit-Pokorny, 2013). An autologous transplant involves the recipient receiving his or her own cells, which have been previously collected and cryopreserved (Niess, 2013).
   C. The Foundation for the Accreditation of Cellular Therapy (FACT) was formed in 1996 by the American Society for Blood and Marrow Transplantation and the International Society for Cellular Therapy to standardize quality practices in transplant centers. Participating in the FACT accreditation process is voluntary and indicates a commitment to providing the highest level of care to transplant recipients. This chapter explores key aspects of the preparation necessary for donors and recipients prior to HSCT. Issues examined include recipient eligibility and management; donor selection and care; and stem cell mobilization, collection, and storage (FACT, 2012). Educational requirements of both recipients and donors also are addressed. Bone marrow transplant nurses are in an ideal position to meet the complex needs of patients on both ends of the HSCT spectrum.

II. Recipient eligibility and management (Cohen, Jenkins, Holston, & Carlson, 2013; FACT, 2012; Harris, 2010; Mitchell, 2009; Niess, 2013)

A. Eligibility criteria: The HSCT process is no easy undertaking. Many factors are considered when determining whether a patient is a transplant candidate, and if so, for which type of transplant. Nonmyeloablative regimens have increased the opportunities for transplants in individuals older than age 65. Comorbidities, stage of cancer, performance status, and donor availability are all assessed when choosing a patient's treatment plan.

B. When determining eligibility, one of the first criterion to consider is whether the patient's disease is chemotherapy sensitive; this is more of a concern with autologous transplants.

C. In addition, it must be established that the patient has acceptable organ function and is free of life-threatening viral exposures or diseases.

D. An assessment of the patient's ability to comply with the regimen, including an assessment of available support systems, is essential.

E. Recipient evaluation and management: FACT has developed specific requirements for recipient evaluation prior to transplant. These requirements assess for adequate organ function, baseline disease status, and general health status. These must be evaluated with blood, urine, and other tests, which vary per institution.

1. Complete blood count with differential
2. Chemistry panel
   a) Electrolytes
   b) Liver and kidney function tests
3. Tests for multiple infectious diseases
   a) Hepatitis B and C
   b) HIV
   c) Human T-cell leukemia virus type 1
   d) Cytomegalovirus
   e) Herpes simplex virus and varicella-zoster virus
4. Other necessary laboratory tests
   a) Pregnancy testing for women of childbearing age
   b) ABO/Rh testing
   c) HLA testing for an allogeneic HSCT (allo-HSCT)
   d) Serology and rapid plasma reagin testing (FACT, 2012)

F. In general, common tests can evaluate organ function.

1. Multigated acquisition scan: Ideally, recipients will begin the transplant process with an ejection fraction of 50% or greater.
2. Echocardiogram
3. Electrocardiogram

G. Disease evaluation: Potential recipients undergo a complete assessment of their disease, which varies according to diagnosis.

1. Bone marrow aspirate and biopsy
2. Lumbar puncture
3. Computed tomography and/or magnetic resonance imaging scans
4. Bone scans or bone survey to assess skeletal involvement
5. Tumor markers
6. Depending on the diagnosis, patients may require a positron-emission tomography scan, as well as 24-hour urine electrophoresis, quantitative immunoglobulin tests, and urine catecholamines.

H. A comprehensive physical, psychosocial, and financial evaluation is required before patients can undergo transplantation.

      1. Physical
        a) Patients with significant medical issues (e.g., uncontrolled diabetes, active infections) may not be candidates for HSCT.
        b) Performance status is assessed, with the ideal candidate being able to independently carry out activities of daily living.
        c) Because neutropenia and mucositis are associated with the preparative regimen, a thorough dental examination is warranted to identify any early abscesses or issues with poor dentition that may become problematic during the transplant process.
      2. Psychosocial
        a) Assessment of coping skills
        b) Identification of potential problems, such as alcohol or drug abuse
        c) Identification of the family member or caregiver who will support the patient throughout the transplant process is critical.
      3. Financial: Because of the costly nature of HSCT, financial resources also are evaluated, including insurance coverage and other sources of payment.

III. Recipient and caregiver pretransplant education
    A. Nurses are in an optimal position to provide education to recipients and caregivers throughout the transplant process. Health literacy is defined as "the degree to which an individual has the capacity to obtain, communicate, process, and understand basic health information and services to make appropriate health decisions" (Institute of Medicine, 2004, p. 32). Cohen et al. (2013) conducted a qualitative study to gain perspective on the health literacy of stem cell transplant recipients. Their findings concluded that HSCT recipients often are overwhelmed and confused by the education they receive from healthcare teams. Considerations for teaching include the following:
      1. Patients with low health literacy commonly struggle to decipher the complex information provided by medical professionals. An ongoing evaluation of the patient's and caregiver's level of understanding must be conducted, and the nurse may be able to provide education in simple layman's terms to enhance comprehension.
      2. It is not uncommon for patients and family members to require multiple teaching sessions. Some patients may have undergone a transplantation in the past and have fewer educational needs.
    B. Education typically begins with an overview of the rationale, risks, and benefits of transplantation. Subsequent teaching topics include the following:
      1. Side effect identification
      2. Symptoms associated with transplant
      3. Infection identification, control, and prevention
      4. Care of the central venous catheter
      5. Review of the medication regimen
      6. It is important for transplant recipients to have a full understanding of the method being used to collect stem cells, including risks associated with anesthesia for those undergoing a bone marrow harvest and the side effects associated with mobilization drugs.

IV. Donor selection and care (Brunstein, Baker, & Wagner, 2007; Christopher, 2000; Confer & Miller, 2007; FACT, 2012; Glasgow & Bello, 2007; Harris, 2010; National Marrow Donor Program [NMDP], n.d.-a; Niess, 2013; Schmit-Pokorny, 2013; Wilkins & Woodgate, 2007)

A. Donor selection for allo-HSCT candidates
   1. Histocompatibility testing: The first step in selecting a donor for an allo-HSCT is to conduct histocompatibility testing or tissue typing to evaluate the HLA match between the donor's and recipient's antigens.
      a) HLAs are glycoproteins that reside on the surface of cells located on chromosome 6 and play a major role in the immune system's ability to recognize self versus nonself. HLAs are unique to each person, and their major action is to produce immune cells that destroy antigens. In the case of allo-HSCT, when donor cells with a different type of HLA from the recipient are infused, the T lymphocytes in the donor graft may perceive the patient's tissues as foreign. This can mount an immune response known as GVHD.
      b) Although an HLA match between the donor and recipient is not essential, it is associated with better outcomes and less risk of GVHD.
   2. ABO blood-type compatibility: Blood-type compatibility between the donor and recipient is not imperative. When bone marrow is collected, red blood cells (RBCs) can be filtered out to prevent RBC lysis after bone marrow infusion. After transplant, the recipient will eventually seroconvert to the donor's blood type.
B. Considerations in choosing the best donor for allo-HSCT
   1. Age of the donor and recipient
   2. HLA typing
   3. Type and stage of underlying disease (cancer or noncancer)
   4. The ideal scenario involves the patient receiving cells from a matched related donor (MRD) (typically a sibling).
   5. Receiving cells from an MRD leads to an increased likelihood of engraftment and less chance of complications. In cases where more than one related HLA-matched donor exists, additional factors are considered to select the most suitable donor.
      a) Family social dynamics
      b) Donor health concerns
      c) Cytomegalovirus serostatus
      d) Other logistics, such as travel and proximity to the recipient
   6. NMDP can be used to identify a matched donor.
      a) Approximately 70% of patients who require an allo-HSCT do not have a suitable MRD (NMDP, n.d.-a; Niess, 2013). These patients typically turn to NDMP to seek an appropriate donor.
      b) NMDP (n.d.-a) is a global network with more than 12 million volunteers registered as potential bone marrow donors and more than 200,000 registered umbilical cord blood (UCB) units.
      c) Providers search the registry to locate donors with HLA markers that match those of their patients. Of the individuals who are able to find a match through NMDP, about 56% will have more than 10 suitably matched donors (Confer & Miller, 2007).
      d) When multiple suitable matched unrelated donors exist, the healthcare team evaluates other criteria to choose the optimal donor. Confer and Miller (2007) determined the following.
         (1) An ideal donor would be a young male with a heavier weight.

(2) Providers tend to prefer male donors because of their relatively larger body size and ability to provide a larger stem cell donation.

(3) In the case of female donors, younger age and larger body size are preferable.

(4) In addition, because of the link between a history of previous pregnancies and a greater risk of GVHD, women with no prior pregnancies are preferred as donors.

7. Minority donors: A person usually is more likely to have an HLA match with someone from the same ethnic or racial background because HLA markers are inherited. Certain combinations of HLA markers are more common in some racial groups than others. Unfortunately, the majority of hematopoietic stem cell donors are Caucasian; fewer donors are of Hispanic or African American heritage.

   a) Glasgow and Bello (2007) found that several factors influence the likelihood of African Americans becoming bone marrow donors, including a mistrust of the U.S. healthcare system, concerns about donor expenses, and fears of getting an infection when donating. However, African Americans who were more likely to donate stated that the positive feeling associated with helping another person was a major motivating factor.

   b) NMDP strives to encourage individuals from all ethnic backgrounds to serve as donors, and intense outreach efforts to recruit diverse donors are underway.

8. UCB: Among patients who lack a suitable sibling donor, about 50% will have difficulty being matched with a donor through NMDP. In particular, patients who have rare HLA typing (e.g., ethnic minorities) may struggle to locate a suitable donor. Patients unable to find a matched donor may be able to undergo transplant with a haploidentical-related donor. Some studies have shown success with this approach, but more research is needed. Another possibility for patients struggling to find a donor is using UCB for a transplant.

   a) UCB transplantations are now frequently performed successfully in children.

   b) For adult recipients, adequate cell yield is an important factor with UCB transplantation.

   c) Double UCB transplantation, in which cord blood from more than one donor is used, is described in the literature as a safe option for adults who might otherwise not have a suitable cord blood sample available to them. UCB is evaluated at the time of collection for HLA typing, infectious disease, and cellular content.

C. Donor evaluation: The U.S. Food and Drug Administration regulations require allogeneic donors to undergo a complete evaluation that includes risk factor screening, review of medical records, a complete physical examination, and testing for pertinent communicable diseases. To avoid bias, FACT requires that the provider conducting the donor's health assessment be someone other than the intended recipient's primary transplant physician. The goal of the assessment is to rule out any health problems that could be a risk to the recipient or lead to adverse events for the donor during the donation process.

1. Blood samples are obtained from potential donors to assess for infectious diseases. Testing for infectious diseases should occur within 30 days prior to collection of hematopoietic stem cells. In addition, FACT guidelines state that a complete medical history should be obtained from potential donors, including vaccination and travel history, prior blood transfusions, and past history of malignant disease.

   2. Appropriate questions should be asked to determine whether a risk of transmission of any communicable diseases exists to the recipient.
      a) HIV
      b) Hepatitis
      c) Syphilis
      d) Cytomegalovirus
      e) Human T-lymphotropic virus
      f) Chagas disease (American trypanosomiasis)
      g) West Nile virus
   3. FACT guidelines require that all female donors of childbearing age have a pregnancy test within seven days prior to stem cell mobilization or collection or initiation of the recipient's preparative regimen (whichever occurs first).

V. Pediatric concerns: See Figure 3-1 for specific issues related to pretransplant care of children. Pediatric siblings of patients requiring a stem cell transplant may find themselves facing the prospect of serving as a donor and even being pressured by parents anxious to find treatment for their sick child. The psychosocial needs of sibling donors must be assessed throughout the transplant process.
   A. Wilkins and Woodgate (2007) conducted a qualitative study to examine the lived experience of siblings of bone marrow transplant patients. Some of the siblings served as donors while others did not. Common themes that arose during the study were a view of transplant by the siblings as an "interruption of family life," the view of life during the transplant process as no longer being "normal," and some siblings feeling isolated from their family.
   B. Nurses need to be aware of the special needs of sibling donors. Although minors cannot consent for themselves, they can provide assent and should be educated about every aspect of the donation process.
   C. Nurses and members of the multidisciplinary team must provide teaching at a level that is developmentally appropriate. Additionally, pediatric donors need to be given the opportunity to ask questions and voice their fears and anxieties.
      1. FACT recommends that a donor advocate be available to represent pediatric allogeneic donors.
      2. The advocate's role is to ensure that the donor understands the risks and benefits associated with donation and that the decision to donate is made without pressure and with adequate information.
      3. The donor advocate should be focused on the best interests of the child donor and should not be part of the recipient's direct care team.

VI. Donor preparation: FACT guidelines state that donors must receive detailed information about the donation process and undergo informed consent.
   A. Donors must be given the opportunity to ask questions and be reassured that they have the right to refuse to donate.
   B. To avoid the impression of coercion, the provider obtaining informed consent should be someone other than the intended recipient's primary transplant physician.
   C. The informed consent discussion must be documented.
   D. Donors also need to review the risks of donation, including the possible need for a central venous access device, the side effects of mobilization, and the risks associated with anesthesia in the case of bone marrow harvest.

Figure 3-1. Special Considerations for Pediatric Pretransplant Care

Recipient Preparation
- For children younger than age 18, consent for transplant needs to be obtained from the parent or guardian. However, children may sign an assent form that indicates their agreement with the plan.
- Child life specialists may be able to assist with the unique educational needs of children undergoing transplantation. Teaching should be geared toward the child's developmental stage.
- The Foundation for the Accreditation of Cellular Therapy requires that a donor advocate represent pediatric donors.

Donor Evaluation
- Because the parent or guardian gives consent for a child to donate stem cells to a sibling, care must be taken to avoid coercion.
- A thorough psychosocial and developmental assessment must take place for all pediatric donors.
- Wilkins and Woodgate (2007) found that feeling an interruption in family life and feeling isolated were common among siblings of transplant recipients.
- Umbilical cord blood (UCB) often is used for pediatric transplant recipients with success. UCB is processed immediately after harvesting and is quickly available when needed. In addition, graft-versus-host disease is less common in patients receiving UCB transplants.
- The National Marrow Donor Program will not accept individuals younger than age 18 to serve as an unrelated donor because legal informed consent is required. Pediatric stem cell donation is typically limited to sibling donation and autologous transplant.

Stem Cell Mobilization
- In the allogeneic setting, children older than age 13 typically undergo mobilization similar to adult donors.
- Some centers may be reluctant to collect stem cells via mobilization in patients younger than age 13; rather, cells typically are collected via bone marrow harvest.
- However, the use of granulocyte–colony-stimulating factor, chemotherapy, and plerixafor for mobilization in pediatric patients younger than age 13 undergoing autologous transplantation has been described in the literature.

Stem Cell Collection
- Care must be taken during apheresis to avoid excessive blood loss in children. Volume of blood processed must be based on the child's weight. Based on the child's tolerance, 200–250 ml/kg typically may be processed.
- To decrease blood loss during priming, an apheresis machine and tubing may be preprimed with irradiated red blood cells.
- Weight-based dosing of calcium gluconate may be used to prevent hypocalcemia.
- Few centers will use mobilization to harvest stem cells from sibling donors younger than age 13.

Note. Based on information from Emir et al., 2014; Foundation for the Accreditation of Cellular Therapy, 2012; National Marrow Donor Program, n.d.-b; Schmit-Pokorny, 2013; Wilkins & Woodgate, 2007.

    E. The medical team should educate donors about the diagnostic and laboratory tests that they will be required to undergo.

    F. Donors should be given information about the collection process, including potential risks and complications and possible outcomes that they or the recipient may experience.

    G. Donors must be taught how to seek medical attention if they have concerns or questions after collection.

    H. Nurses should be aware that serving as a stem cell donor can be a stressful experience. Christopher (2000) conducted a qualitative study to examine the experience of donating stem cells to a relative. Although most participants stated that they would donate cells again if given the opportunity, many admitted that stress was associated with donating and that they had concerns about negative outcomes for the recipient. Christopher concluded that formal donor support programs should be available and that donors should receive adequate education as well as an assessment of their coping skills.

VII. Stem cell procurement (Bensinger, DiPersio, & McCarty, 2009; Bishop et al., 1997; Camp-Sorrell, 2011; Devine, Tierney, Schmit-Pokorny, & McDermott, 2010; Devine et al., 2008; Emir et al., 2014; Faiman, Miceli, Noonan, & Lilleby, 2013; FACT, 2012; Harris, 2010; Mitchell, 2009; National Institutes of Health, n.d.-b, n.d.-c, n.d.-d; NMDP, n.d.-b; Niess, 2013; Sanofi-Aventis, 2013; Schmit-Pokorny, 2013)

A. The method used to obtain stem cells depends on the type of transplant the patient will receive. Cells may be either harvested from the bone marrow or collected from the peripheral blood using a technique called *apheresis* by first using stem cell mobilization.

B. Peripheral blood: The majority of transplants today (about 70%) are carried out using peripherally collected stem cells.

1. Advantages of using peripheral stem cells versus bone marrow cells
   a) Engraftment occurs faster because of a greater maturity of cells.
   b) No anesthesia risk exists because anesthesia is not required to collect peripheral cells.
   c) Stem cells collected peripherally may have a decreased likelihood of being contaminated with tumor cells.

2. The main disadvantage for recipients of peripheral stem cells is a higher risk of developing chronic GVHD. However, the T-lymphocyte cells responsible for causing GVHD may also be responsible for a desired graft-versus-tumor effect.
   a) Some patients do not require this added benefit, including those receiving a transplant for sickle-cell anemia or aplastic anemia.
   b) These patients may benefit from receiving cells harvested from the donor's bone marrow to reduce the risk of GVHD.

3. The success of stem cell procurement is measured by the number of CD34+ cells obtained. CD34+ is a protein expressed on the surface of hematopoietic stem cells found in the bone marrow and UCB. Studies have linked higher stem cell doses with increased patient survival rates and more rapid engraftment. Therefore, the mobilization strategy used is of utmost importance.

C. Stem cell mobilization

1. Mobilization is the process by which hematopoietic stem cells are released from the bone marrow into the peripherally circulating blood. Medications are used to stimulate production of hematopoietic cells and drive stem cells into the peripheral system. The goal of mobilization is to move an adequate number of hematopoietic stem cells into the peripheral blood capable of regeneration so that the patient can achieve engraftment following transplant. Stem cell mobilization is a technique that can be used for both autologous transplantation, which involves harvesting cells from the patient for future use, and allogeneic transplantation, which involves harvesting cells from a donor for use by another patient.

2. Factors that affect the success of mobilization efforts for patients undergoing autologous transplantation
   a) Exposure to prior chemotherapy and radiation

  b) Patient age

  c) Gender

  d) Previous mobilization attempts

  e) Whether the disease involves the bone marrow

3. The main classes of drugs used to mobilize stem cells into the peripheral blood are hematopoietic growth factors, chemotherapy, and chemokine antagonists. These medications are discussed later in this chapter, and pertinent information related to specific drugs can be found in Table 3-1.

  a) Hematopoietic growth factors: One of the most common approaches for stem cell mobilization involves the use of hematopoietic growth factors, or cytokines. The two cytokines currently approved for stem cell mobilization are filgrastim, which is a granulocyte–colony-stimulating factor (G-CSF), and sargramostim, which is a granulocyte macrophage–colony-stimulating factor (GM-CSF).

   (1) G-CSF (filgrastim): G-CSF is a glycoprotein that stimulates production of hematopoietic cells by binding to certain cell surface receptors and is most commonly used for stem cell mobilization.

    (a) G-CSF is commonly administered via daily subcutaneous (SC) injections. A typical dose of G-CSF is 10 mcg/kg per day; however, doses may range up to 32 mcg/kg per day.

    (b) Stem cell collection begins after four to five days of G-CSF injections. The ideal duration for G-CSF administration and the best day to begin stem cell collection have not been fully determined.

    (c) Overall, G-CSF is well tolerated. However, common side effects of this drug include bone pain, headache, fatigue, muscle aches, nausea and vomiting, and stomach pain. Rare but serious cases of splenic rupture, myocardial infarction, and acute respiratory distress syndrome have been observed.

   (2) GM-CSF (sargramostim): GM-CSF is approved but rarely used today for mobilization because of low stem cell yields when compared to other modalities (such as plerixafor and G-CSF), as well as an increased occurrence of mild and severe adverse events compared to G-CSF.

    (a) Studies in the 1980s and 1990s demonstrated an increase in the number of circulating progenitor cells after patients received GM-CSF. GM-CSF has a similar mechanism of action to G-CSF, working on cell receptor sites to stimulate the proliferation of progenitor stem cells. Later studies showed that G-CSF was superior to GM-CSF in mobilizing stem cells, while also demonstrating increased toxicity with GM-CSF. However, GM-CSF is still approved for stem cell mobilization.

    (b) Common dosing is 250 mcg/m^2 per day given as a continuous IV infusion or a daily SC injection. Bone pain is common with this medication as well as other adverse events.

  b) Chemotherapy and hematopoietic growth factors: Prior to the development of cytokines for stem cell mobilization, a brief, predictable increase in circulating stem cells was observed after the administration of myelosuppressive chemotherapy. This is because chemotherapy agents such as

Table 3-1. Medications Used for Mobilization of Stem Cells

Drug Class	Drug Name	Mechanism of Action	Administration	Special Considerations
Hematopoietic growth factors	Granulocyte–colony-stimulating factor (G-CSF) (filgrastim)	A glycoprotein that stimulates the production of hematopoietic cells by binding to certain cell surface receptors. Leads to increased peripheral circulation of progenitor cells. Median time to engraftment with G-CSF mobilization is 11 days. May be given along with chemotherapy to mobilize progenitor cells.	Daily subcutaneous (SC) injections of 10–32 mcg/kg/day beginning at least 4 days before first apheresis and continuing until last apheresis session. Some providers choose to give twice-daily injections.	Most common growth factor used for mobilization. Bone pain, fatigue, muscle aches, nausea and vomiting, and stomach aches are the most common side effects. Allergic reactions are rare, but patient should be monitored for rash, itching, and respiratory distress. Fatal cases of splenic rupture, myocardial infarctions, and cerebral ischemia have been described. Acute respiratory distress syndrome has occurred in patients receiving G-CSF. Patients should be monitored for respiratory distress.
	Granulocyte macrophage–colony-stimulating factor (GM-CSF) (sargramostim)	A glycoprotein that causes partially committed progenitor cells to divide and differentiate into neutrophils, monocytes/macrophages, and dendritic cells. Can also activate mature granulocytes and macrophages. May be given along with chemotherapy to mobilize progenitor cells.	Recommended dose is 250 mcg/m²/day IV over 24 hours, or SC once daily. Doses may vary. Dose should continue throughout the time frame of stem cell collection.	Used less frequently than G-CSF because of lower stem cell yields and increased risk of adverse events. Arthralgias, bone pain, muscle aches, and fever/chills are associated with GM-CSF. Severe adverse events that have occurred include supraventricular arrhythmias, immune hypersensitivity reactions, and dyspnea.

(Continued on next page)

Table 3-1. Medications Used for Mobilization of Stem Cells (Continued)

Drug Class	Drug Name	Mechanism of Action	Administration	Special Considerations
Hematopoietic growth factors (cont.)	Pegylated G-CSF (pegfilgrastim)*	A longer-lasting form of G-CSF. Stimulates production of hematopoietic cells by binding to certain cell surface receptors. More research is needed to determine the role of pegylated G-CSF with hematopoietic stem cell mobilization.	SC injection. Doses vary widely in studies. Although some researchers have prescribed 6 mg or 12 mg daily, others have ordered daily doses of 8 mg/kg.	Not currently approved for mobilization of stem cells. More investigation is needed. Bone and extremity pain are most common adverse events. Injection site and allergic reactions have also been reported. Rare reports of splenic rupture and acute respiratory distress syndrome.
	Recombinant human erythropoietin (EPO) (epoetin alpha)	Mechanism of action is unclear. EPO typically is used to stimulate production of red blood cells. However, it has been observed that patients who receive EPO in addition to G-CSF have an increase in circulating stem cells, even from outside the erythropoietic lineages.	Administered SC. Doses vary. 3–4 daily concomitant doses of EPO 150 IU/kg SC, or 200 units/day, along with G-CSF.	Not currently approved for mobilization of stem cells. More investigation is needed. Generally, EPO is not considered an efficient method for mobilization. Black box warnings include risk of myocardial infarction, stroke, and thromboembolism. Common side effects include abdominal pain and edema.
Chemotherapy	Cyclophosphamide	Chemotherapy destroys cells that divide rapidly, including white blood cells. After the nadir, or low point, resolves, a transient increase in circulating stem cells occurs. These cells can be harvested for stem cell transplant. Administered concurrently with G-CSF or GM-CSF to mobilize stem cells.	Typically given IV but may also be given orally. Doses range between 1.5–7 g/m^2, or chemotherapy dose used to treat the specific cancer.	Most common chemotherapy used for mobilization. However, the chemotherapy regimen specific to the patient's cancer may be used for mobilization. Common side effects include nausea/vomiting, myelosuppression, and impaired fertility. Hemorrhagic cystitis also may occur.

(Continued on next page)

Table 3-1. Medications Used for Mobilization of Stem Cells (Continued)

Drug Class	Drug Name	Mechanism of Action	Administration	Special Considerations
Chemokine antagonists	Plerixafor	Blocks the interaction between the chemokine receptor CXCR4 and stromal-derived factor-1, causing stem cells to be released from the bone marrow into the circulating blood. Used with G-CSF to mobilize hematopoietic stem cells for transplant in patients with non-Hodgkin lymphoma and multiple myeloma.	Treatment with plerixafor is started after patient has received G-CSF for 4 days. Dose is 0.24 mg/kg administered by SC injection about 11 hours before initial apheresis. Plerixafor dose may be repeated for up to 4 consecutive days.	The most common side effects of this drug are nausea and vomiting, fatigue, diarrhea, headache, body aches, and injection site reactions. Blood counts should be monitored because of risk for thrombocytopenia and increased circulating leukocytes. Rarely, splenic rupture has occurred. May cause fetal harm.

* The use of pegfilgrastim for stem cell harvest remains investigational.

Note. Based on information from Bensinger et al., 2009; National Institutes of Health, n.d.-a, n.d.-b, n.d.-c, n.d.-d; Sanofi-Aventis, 2013; Schmit-Pokorny, 2013.

cyclophosphamide and paclitaxel cause a reduction in the production of blood cells, which stimulates hematopoietic recovery. Later, it was discovered that combining chemotherapy with G-CSF or GM-CSF, a technique known as *chemomobilization*, improved CD34+ yields compared with using growth factors alone.

(1) Common chemotherapy agents used for mobilization include cyclophosphamide, paclitaxel, etoposide, and cytarabine.

(2) Advantages of using chemotherapy to mobilize stem cells
    (a) Improved mobilization
    (b) A possibility of fewer apheresis procedures
    (c) More rapid engraftment
    (d) Increased survival
    (e) Chemotherapy may reduce the risk of tumor cell contamination of the graft. However, no clear consensus currently exists in the literature about whether a reduction in tumor burden leads to an improved survival benefit for patients.

(3) Disadvantages of using chemotherapy to mobilize stem cells
    (a) Patients may need to be hospitalized to receive chemotherapy.
    (b) The side effects and toxicities associated with chemotherapy are a concern, especially the risk of infection associated with neutropenia.
    (c) Hemorrhagic cystitis, cardiac toxicity, and risk of anaphylactic reactions are also associated with using chemotherapy for mobilization.
    (d) Given the possible long-term effects of chemotherapy on the bone marrow microenvironment, as well as issues with delayed engraftment associated with chemomobilization, it is unclear whether the risks of using chemotherapy for mobilization outweigh the benefits.
    (e) Scheduling apheresis may be difficult because of variability in the time to recovery of white blood cells (WBCs) following chemotherapy. Patients may take 10–18 days to reach the peak production of hematopoietic cells after receiving chemotherapy.
    (f) It also has been noted that using chemotherapy to mobilize stem cells causes an extreme decrease in T cells, which could have a negative impact on immunity.
    (g) Common side effects of cyclophosphamide, a chemotherapy used for mobilization, include nausea and vomiting, myelosuppression, fatigue, reproductive impairment, and alopecia. Hemorrhagic cystitis also may occur with higher doses, but cystitis is not common at the doses typically used for mobilization. It is important to remind patients to drink plenty of fluids and void frequently to avoid bladder irritation.

c) Chemokine antagonists: Chemokines are small proteins produced by both hematopoietic and nonhematopoietic cells that regulate cellular movement.
    (1) Chemokine antagonists directly induce mobilization of stem cells by working as an antagonist between the chemokine stromal-derived factor-1 and its receptor, CXCR4. Plerixafor is a type of chemokine antagonist that was approved in 2008 for mobilization of stem cells in

patients undergoing transplantation for non-Hodgkin lymphoma and multiple myeloma.

(2) When used with G-CSF, plerixafor has demonstrated the ability to rapidly and predictably increase the number of CD34+ cells yielded each day of apheresis. Some studies have shown that plerixafor used in combination with G-CSF mobilizes more stem cells than using G-CSF alone. Additionally, plerixafor has been linked with fewer mobilization failures.

(3) Administration of plerixafor begins on the evening of the fourth dose of G-CSF. Plerixafor should be given approximately 11 hours before the first apheresis procedure at a dose of 0.24 mg/kg SC. Therapy with plerixafor may be repeated at the same dose for four consecutive days.

(4) Plerixafor is generally well tolerated. However, common hematologic side effects include leukocytosis and thrombocytopenia. Other side effects include nausea, erythema at the injection site, dizziness, diarrhea, and fatigue.

D. Stem cell collection and storage: A variety of methods are used to collect stem cells, depending on the type of transplant and disease characteristics. Although some donors still undergo bone marrow harvest, the majority of stem cells are collected by mobilization.

1. Donor preparation

   a) The collection procedure must be explained in a manner that the donor is able to understand. The informed consent needs to include, at minimum, the risks and benefits of the procedure, tests and procedures that will be performed on the donor, the right of the donor (or parent of the donor, in the case of a minor) to review the results of any tests in accordance with applicable laws and regulations, and protection of confidentiality and personal medical information. Donors should be given the opportunity to ask questions and be notified of their right to refuse to donate. Allogeneic donors should be educated about the possible consequences to the recipient of their refusal.

   b) Informed consent from allogeneic donors must be clearly documented and should be obtained by a licensed healthcare professional other than the recipient's transplant physician.

2. A bone marrow harvest is a surgical procedure in which large-bore needles are inserted into the pelvic bone to withdraw marrow.

   a) The patient is placed under general anesthesia while multiple aspirations of bone marrow are taken from the posterior iliac crest.

   b) If an adequate number of cells are not obtained from the posterior iliac crest, additional marrow may be harvested from the sternum or the anterior iliac crests.

   c) An anticoagulant is added to the bone marrow to prevent clotting, and the specimen is filtered to remove bone chips, blood clots, fat cells, and debris.

   d) A total of 1–2 L of marrow volume is typically obtained. The goal is to collect a total of $2-3 \times 10^8$ nucleated cells per kg of the recipient's body weight.

   e) Bone marrow donation is typically a same-day procedure, but donors are occasionally admitted overnight for observation.

   f) Typical side effects of bone marrow donation include back and hip pain, fatigue, and throat pain.

   g) Donors may need analgesia for pain at the collection site.
   h) Other side effects that may occur are headache, dizziness, and loss of appetite.
   i) Donors typically make a full recovery within a few weeks after donation.
3. Peripheral blood stem cell collection is a procedure in which cells are harvested from the peripheral blood after mobilization by using a process called *leukapheresis*, or apheresis. Deciding when to begin apheresis involves many factors.
   a) The total WBC count including absolute neutrophil count
   b) Circulating CD34+ cells
   c) The number of days that cytokines have been administered prior to apheresis
4. Apheresis involves using a cell separator device to collect stem cells and return the remaining plasma and cells to the donor's bloodstream. Figure 3-2 shows an apheresis machine.
   a) The procedure takes approximately three to four hours.
   b) The number of apheresis sessions required is determined by the number of progenitor cells harvested during each procedure.
   c) The goal is to collect 5×10^6 CD34+ cells per kg of the recipient's body weight.
   d) Some patients require multiple apheresis sessions to obtain the necessary number of cells. Patients should be assessed prior to apheresis to determine their ability to tolerate the procedure.
   e) FACT guidelines mandate that a complete blood count, including platelet count, be obtained prior to each apheresis procedure (FACT, 2012).
5. Common symptoms experienced during leukapheresis
   a) The donor may experience hypocalcemia during apheresis because the sodium citrate used to prevent blood from clotting in the apheresis machine binds to ionized calcium, causing a drop in the serum calcium. Common symptoms of hypocalcemia include fatigue, chills, tingling in the lips and extremities, and dizziness. A typical strategy for preventing hypocalcemia in patients undergoing leukapheresis is to take an oral calcium supplement and increase the intake of foods rich in calcium.
   b) Other possible side effects associated with apheresis include hypovolemia, thrombocytopenia, chills, and headaches. Patients are monitored carefully throughout the procedure and treated appropriately.
E. Vascular access: For patients having their own stem cells harvested for an autologous transplant, cells usually are collected using a large-bore apheresis or hemodialysis catheter. A peripheral catheter may be used, but this may not be the best option for patients with fragile or sclerosed veins. Frequent site changes caused by issues with maintaining peripheral IV access may exhaust suitable options for peripheral veins.
   1. Advantages of central venous catheter access
      a) Fewer peripheral blood draws and venipunctures
      b) Provides the ability to use the catheter for both apheresis and subsequent therapy including chemotherapy, stem cell infusions, supportive hydration, antibiotics, and blood transfusions. Figure 3-3 shows an example of a cuffed, tunneled, large-bore central venous catheter that can be used for apheresis, as well as for chemotherapy.
   2. Disadvantages of central venous catheter access
      a) Increased risk of infection
      b) More costly and invasive insertion procedure

Figure 3-2. Apheresis Machine

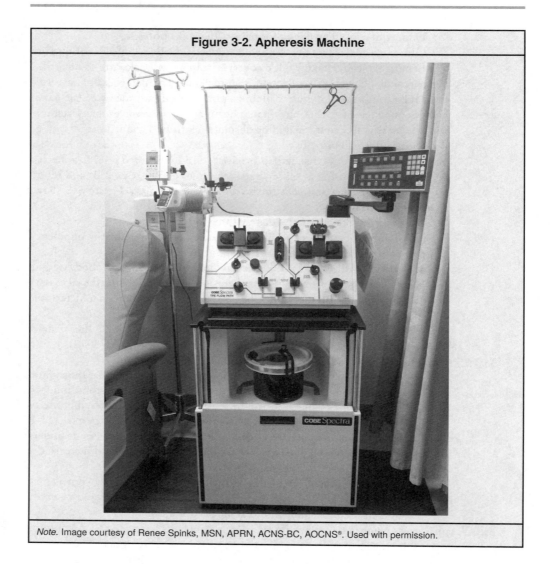

Note. Image courtesy of Renee Spinks, MSN, APRN, ACNS-BC, AOCNS®. Used with permission.

---

       c) Catheter-associated thrombosis

F. Peripheral catheters are commonly used for donor apheresis.
    1. Donors often provide cells for an allogeneic transplant via a peripheral IV inserted in an antecubital vein.
    2. If IV access cannot be obtained or maintained, an apheresis catheter may be placed in the jugular vein for collection.

G. Pediatric stem cell collections
    1. Children older than age 13 serving as stem cell donors often will undergo mobilization and collection similar to an adult donor.
    2. Transplant centers may be reluctant to perform mobilization on children younger than age 13. Instead, patients of this age often will undergo a bone marrow harvest under anesthesia. However, the use of medications, including G-CSF, che-

motherapy, and chemokine antagonists to mobilize stem cells in very young children, has been described in the literature (Emir et al., 2014).

   3. When collecting cells from pediatric donors via apheresis, care must be taken to avoid excessive blood loss.

   4. FACT requires that clinicians adjust collection methods to take into account the age and size of the child.

     a) The volume of the blood processed must be based on the child's weight. Depending on the child's tolerance of the procedure, 200–250 ml/kg typically may be processed.

     b) To decrease blood loss, the apheresis machine may be preprimed with irradiated blood cells.

     c) The patient must be carefully assessed for hypoglycemia, and a weight-based approach must be used to replace calcium.

H. UCB collection: Donating UCB, or electing to have cord blood harvested for future use within one's own family, is considered a safe procedure and poses no risk to the mother or infant. However, UCB collection must be done in such a way as to avoid disturbing the labor, delivery, and postpartum period. UCB may be collected by removing the placenta from the delivery room and obtaining blood from the umbilical cord and placenta with a needle using aseptic technique. Alternatively, blood may be collected from the placenta while it is still in utero (after the baby is born but before placenta delivery).

   1. Advantages of using UCB for an HSCT include quick access to cord blood units when needed and decreased incidence and severity of GVHD when compared to a transplant using peripheral blood stem cells. Lastly, UCB can be used for patients with rare tissue types, including ethnic minorities, because it does not have to be as closely matched to the patient as marrow donor cells.

   2. An important disadvantage of using UCB for transplantation is the possibility of transferring an undiagnosed genetic disease to the recipient. Another risk is

---

Figure 3-3. A Large-Bore, Tunneled, Cuffed Catheter

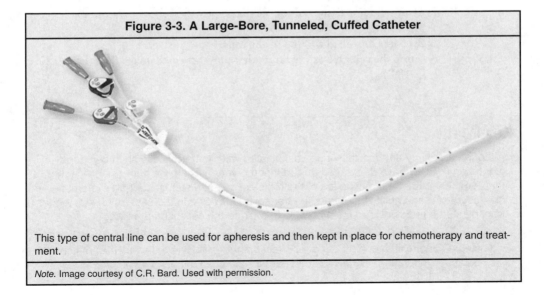

This type of central line can be used for apheresis and then kept in place for chemotherapy and treatment.

Note. Image courtesy of C.R. Bard. Used with permission.

the accidental contamination of the cord blood product with microbes or maternal T lymphocytes.

I. Storage of stem cells: After collection, cells intended for an autologous transplant are typically frozen and stored until after the patient has undergone high-dose chemotherapy. Cells harvested for an allogeneic transplant may be infused immediately, refrigerated in order to be used the following day, or frozen. Cells not intended for immediate use typically are transported to a long-term storage facility.

1. FACT requires that bone marrow collection facilities create processes to ensure that cellular therapy products are stored in such a way that their integrity and potency are maintained and that products are not released before proper criteria have been met. In addition, careful records must be maintained to keep track of the cellular product from the donor to the recipient. Contamination and errors must be avoided.

2. UCB is either immediately cryopreserved and stored for use by the donor or donated to a registry bank for an allogeneic recipient. The amount of time that UCB can be stored while remaining viable currently is unknown.

3. After collection, stem cells are processed prior to infusing or freezing. Processing includes counting the number of CD34+ cells obtained, testing for sterility, blood typing, and checking for infectious diseases. The fluid volume of the product is typically reduced to minimize the amount of cryoprotectant that is needed, as it can lead to increased infusion-related toxicities. Product intended for allogeneic transplant may be red-cell depleted if an ABO mismatch is present between the donor and recipient.

4. Cryopreservation: The majority of the time, cells intended for autologous transplant are cryopreserved. Allogeneic product also is occasionally cryopreserved. Cryopreservation involves a number of key steps.

   a) Reduce the number of mature blood cells in the sample.

   b) Protect the cells from ice crystal formation and dehydration during freezing by using a cryoprotectant such as dimethyl sulfoxide.

   c) Add plasma protein to the product to prevent cell injury.

   d) Add saline or tissue culture media to provide cell suspension and serve as a diluent.

   e) Ensure controlled cooling of the cells.

   f) Store the cells at a temperature that prevents cell damage (less than $-120°C$ [$-184°F$]).

Key Points

- Although morbidity and mortality rates associated with hematopoietic stem cell transplantation (HSCT) have decreased throughout the years, it is still a high-risk procedure that requires a thorough evaluation of the recipient's health status, support system, financial resources, and ability to tolerate the transplant process. In the case of an autologous transplant, the recipient also must be able to tolerate the collection process.

- In the case of patients undergoing allogeneic transplant, the best possibility of success lies in finding a donor with a perfect or near-perfect human leukocyte antigen (HLA) match with the recipient. Depending on the scenario, partially matched donors may be utilized.

- The Foundation for the Accreditation of Cellular Therapy was founded in 1996 by the American Society for Blood and Marrow Transplantation and the International Society for Cellular Therapy. This voluntary inspection and accreditation program aims to improve quality in all phases of the transplant process, including donor and recipient evaluation, stem cell collection and processing, and transplantation.

- The goal of the donor evaluation is to identify potential risks to the recipient, as well as any health problems that may pose a risk to the donor during the collection process. Potential donors must undergo an extensive evaluation, including laboratory testing, history and physical, cardiac function testing, and a psychosocial evaluation. HLA typing is performed to determine whether the donor and recipient are suitably matched.

- The majority of individuals donating cells for HSCT now undergo peripheral stem cell mobilization and collection rather than bone marrow harvest. Benefits of obtaining peripheral cells include more rapid engraftment, lack of anesthesia for collection, and decreased risk of tumor contamination of the collected cells. A major drawback of using peripheral cells is the increased risk of the recipient developing chronic graft-versus-host disease (GVHD) (in the case of allogeneic transplant).

- Some donors continue to undergo bone marrow harvest under anesthesia—namely, pediatric donors and those who do not need the graft-versus-tumor effect that accompanies GVHD (e.g., patients with aplastic anemia and sickle-cell anemia).

- Pediatric donors have special concerns that must be addressed. Although parents provide informed consent for minors, coercion of the donor to assent must be avoided. Education must be geared toward the child's developmental level, and an advocate for the donor should be appointed.

- Mobilization involves using medications to stimulate the production of hematopoietic cells and drive stem cells into the peripheral blood. Common medications used to mobilize cells include hematopoietic growth factors (also known as cytokines), chemotherapy, and chemokine antagonists.

- Apheresis is the process used to collect stem cells from the peripheral blood. A catheter is placed into the bloodstream, and blood is withdrawn and separated by a machine. The portion of the blood containing the progenitor cells is removed, and the remaining blood is reinfused.

- After stem cells are collected from bone marrow, peripheral blood, or umbilical cord blood, they are processed to check for infectious diseases, blood type, and sterility.

- Umbilical cord donation offers a chance of transplantation to those with rare HLA types, including ethnic minorities, who might not otherwise be able to find a match.

- Cells may be infused fresh immediately after collection (allogeneic transplant) or cryopreserved and frozen (autologous transplant). Cryopreservation involves taking specific steps to increase the likelihood that the cells will remain viable after freezing.

- A key predictor of HSCT outcome is the number of CD34+ cells obtained via collection. Donors with a large body size typically yield a larger volume of cells. Combining growth factors with chemotherapy or plerixafor (a chemokine antagonist) is associated with a higher stem cell yield than using growth factors alone. Research is still underway to identify optimal strategies for mobilizing stem cells with existing medications, as well as novel agents.

References

Bensinger, W., DiPersio, J.F., & McCarty, J.M. (2009). Improving stem cell mobilization strategies: Future directions. *Bone Marrow Transplantation, 43,* 181–195. doi:10.1038/bmt.2008.410

Bishop, M.R., Tarantolo, S.R., Jackson, J.D., Anderson, J.R., Schmit-Pokorny, K., Zacharias, D., … Kessinger, A. (1997). Allogeneic-blood stem-cell collection following mobilization with low-dose granulocyte colony-stimulating factor. *Journal of Clinical Oncology, 15,* 1601–1607.

Brunstein, C.G., Baker, K.S., & Wagner, J.E. (2007). Umbilical cord blood transplantation for myeloid malignancies. *Current Opinion in Hematology, 14,* 162–169. doi:10.1097/MOH.0b013e32802f7da4

Camp-Sorrell, D. (Ed.). (2011). *Access device guidelines: Recommendations for nursing practice and education* (3rd ed.). Pittsburgh, PA: Oncology Nursing Society.

Christopher, K.A. (2000). The experience of donating bone marrow to a relative. *Oncology Nursing Forum, 27,* 693–700.

Cohen, M.Z., Jenkins, D., Holston, E.C., & Carlson, E.D. (2013). Understanding health literacy in patients receiving hematopoietic stem cell transplantation. *Oncology Nursing Forum, 40,* 508–515. doi:10.1188/13.ONF.508-515

Confer, D.L., & Miller, J.P. (2007). Optimal donor selection: Beyond HLA. *Biology of Blood and Marrow Transplantation, 13*(Suppl. 1), 83–86. doi:10.1016/j.bbmt.2006.10.011

Devine, H., Tierney, D.K., Schmit-Pokorny, K., & McDermott, K. (2010). Mobilization of hematopoietic stem cells for use in autologous transplantation. *Clinical Journal of Oncology Nursing, 14,* 212–222. doi:10.1188/10.CJON.212-222

Devine, S.M., Vij, R., Rettig, M., Todt, L., McGlauchlen, K., Fisher, N., … DiPersio, J.F. (2008). Rapid mobilization of functional donor hematopoietic cells without G-CSF using AMD3100, an antagonist of the CXCR4/SDF-1 interaction. *Blood, 112,* 990–998. doi:10.1182/blood-2007-12-130179

Emir, S., Demir, H.A., Aksu, T., Kara, A., Özgüner, M., & Tunç, B. (2014). Use of plerixafor for peripheral blood stem cell mobilization failure in children. *Transfusion and Apheresis Science, 50,* 214–218. doi:10.1016/j.transci.2013.12.017

Faiman, B., Miceli, T., Noonan, K., & Lilleby, K. (2013). Clinical updates in blood and marrow transplantation in multiple myeloma. *Clinical Journal of Oncology Nursing, 17*(6, Suppl.), 33–41. doi:10.1188/13.CJON.S2.33-41

Foundation for the Accreditation of Cellular Therapy. (2012). *FACT-JACIE international standards for cellular therapy product collection, processing, and administration* [Version 5.3]. Omaha, NE: Author.

Glasgow, M.E.S., & Bello, G. (2007). Bone marrow donation: Factors influencing intentions in African Americans. *Oncology Nursing Forum, 34,* 369–377. doi:10.1188/07.ONF.369-377

Harris, D.J. (2010). Transplantation. In J. Eggert (Ed.), *Cancer basics* (pp. 317–342). Pittsburgh, PA: Oncology Nursing Society.

Institute of Medicine. (2004). *Health literacy: A prescription to end confusion.* Washington, DC: National Academies Press.

Mitchell, S.A. (2009). Hematopoietic stem cell transplantation. In S. Newton, M. Hickey, & J. Marrs (Eds.), *Mosby's oncology nursing advisor: A comprehensive guide to clinical practice* (pp. 142–160). St. Louis, MO: Elsevier Mosby.

National Institutes of Health. (n.d.-a). Cyclophosphamide: Cyclophosphamide injection, powder, for solution. Retrieved from http://dailymed.nlm.nih.gov/dailymed/drugInfo.cfm?setid=6bae5c14-9e87-4fb6-ae9c-4d875c1ecffe

National Institutes of Health. (n.d.-b). Leukine: Sargramostim injection, powder, for solution. Retrieved from http://dailymed.nlm.nih.gov/dailymed/drugInfo.cfm?setid=c96afe62-f0cf-4d4b-b57d-194a8ec12389

National Institutes of Health. (n.d.-c). Mozobil: Plerixafor solution. Retrieved from http://dailymed.nlm.nih.gov/dailymed/drugInfo.cfm?setid=a56b1b78-0ae2-41b4-9c76-98ad9d439199

National Institutes of Health. (n.d.-d). Neupogen: Filgrastim injection, solution. Retrieved from http://dailymed.nlm.nih.gov/dailymed/drugInfo.cfm?setid=3bc802bd-76b4-4f45-8571-a436ec26228e

National Marrow Donor Program. (n.d.-a). About Be The Match. Retrieved from http://marrow.org/about-us

National Marrow Donor Program. (n.d.-b). Transplant basics. Retrieved from https://bethematch.org/transplant-basics

Niess, D. (2013). Basic concepts of transplantation. In S.A. Ezzone (Ed.), *Hematopoietic stem cell transplantation: A manual for nursing practice* (2nd ed., pp. 13–21). Pittsburgh, PA: Oncology Nursing Society.

Sanofi-Aventis. (2013). About Mozobil. Retrieved from http://www.mozobil.com/healthcare/about

Schmit-Pokorny, K. (2013). Stem cell collection. In S.A. Ezzone (Ed.), *Hematopoietic stem cell transplantation: A manual for nursing practice* (2nd ed., pp. 23–46). Pittsburgh, PA: Oncology Nursing Society.

Wilkins, K.L., & Woodgate, R.L. (2007). An interruption in family life: Siblings' lived experience as they transition through the pediatric bone marrow transplant trajectory [Online exclusive]. *Oncology Nursing Forum, 34,* E28–E35. doi:10.1188/07.ONF.E28-E35

Study Questions

1. S.J. is about to undergo leukapheresis in preparation for an autologous transplant. The nurse informs her that she may experience tingling in her lips and extremities during the procedure. Which statement best explains this symptom?
   A. Numbness and tingling are signs of a hypersensitivity reaction to the medications commonly used for mobilization.
   B. Paresthesia of the mouth and extremities may occur during leukapheresis because the sodium citrate added to the blood to prevent clotting binds ionized calcium, causing serum hypocalcemia.
   C. Patients often experience numbness and tingling as a result of the cooling of blood while circulating in the apheresis machine.
   D. Paresthesia of the mouth and extremities is a sign that too much blood is being processed and that the procedure should be stopped.

2. Plerixafor works to mobilize hematopoietic stem cells by which of the following mechanisms of action?
   A. The drop in white blood cells after receiving plerixafor leads to a transient, predictable increase in circulating progenitor cells, which can be collected for hematopoietic stem cell transplantation.
   B. Plerixafor works by binding to certain cell surface receptors to stimulate the division and differentiation of progenitor stem cells.
   C. Plerixafor blocks the interaction between the chemokine receptor CXCR4 and stromal-derived factor-1, causing stem cells to be released from the bone marrow into the circulating blood.
   D. Plerixafor is used with chemotherapy to increase the number of circulating progenitor cells.

3. P.J. is a 10-year-old female who requires an allogeneic transplant for leukemia. It is determined that the patient's younger sister is a perfect human leukocyte antigen match. Plans are made to begin the collection process as soon as possible. Which of the following is the best strategy for the nurse to support the pediatric donor through the donation process?
   A. Direct all teaching efforts to the parents to avoid causing the donor unnecessary stress.
   B. Avoid approaching the donor to obtain assent for the procedure because the parents have already given consent and the transplant should take place as soon as possible.
   C. Refer the family to a psychologist to manage all of the donor's psychosocial needs after the transplant has taken place.
   D. Provide frequent teaching for the donor that is geared toward her developmental level, while giving her the opportunity to ask questions.

CHAPTER 4

Transplant Preparative Regimens, Cellular Infusion, Acute Complications, and Engraftment

Heather Koniarczyk, MSN, NP-C, AOCNP®, and
Christina Ferraro, MSN, RN, NP-C, OCN®, BMTCN®

I. Introduction
   A. Hematopoietic stem cell transplantation (HSCT) is a procedure used to control or cure many conditions (primarily malignant). The preparative or conditioning regimen can range from a single dose of chemotherapy to a combination of multiple chemotherapy drugs, biotherapy drugs, and/or radiation.
   B. Side effects from the preparative regimen and cellular product infusion vary among patients.
   C. This chapter will discuss preparative regimens, acute complications, cellular infusions, and engraftment.

II. Transplant conditioning regimens (Gratwohl & Carreras, 2012; Gyurkocza & Sandmaier, 2014)
   A. Preparative regimens are an essential part of HSCT when treating malignant diseases. The goal of preparative regimens is to eradicate residual disease and/or to provide immunosuppression, thus preventing graft rejection.
   B. Not all malignancies treated with HSCT are chemotherapy sensitive; therefore, not all patients receive the benefit of cytoreduction from the conditioning chemotherapy regimens. Conditioning regimens prepare recipients' bone marrow to accept new donor cells, while preserving function of nonhematologic organs in addition to treating residual disease.
   C. Preparative regimens consist of single doses of chemotherapy, several chemotherapies given over multiple days, or a combination of chemotherapy, biotherapy, and/or radiation.

III. History of conditioning regimens (Antin & Raley, 2013; Bubalo, 2011; Gratwohl & Carreras, 2012; Gyurkocza & Sandmaier, 2014; Lally, 2008)

A. The HSCT process was first used as a treatment for radiation exposure and atomic bomb accidents. Therefore, total body irradiation (TBI) was the first conditioning regimen used for patients undergoing transplantation. The first successful transplant was performed in 1956 by Dr. E. Donnall Thomas, who used radiation therapy as a conditioning regimen. The transplant involved identical twins, one of whom had leukemia.

B. In the beginning, TBI alone was successful in achieving marrow ablation and allowed for engraftment. However, it did not provide long-term disease control for patients with leukemia.

C. Researchers began to look at other treatments to add to TBI that would increase disease control.

D. Cyclophosphamide was the first traditional chemotherapy drug studied to be used as a conditioning agent prior to transplant. When cyclophosphamide was given in combination with TBI, patients had a statistically significant increase in disease-free survival.

E. TBI was replaced with other radiomimetic or high-dose, leukemia-specific chemotherapy, including busulfan, etoposide, cytarabine, carmustine, and melphalan. Studies have shown that these drugs were effective in not only controlling the cancer but also minimizing dose-limiting toxicities and reducing the risk of rejection, relapse, and treatment-related mortality.

F. Although the TBI dosing has been adjusted, no studies have shown that one dose of TBI is superior to another in disease-free survival or overall survival. In actuality, higher doses of TBI have been associated with an increase in transplant-related mortality.

IV. Types of preparative regimens (Antin & Raley, 2013; Bubalo, 2011; Gratwohl & Carreras, 2012; Gyurkocza & Sandmaier, 2014)

A. The decision to use a certain conditioning regimen is based on several patient-specific findings.
1. Type of malignancy or condition
2. Disease status
3. Number of comorbid conditions
4. Allogeneic HSCT (allo-HSCT): Donor availability, number of human leukocyte antigen (HLA) mismatches, and type of donor cells requested

B. Preparative regimens range in intensity; the highest intensity is myeloablative, and the lower intensity are nonmyeloablative and reduced-intensity conditioning (RIC) regimens (see Figure 4-1).
1. Myeloablative regimens consist of lethal doses of chemotherapy, usually single or multiple alkylating agents, with or without TBI. Patients require stem cell support from either themselves or a donor, because autologous hematologic recovery is improbable.
2. Although nonmyeloablative regimens do not require stem cell support, it is given with the goal of generating a new graft, or immune system. In this setting, autologous hematologic recovery is likely. Myelosuppression is reversible and usually occurs within 28 days without stem cell support.
3. RIC regimens are treatments that do not fit with either definition for myeloablative or nonmyeloablative. These conditioning regimens cause cytopenias, which can be prolonged and necessitate stem cell support.

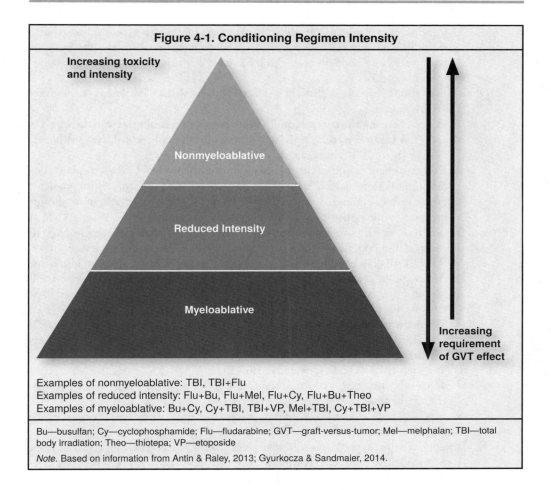

Figure 4-1. Conditioning Regimen Intensity

Increasing toxicity and intensity

Nonmyeloablative

Reduced Intensity

Myeloablative

Increasing requirement of GVT effect

Examples of nonmyeloablative: TBI, TBI+Flu
Examples of reduced intensity: Flu+Bu, Flu+Mel, Flu+Cy, Flu+Bu+Theo
Examples of myeloablative: Bu+Cy, Cy+TBI, TBI+VP, Mel+TBI, Cy+TBI+VP

Bu—busulfan; Cy—cyclophosphamide; Flu—fludarabine; GVT—graft-versus-tumor; Mel—melphalan; TBI—total body irradiation; Theo—thiotepa; VP—etoposide

Note. Based on information from Antin & Raley, 2013; Gyurkocza & Sandmaier, 2014.

    a) Doses of RIC typically are about 30% less than myeloablative regimens and result in mixed chimerism—the presence of both donor and recipient hematopoietic cell lines in the recipient—in a proportion of patients when initially checked. Again, stem cell support is given with the goal of generating a new graft, or immune system.

    b) Chimerism is evaluated by testing genetic markers to confirm engraftment and to distinguish the donor from the recipient.

    c) Currently, patients experience higher relapse rates with RIC and nonmyeloablative regimens compared to myeloablative treatments. RIC and nonmyeloablative transplants allow access to transplant for patients who might not be eligible for fully ablative transplants because of increased age and comorbidities (e.g., renal, hepatic, or cardiac disease).

    d) RIC regimens offer lower rates of nonhematologic toxicity.

  C. In general, patients who are in remission prior to transplant have a lower incidence of relapse.

    1. Patients with high-risk hematologic disease should be evaluated for transplant in first remission to allow for better outcomes after transplant.

2. Randomized phase III trials comparing regimens are lacking, but studies recently have pointed to a significant benefit in survival for healthy patients with well-controlled disease who received myeloablative transplant in hematologic cancers.

D. Considerations (Cheuk, 2013; Gratwohl & Carreras, 2012; Gyurkocza & Sandmaier, 2014)

1. When choosing the correct conditioning regimen, risk of graft-versus-host disease (GVHD), infection, toxicities, and relapse must be considered. Whether GVHD is a goal of therapy must also be considered.

2. RIC transplant conditioning regimens differ from myeloablative transplant conditioning regimens. RIC chemotherapy and radiation do not seek to eradicate tumor cells using high doses of chemotherapy but seek to achieve immunosuppression to allow the donor's immune system to engraft.

3. Graft-versus-tumor (GVT) effect is dependent on the conditioning regimen, graft composition, engraftment, and use of post-transplant donor lymphocyte infusion (DLI). DLIs can be infused after allo-HSCT to improve total donor chimerism.

4. Although the complete mechanism of GVHD is unknown, thymus-derived cells (T cells) are part of the regulation of the immune response, which causes acute and chronic GVHD.

5. The maturity of T cells depends on the source of the hematopoietic stem cells. Umbilical cord blood (UCB) units have the least mature T cells, and peripherally derived cells have the most mature T cells.

6. The maturity of T cells determines how likely GVHD is to occur.

7. T cells also are a major contributing factor to engraftment; the more T cells present, the less likely graft failure is to occur.

8. Peripheral blood stem cells engraft faster than bone marrow stem cells, which engraft faster than UCB units.

E. Autologous hematopoietic stem cell transplant (AHSCT) conditioning chemotherapy

1. Myeloablative regimens (Antin & Raley, 2013; Bubalo, 2011; Gratwohl & Carreras, 2012; Gyurkocza & Sandmaier, 2014)

a) Melphalan is the primary choice for multiple myeloma and amyloidosis. Others regimen combinations used include melphalan and TBI; fludarabine and melphalan; and busulfan and cyclophosphamide.

b) Carmustine, etoposide, cytarabine, and melphalan (BEAM); and busulfan, etoposide, and cyclophosphamide are the primary regimens used for patients with lymphoma or acute myeloid leukemia. Other regimen combinations include TBI, cyclophosphamide, and etoposide; thiotepa, busulfan, and melphalan; cyclophosphamide, carmustine, and etoposide; and busulfan and cyclophosphamide.

c) Carboplatin, ifosfamide, and etoposide; and etoposide and carboplatin are regimens used for relapsed or refractory germ cell tumors.

d) Radioimmunotherapy and monoclonal antibodies are being used in clinical trials to evaluate their efficacy in conditioning regimens for transplants, such as ibritumomab tiuxetan, tositumomab, and rituximab.

2. The basis for AHSCT in most cancers is to use high-intensity chemotherapy to treat the underlying disease. Nonmyeloablative AHSCTs are not therapeutic and are therefore not performed.

F. Allo-HSCT chemotherapy

    1. Myeloablative regimens (Antin & Raley, 2013; Bubalo, 2011; Gratwohl & Carreras, 2012; Gyurkocza & Sandmaier, 2014)

        a) Cyclophosphamide and antithymocyte globulin (ATG), with or without TBI, is used in aplastic anemia.

        b) TBI and etoposide; cyclophosphamide and TBI; and busulfan and fludarabine are administered to patients with leukemia, myelodysplastic syndrome (MDS), or lymphoma.

        c) Busulfan (IV or PO) and cyclophosphamide is administered to patients with myeloid leukemias, non-Hodgkin lymphoma, and MDS.

    2. Nonmyeloablative and RIC regimens (Antin & Raley, 2013; Bubalo, 2011; Gratwohl & Carreras, 2012; Gyurkocza & Sandmaier, 2014): TBI and fludarabine; fludarabine and cyclophosphamide; and busulfan and fludarabine can be used in all diseases.

G. TBI (Antin & Raley, 2013; Bubalo, 2011; Gratwohl & Carreras, 2012; Gyurkocza & Sandmaier, 2014)

    1. Process

        a) TBI is used in conjunction with chemotherapy mainly in myeloablative allo-HSCT to prevent the rejection of new cells and promote tumor kill.

        b) Toxicities increase when given in a single dose versus multiple fractions.

        c) Doses are delivered homogeneously over the entire body, penetrating hard-to-reach areas, such as the central nervous system (CNS) and testes. Based on institutional protocol, patients may be required to stand for the procedure.

        d) Measurements and simulations of the radiation are done prior to the actual treatment to determine the correct dose and position of the machine that is administering the dose of radiation.

        e) Shields are used to prevent increased toxicities and potential long-term side effects to specific organs (e.g., heart, lungs).

        f) AHSCT patients do not encounter graft rejection and therefore do not require additional immune suppression.

    2. Dosing

        a) Myeloablative doses range between 12 and 15 Gy and are delivered over 8–12 fractions for three to four days.

        b) RIC doses range between 2 and 8 Gy over 1–4 fractions and can be given in single or multiple days.

    3. Acute side effects

        a) Gastrointestinal (GI)

            (1) Nausea and vomiting

            (2) Gastroenteritis

            (3) Mucositis

            (4) Dermatitis

            (5) Fatigue

        b) Pulmonary

            (1) Pneumothorax

            (2) Pulmonary infection

            (3) Idiopathic pneumonia syndrome

            (4) Hemorrhage

            (5) Edema

    c) Hepatic sinusoidal obstruction syndrome (SOS), formerly known as veno-occlusive disease

      (1) An increased risk of SOS occurs with prior hepatic injury, TBI administration after cyclophosphamide, poor performance status, and alternative donors.

      (2) Treatment in mild cases of SOS is not necessary, but the use of defibrotide may reduce the process in severe cases. This is currently being studied in the United States.

  4. Long-term side effects

    a) Sterility

    b) Cataracts

    c) Growth failure

    d) Thyroid dysfunction

    e) Gonadal failure

    f) Renal dysfunction

  5. Treatments

    a) IV fluids

    b) Electrolyte management

    c) Antidiarrheal agents

    d) Antiemetic agents

    e) Analgesics

    f) Antibiotics (for infection prevention)

  6. Patient education

    a) Frequent mouth care: Keep oral mucosa moist and clean to decrease mouth acidity and risk of infections such as yeast infection.

    b) Patients should be instructed on managing fatigue.

    c) Patients receiving radiation should avoid lotions, creams, deodorants, or any topical medication because they can increase skin injury, unless given per the radiation department.

    d) Education on relaxation and stress reduction techniques during treatment also should be reviewed and provided to patients.

  7. Nursing considerations: Patient education regarding sperm banking prior to transplant, routine eye checkups, and routine follow-up with primary care provider

V. Chemotherapy and side effects (Antin & Raley, 2013; Bubalo, 2011; Gratwohl & Carreras, 2012; Gyurkocza & Sandmaier, 2014)

  A. Conditioning regimens are designed to allow for higher doses of chemotherapy from different drug classes to be given without having the same side effect profile. Two drugs with similar high-risk toxicity profiles are not given in the same regimen.

  B. All chemotherapies work in a similar fashion by attacking all fast-growing cells in the body, including tumor cells and the cells lining the GI tract, skin, and bone marrow.

  C. Side effects exist that are commonly shared by all chemotherapies used in stem cell transplant conditioning regimens. Most patients experience these side effects, but the symptoms vary according to the intensity of the treatment and can be worse than with traditional doses of chemotherapy.

    1. Nausea and vomiting

    2. Diarrhea

    3. Constipation

    4. Myelosuppression
    5. Alopecia
    6. Dermatitis
    7. Mucositis/colitis/proctitis
D. Nursing considerations
    1. Monitor and assess patients for transplant-related side effects. Educate patients on the identification and prompt reporting of side effects.
    2. Review with and educate patients on early signs and symptoms of infection.
    3. Encourage activity before, during, and after treatment to combat fatigue.
    4. Encourage fluid intake to prevent dehydration and to increase urinary output, which can help reduce the risk of hematuria in patients receiving cyclophosphamide.
    5. Nurses should provide patient education on specific side effects of each part of the conditioning regimen and how the team will attempt to minimize toxicities. For example, a regimen containing busulfan would not be used in combination with carmustine (BCNU) because of the high risk of lung toxicity from both drugs.
E. ATG (Antin & Raley, 2013; Bubalo, 2011)
    1. Immunosuppressive agent that inhibits thymus-dependent human T cells and other immune cells, such as natural killer (NK) cells and dendritic cells, which are involved in cellular-mediated immunity
    2. Used to deplete residual host T cells and reduce the effective dose of infused T cells with the graft in myeloablative, nonmyeloablative, and RIC transplants for aplastic anemia
    3. Premedications are administered prior to infusion (usually acetaminophen and diphenhydramine with or without corticosteroids) to manage side effects from cytokine release syndrome.
    4. Infusions are started slowly and increased as tolerated.
        a) Acute side effects
            (1) Fevers
            (2) Chills
            (3) Hypotension
            (4) Fluid overload and third spacing
        b) Life-threatening side effects
            (1) Pulmonary edema
            (2) Pre-renal azotemia
            (3) Hepatic dysfunction
            (4) Serum sickness skin rash
            (5) Joint pain that impedes mobility
F. BCNU (Antin & Raley, 2013; Bubalo, 2011)
    1. Causes DNA cross-links and strand breaks
    2. Inhibits DNA repair and causes carbamylation of cellular proteins to destroy cells
    3. Crosses the blood-brain barrier (because of lipid-solubility)
    4. Requires pre- and post-hydration
        a) Acute side effects
            (1) GI: Nausea and vomiting and reversible hepatic dysfunction
            (2) Infusion reactions (e.g., hypotension because of drug being delivered in an ethanol-based fluid)
        b) Long-term side effects
            (1) Nephrotoxicity

        (a) Laboratory signs of nephrotoxicity include elevation in serum creatinine and blood urea nitrogen levels.

        (b) Elevated creatinine is treated with hydration and by eliminating agents that can cause high creatinine levels.

    (2) Pulmonary toxicity

        (a) Symptoms of pulmonary toxicity may include cough, dyspnea, tachypnea, and restrictive ventilation deficiency.

        (b) Patients with abnormal pulmonary function tests prior to transplant or with past exposure to other chemotherapies that affect the lungs or TBI are at great risk for pulmonary toxicity.

        (c) Acute lung injury, with an onset of generally 10–30 days after infusion, can be treated with corticosteroids. Early detection and treatment is imperative to preventing long-term complications and decreased quality of life for patients. Acute lung injury can be fatal if the patient does not respond to steroids.

G. Busulfan (Antin & Raley, 2013; Bubalo, 2011)

  1. Busulfan is an alkylating agent that forms carbonium ions through the release of methane sulfonate group. This causes alkylation of the DNA, a nonspecific phase that acts on the granulocyte precursors in the bone marrow, causing myelosuppression. It is then metabolized by the liver and excreted in the urine.

  2. Busulfan crosses the blood-brain barrier, therefore increasing the risk of seizures. Antiepileptic drugs can be used as prophylaxis in patients at high risk for seizures.

  3. Busulfan dosing is based on prior research and drug pharmacokinetics. Pharmacokinetic-targeted therapy is ideal for delivering the appropriate dose of medication to the patient.

  4. Busulfan may be given either IV or PO. When giving busulfan orally, the nurse should instruct the patient to take it on an empty stomach. If emesis occurs, an additional dose of busulfan may be necessary. According to the manufacturer, if emesis occurs within 30 minutes or if fragments of tablets/capsules are found in vomitus, 50% of the dose can be readministered.

  5. Acute side effects

    a) Neurotoxicity: Because busulfan can increase the risk of seizures, antiseizure medications often are administered on busulfan infusion days.

    b) GI-related side effects

      (1) Nausea and vomiting

      (2) Diarrhea

      (3) Stomatitis

      (4) Anorexia

      (5) Hepatitis

      (6) SOS

    c) Dermatologic-related side effects

      (1) Hyperpigmentation

      (2) Rash

      (3) Alopecia (sometimes permanent)

  6. Long-term effects

    a) Pulmonary fibrosis (4–10 years post-therapy)

    b) Sexual dysfunction

      (1) Sterility

(2) Menopause

c) Birth defects: Busulfan is a potential teratogen.

H. Carboplatin (Bubalo, 2011; Lexicomp, 2014b)

1. Carboplatin is an alkylating agent that covalently binds to DNA, interfering with the production of interstrand DNA cross-links. Because carboplatin is excreted in the urine, it is important to maintain hydration throughout infusion.

2. Antiemetic premedication is necessary.

3. Acute side effects

 a) Electrolyte disturbance

 b) Delayed nausea and vomiting

 c) Renal insufficiency

 d) Acidosis

 e) Hypernatremia

4. Long-term side effects

 a) Nonreversible ototoxicity

 b) Neurotoxicity (e.g., peripheral neuropathy)

I. Cyclophosphamide (Antin & Raley, 2013; Bubalo, 2011)

1. Cyclophosphamide is an alkylating agent that forms carbonium ions through the release of a methane sulfonate group. This causes alkylation of DNA.

2. Cyclophosphamide does not act on a specific phase of the cell cycle.

3. Cyclophosphamide is inactive until the liver and serum enzymes convert it to the active form that is then excreted by the kidneys.

4. Nursing considerations

 a) Monitor intake and output closely and use diuretics as needed to maintain euvolemia.

 b) Monitor electrolytes daily.

 c) Monitor urinalysis for microscopic hematuria when the patient receives high-dose cyclophosphamide.

5. Acute side effects

 a) Histamine reaction: Burning in the nose or jaw, facial pain, tingling lips

  (1) Premedication of diphenhydramine is sometimes administered but not always common practice.

  (2) Granisetron and dexamethasone are routinely given as premedications for emetogenic side effects.

 b) Cardiac (rare complications): Cardiomyopathy, hemorrhagic myocardial necrosis, and coronary artery vasculitis

  (1) Check for signs of cardiac tamponade, congestive heart failure, or arrhythmias.

  (2) An electrocardiogram and a baseline echocardiogram should be done prior to administration.

 c) Genitourinary: Hemorrhagic cystitis

  (1) Prevention is the key to this side effect.

  (2) Increased hydration and administration of mesna decrease this risk and often are required in most institutional protocols.

 d) Endocrine: Syndrome of inappropriate antidiuretic hormone secretion (SIADH) is characterized by excessive release of antidiuretic hormone from the posterior pituitary gland, leading to water retention and causing hyponatremia and possibly seizures.

    e) GI: Nausea and vomiting, diarrhea

    f) Skin: Alopecia, hyperpigmentation, ridging of nail beds

    g) Pulmonary: Rare pneumonitis, fibrosis. Treatment includes corticosteroids.

  J. Cytarabine (Bubalo, 2011; Lexicomp, 2014c)

    1. Cytarabine is an antimetabolite that inhibits DNA synthesis in the S phase of the cell cycle. Cytarabine is metabolized by the liver and excreted in the urine.

    2. Acute side effects

      a) Mucositis

      b) Ataxia

      c) Nystagmus

      d) Slurred speech and gait changes as a result of cerebellar dysfunction

      e) Chemical conjunctivitis

      f) Acral erythema or generalized dermatitis

      g) Biliary stasis

      h) Elevated liver function tests

      i) Fever

      j) Myalgia

      k) Bone pain

      l) Chest pain

      m) Capillary leak syndrome

  K. Etoposide (Antin & Raley, 2013; Bubalo, 2011)

    1. Etoposide is a plant alkaloid that inhibits synthesis of DNA in the S phase and G_2 phase by inhibiting type II topoisomerase. These cells are unable to enter mitosis, and single-strand breaks in DNA also are noted. Etoposide is excreted in the urine and bile.

    2. Because of the rare occurrence of acute anaphylactic reactions, it is important to premedicate the patient with diphenhydramine, corticosteroids, and fluid bolus if high doses are administered with a rapid infusion.

    3. Acute side effects

      a) Anaphylaxis

      b) Hypotension

      c) Fever

      d) Nausea and vomiting

      e) Large-volume diarrhea

      f) Hepatitis

      g) Stomatitis

      h) Metabolic acidosis

      i) Rash

      j) Plantar and palmar burning

      k) Peripheral neuropathy

      l) Myocardial infarction in those who have had prior mediastinal radiation

  L. Fludarabine phosphate (Antin & Raley, 2013; Bubalo, 2011)

    1. Fludarabine inhibits DNA-polymerase-alpha, ribonucleotide reductase, which inhibits DNA synthesis. Fludarabine is eliminated by the kidneys.

    2. Acute side effects

      a) GI: Nausea and vomiting, diarrhea

      b) Dermatologic: Alopecia

  M. Ifosfamide (Lexicomp, 2014d)

       1. Ifosfamide binds to the nucleic acids and other intracellular structures, causing cross-linking of DNA strands. This inhibits protein synthesis and DNA synthesis. Ifosfamide is metabolized in the liver and excreted in the urine.

       2. Acute side effects

          a) Nausea and vomiting

          b) Metabolic acidosis

          c) Alopecia

          d) Encephalopathy

          e) Hemorrhagic cystitis

          f) Pulmonary toxicities

N. Melphalan (Antin & Raley, 2013; Bubalo, 2011)

       1. Melphalan is an alkylating agent that prevents cell replication by causing breaks and cross-links in the DNA strand, which causes miscoding and breakage to the DNA nonspecific phases of the cell cycle. Melphalan is excreted in the feces and urine.

       2. Melphalan requires dose reduction in patients with a decreased creatinine clearance.

       3. Cryotherapy (e.g., sucking on ice chips) is encouraged for patients prior to melphalan administration and for at least 30 minutes after infusion completion to decrease blood flow to oral mucosa. Cryotherapy has been shown to prevent or lessen the severity of chemotherapy-related oral mucositis.

       4. Acute side effects

          a) Nausea and vomiting, stomatitis

          b) Skin rash

       5. Long-term side effects: Interstitial pneumonitis and fibrosis, which often is reversible with corticosteroids

O. Thiotepa (Bubalo, 2011; Lexicomp, 2014e)

       1. Thiotepa is an alkylating agent that reacts with DNA phosphate groups and produces cross-linking of DNA strands. Reactivity is enhanced at a low serum pH. Thiotepa is metabolized in the liver and excreted in sweat and urine.

       2. Patients should shower two to three times daily during and for 24 hours after infusion of thiotepa.

       3. Acute side effects

          a) Nausea and vomiting

          b) Mental status decline with CNS changes

          c) Headache

          d) Mucositis

          e) Skin desquamation: Topical steroid creams are used to treat skin desquamation.

          f) Elevated liver enzymes

       4. Long-term side effects

          a) Pulmonary toxicities

          b) SOS

P. Specific conditioning regimen considerations

       1. T cells and conditioning regimens (Gratwohl & Carreras, 2012)

          a) Donor T cells are a specific component necessary for engraftment because of their soluble factors and their direct effect on residual host T cells. T cells also are a very important factor in GVT effect. GVT occurs when the donor T cells and/or immune system recognize the recipient's underlying disease as being abnormal and destroy those cells.

          b) GVHD occurs when the immune reaction extends to the recipient's normal tissues.

   c) T-cell depletion, reduction, and selected techniques to improve engraftment and GVT while decreasing GVHD are in clinical studies.

   d) By inhibiting T cells during the conditioning regimens and post-transplant therapy, GVHD is decreased, but this also can decrease the GVT effect, thus causing an increased risk of disease relapse and graft failure. GVT effect is seen in haploidentical (half-matched related) transplant recipients.

   e) Increasing the dose of radiation suppresses the T cells, thus causing a lower risk of graft failure, but can increase morbidity and treatment-related mortality.

   f) Some centers use post-transplant cyclophosphamide to suppress T-cell activity and to prevent graft failure in patients.

  2. ATG considerations (Gratwohl & Carreras, 2012; Lexicomp, 2014a)

   a) Anti-T-cell globulins are derived from horse, rabbit, or, more rarely, goat and pig polyclonal antibodies.

   b) Anti-T-cell globulins target T cells, bone marrow–derived cells (B cells), NK cells, macrophages, and dendritic cells to prevent GVHD.

   c) ATG also is used in conditioning regimens to prevent graft failure, especially in patients with a high risk of graft rejection, such as UCB transplant, RIC transplant, or mismatched transplant recipients.

   d) Engraftment is enhanced when ATG is used in the conditioning regimen.

   e) Many side effects of ATG exist that must be considered prior to administering it to patients.

   f) Patients must be admitted to the hospital for close monitoring while receiving ATG because of its potential side effects.

  3. Pediatric considerations (Gratwohl & Carreras, 2012)

   a) Children tolerate side effects better than adults.

   b) Growth and development must be taken into consideration when choosing treatment for younger patients who are still growing.

   c) Outcomes of regimens with or without TBI are similar; therefore, TBI should be avoided in smaller children and should never be given to children younger than two years old.

  4. Disease-specific considerations

   a) Severe combined immunodeficiency (SCID) (Gratwohl & Carreras, 2012)

    (1) SCID is a primary immune deficiency of the lymphoid immune system. Chemotherapy-based conditioning regimens prior to transplant are not always necessary except in rare forms of SCID.

    (2) Stem cell transplants in these patients have a unique goal of focusing on the chimerism of lymphocytes.

    (3) Busulfan and cyclophosphamide regimens can be used in these patients to enhance complete donor chimerism and decrease the risk of rejection. If the risk of treatment-related morbidity and mortality is too high, the recipient can forgo chemotherapy conditioning regimens.

   b) Severe aplastic anemia (SAA) (Gratwohl & Carreras, 2012)

    (1) SAA is a disease in which an autoimmune reaction occurs, leaving the patient's bone marrow empty and unable to produce normal immune cells.

    (2) The aim of the conditioning regimen is immunosuppression of the host to allow the new graft to be accepted. There is no benefit of GVT or GVHD, as this disease is not malignant.

      (3) Rejection of donor cells is the biggest challenge in patients with SAA, and adding ATG is thought to decrease the risk and is the current standard.

      (4) Long-term follow-up studies have shown an increased incidence of secondary malignancy in patients who receive TBI in their conditioning regimens. An example of a conditioning regimen includes cyclophosphamide with or without ATG.

   c) Fanconi anemia (FA) (Gratwohl & Carreras, 2012)

      (1) FA is a genetic disorder associated with progressive bone marrow failure, increased risk of leukemia, and other cancers.

      (2) Molecular defects are present in these patients that inhibit DNA repair mechanisms; therefore, RIC regimens must be used.

      (3) TBI is currently used at some centers but carries a high risk of secondary cancers. Thus, busulfan and fludarabine are being evaluated in randomized trials to replace TBI.

      (4) ATG is used to prevent graft failure. An example of a conditioning regimen is cyclophosphamide with or without TBI and ATG.

   d) Lymphoma and myeloma (Giralt & Bensinger, 2013; Gratwohl & Carreras, 2012)

      (1) AHSCTs are more common in patients with lymphoma and myeloma. The conditioning regimens are myeloablative.

      (2) Data have shown that patients with Hodgkin lymphoma and non-Hodgkin lymphoma can be cured with AHSCT.

      (3) In a select group of patients with multiple myeloma, AHSCT can provide a longer progression-free survival but is not considered curative.

      (4) For patients who have aggressive or multiple-relapsed Hodgkin lymphoma and non-Hodgkin lymphoma, RIC allo-HSCT can be used.

      (5) Current data are controversial in using RIC allo-HSCT in patients with multiple myeloma. In this instance, allo-HSCT is recommended only in the context of a clinical trial.

   e) Solid tumors (Gratwohl & Carreras, 2012)

      (1) In the mid-1990s, a great interest circulated around dose-intense, tumor-specific treatment with AHSCT for solid tumors, such as breast cancer. No significant survival benefit has been shown when compared to traditional treatment, although interest in studying AHSCT for metastatic germ cell tumors exists.

      (2) Allo-HSCT in patients with select solid tumors is under investigation.

VI. Hematopoietic stem cell infusion and cryopreserved products (Antin & Raley, 2013; Devine, 2016; Schmit-Pokorny, 2007; Walker-McAdams & Reilly-Burgunder, 2013)

   A. The day of stem cell infusion is considered "day 0" and usually occurs at least 48 hours after the last dose of chemotherapy.

   B. TBI may be given in the morning on the same day of stem cell infusion, as the stem cells will experience no cytotoxic effect.

   C. Key concepts for cryopreserved products

      1. All autologous stem cells are red-cell depleted and then cryopreserved using dimethyl sulfoxide (DMSO).

      a) On day 0, the cells are removed from the freezer, thawed in 37°C (98.6°F) water, and prepared for transfusion.

      b) UCB units also are cryopreserved using DMSO and thawed in a similar fashion.

      c) Related and unrelated allogeneic stem cells also may be cryopreserved if needed at a later date.

      d) The identity of the recipient must be verified against the bag or syringe of stem cells by two witnesses (e.g., nurse, physician, laboratory staff).

      e) It is important to note that a patient should not receive more than 1 ml/kg per day of DMSO. The cells can be washed of DMSO if necessary, or the residual cells can be infused the following day.

  2. Adverse effects during stem cell infusion

      a) The majority of side effects resulting from the transfusion of cryopreserved cells are related to the preservative DMSO. Reactions can last up to 24 hours, including the following:

        (1) Allergic or hypersensitivity reactions

        (2) Hemolytic reactions

        (3) Volume overload

      b) The most frequently experienced symptoms include fever, chills, hypotension, hypertension, tachycardia, bradycardia, cardiac dysrhythmia, chest tightness, dyspnea, nausea and vomiting, and abdominal cramping.

      c) Hematuria can occur from the breakdown of red blood cells (RBCs) in the bag prior to transfusion and usually is nonpathogenic.

      d) Patients also may report a temporary garlic-like odor or taste that is related to DMSO, as it is infused as a portion of the cellular product.

D. Management of acute reactions

  1. Institutional protocols usually exist to manage common adverse reactions during stem cell infusion. Nurses should be aware of their institution's protocols and emergency procedures.

      a) DMSO toxicity

        (1) Intolerance to DMSO in cryopreserved stem cells may be observed. Signs and symptoms of DMSO toxicity include a range of allergic-type symptoms (see Figure 4-2).

        (2) Management

          (a) Minimize the risk of an infusion reaction by premedicating patients with diphenhydramine.

          (b) If a reaction occurs, the nurse should maintain hydration, slow the rate of the cellular infusion, and check vitals frequently.

Figure 4-2. Symptoms of Dimethyl Sulfoxide Toxicity

• Abdominal cramps	• Flushing	• Tachycardia
• Bradycardia	• Hypertension	• Tasting a garlic-like odor
• Chest tightness	• Nausea	• Vomiting
• Dysrhythmias	• Shortness of breath	• Wheezing
• Fever		

Note. Based on information from Antin & Raley, 2013; Schmit-Pokorny, 2007; Walker-McAdams & Reilly-Burgunder, 2013.

  (c) The next bag of cells can be washed of DMSO prior to transfusion.
  (d) Nurses should keep emergency equipment at the bedside.
  (e) Patients should notify the nurse or provider immediately of any abnormal symptoms.
b) Acute hemolytic reaction, also known as major ABO incompatibility
  (1) Signs and symptoms
    (a) Chest and back pain
    (b) Fever
    (c) Chills
    (d) Dyspnea
    (e) Shock
    (f) Abnormal bleeding
    (g) Disseminated intravascular coagulation (DIC)
  (2) Management: The patient may need to receive additional blood products to correct any coagulopathy, such as platelets, fresh frozen plasma, or cryoprecipitate.
    (a) Stop the infusion.
    (b) Call the physician or provider immediately.
    (c) Maintain IV fluids.
    (d) Administer oxygen.
    (e) Keep emergency equipment at the bedside.
c) Allergic reaction
  (1) Signs and symptoms
    (a) Rash
    (b) Urticaria
    (c) Pruritus
    (d) Facial edema
    (e) Pharyngeal or glottic edema
  (2) Management
    (a) Stop the infusion.
    (b) Call the physician or advanced practice provider immediately.
    (c) Administer antihistamines.
    (d) Maintain a patent airway.
    (e) Administer oxygen if needed.
    (f) Administer corticosteroids and epinephrine for severe reactions.
    (g) Keep emergency equipment at the bedside.
d) Anaphylactic reaction
  (1) Signs and symptoms
    (a) Dyspnea
    (b) Bronchospasm
    (c) Hypotension
    (d) Hypoxia
    (e) Pulmonary and facial edema
    (f) Diaphoresis
    (g) Abdominal pain
  (2) Management
    (a) Stop the infusion.
    (b) Call the physician or provider immediately.

      (c) Administer corticosteroids and epinephrine.

      (d) Keep emergency equipment at the bedside.

      (e) Maintain aggressive IV fluids.

      (f) Maintain a patent airway.

      (g) Administer oxygen if needed.

      (h) Maintain adequate hydration and urine output. It is important to minimize the renal complications associated with infusing broken-down RBCs with stem cells. Ensure the administration of pre-medications, such as acetaminophen, lorazepam, diphenhydramine, and/or hydrocortisone to minimize the risk of DMSO-related side effects and allergic hypersensitivity reactions.

      (i) Nurses should perform frequent patient monitoring and report abnormal vital signs, cardiac statuses, and symptoms.

  2. Patient and caregiver education

    a) Provide patients and caregivers with information about the transplant and hematopoietic stem cell infusion process to reduce anxiety. Educate patients about what symptoms may occur and how to report them.

    b) Inform patients to expect a garlic-like taste during the transplant and up to 48 hours post-transplant. Hard candies may be useful to combat the unpleasant taste.

VII. Fresh products (Antin & Raley, 2013; Schmit-Pokorny, 2007; Walker-McAdams & Reilly-Burgunder, 2013)

  A. Allogeneic grafts, other than UCB, are routinely administered quickly after apheresis or bone marrow harvest per institutional protocol.

  B. Once received by the laboratory, the cells are evaluated and may need to be depleted of red cells, plasma, or T cells.

  C. Depleting the product of RBCs or plasma can reduce the incidence of major and minor ABO incompatibilities.

  D. T-cell depletion may reduce the incidence of GVHD, but because a suspicion of increased graft rejection and possible relapse has been linked to this procedure, it is not commonly used.

  E. The cellular product is transfused through a central venous catheter by a nurse with a physician or an advanced practice provider available to intervene in the setting of an adverse reaction.

  F. Adverse effects

    1. Fresh cellular infusions have fewer side effects than cryopreserved cells.

    2. ABO incompatibility can cause acute hemolytic transfusion reaction and is the leading cause of adverse effects in transfusion of fresh cellular allogeneic grafts.

    3. Symptoms of a reaction are similar to those of blood product transfusions and include anaphylaxis, hives, shortness of breath, chest pain, hyper- or hypotension, tachycardia, fever, acute renal failure, chills, and nausea and vomiting.

    4. It is essential to eventually transfuse the entire product regardless of the side effects related to the transfusion. Low cell doses can lead to a lack of engraftment.

    5. Neutropenia, graft failure/rejection, and the need for another transplant may result if the patient is not given a sufficient number of cells.

    6. Supportive medications such as diphenhydramine, hydrocortisone, epinephrine, and bronchodilators, as well as oxygen, can be given. The rate of stem cell infu-

sion also can be reduced. The intensive care unit may be the necessary level of care in rare cases.

G. Nursing management of fresh products
   1. Ensure that the administration of premedications, such as acetaminophen and diphenhydramine, are given to the patient to prevent allergic-type reaction.
   2. According to the Foundation for the Accreditation of Cellular Therapy and Oncology Nursing Society, no standard rules exist as to which type of tubing should be used to infuse the cellular product (filtered or nonfiltered).
   3. Administer the cells based on institutional protocol. The usual duration of infusion is two to four hours or less if the cells are plasma-depleted.
   4. Frequent vital signs and cardiac monitoring should be performed at a minimum of every 30 minutes.
   5. The transplant physician or provider must be notified immediately at the onset of any reactions that may occur to assess the patient, preserve cell viability, prescribe supportive treatments, and implement advanced cardiopulmonary support if needed.
   6. IV fluids are essential in the setting of ABO-incompatible cellular infusions to support the renal system in excretion of hemolyzed cells and ensure that they are running throughout the transfusion.

H. Patient and caregiver education: Provide patients and caregivers with information about the transplant and infusion process to reduce anxiety, as well as to educate patients on what symptoms may occur and how to report them.

VIII. Acute complications
A. Acute complications are those that occur from the time of the conditioning regimen to day 100. These complications are related to the conditioning therapy or result directly from the cellular infusion or graft.
B. Acute tumor lysis syndrome (TLS) (Cope, 2016; Poliquin, 2007; Walker-McAdams & Reilly-Burgunder, 2013; Wilson & Berns, 2014)
   1. TLS is a metabolic emergency that can be detected during the conditioning phase of HSCT but not usually following the transfusion of the graft.
   2. Most transplant patients are in remission when conditioning chemotherapy is initiated, but for those who have a large tumor burden of leukemia or high-grade lymphoma, TLS can be a serious complication. It is possible to develop TLS with the use of steroids alone. Additional risk factors include high lactate dehydrogenase (LDH) and renal dysfunction.
   3. Pathophysiology: TLS occurs with the lysis of malignant cells that reproduce at a rate too fast for renal excretion of the cellular contents. TLS is characterized by the following:
      a) Hyperkalemia
      b) Hyperuricemia
      c) Hyperphosphatemia
      d) Hypocalcemia
      e) Acute renal failure as a result of uric acid or calcium crystals interrupting the function of renal tubules
   4. Frequent monitoring of potassium, uric acid, calcium, phosphorus, LDH, and renal function is essential. Often, laboratory studies are monitored twice per day, at minimum, for those at high risk.

5. Medical management

   a) Preservation of renal function has greatly improved since the initiation of allopurinol prior to chemotherapy or steroids, which prevents uric acid–mediated nephropathy.

   b) Alkalization of urine with sodium bicarbonate should be initiated if hyperuricemia continues despite the use of allopurinol or when recombinant urate oxidase (rasburicase) is unavailable, with a goal to increase the pH level of urine to at least 7.

   c) Hyperkalemia is the most life-threatening component of TLS and should be acted upon immediately. Furosemide and IV glucose, followed by IV insulin and sodium polystyrene sulfonate, are treatments to reduce extracellular potassium.

   d) Hemodialysis may be used to correct hyperkalemia, hyperuricemia, hyperphosphatemia, and hypocalcemia, if supportive measures fail to correct the electrolyte and metabolic abnormalities.

6. Nursing management: Early identification of patients at risk for TLS (high low-density lipoprotein, high tumor burden) is essential, as well as careful assessment of laboratory values, fluid status, urine output, and symptoms of hyperkalemia, hyperuricemia, hyperphosphatemia, and hypocalcemia.

C. ABO incompatibilities and hemolysis (Antin & Raley, 2013; Carreras, 2012)

1. Whenever possible, donors and recipients are matched in regard to ABO blood type. HLA and ABO typing are unrelated; therefore, it is not always possible to have an ABO match with the best HLA-typed donor.

2. Transfusion complications may occur during or immediately after the cellular infusion or can be delayed.

3. ABO incompatibility and hemolysis are more of a concern in nonmyeloablative and RIC allo-HSCT.

4. Major ABO incompatibilities: The donor has A, B, or AB blood type and the recipient has type O.

   a) The recipient already has antibodies against A, B, and AB blood, and unmodified cellular infusion can cause a rapid and fatal acute hemolytic reaction.

   b) Other risks of major ABO mismatches can be the development of red cell aplasia or a prolonged failure of erythropoiesis.

   c) The risks of major ABO incompatibility can be overcome by red-cell depletion of the cellular product in the laboratory prior to transfusion into the recipient, along with significant IV fluid support to promote cellular debris excretion.

5. Minor ABO incompatibilities: The recipient is type A, B, or AB and the donor is type O.

   a) The recipient is at risk for acute and delayed hemolytic reactions after the product is transfused.

   b) The type O donor has natural antibodies to A or B blood types, putting the recipient at risk for acute hemolysis.

   c) Delayed hemolysis can occur once the graft produces anti-A and anti-B antibodies to the recipient's current blood type of A, B, or AB. Usually, the recipient has a mixed blood type for a period of time. In this case, it often is helpful to reduce the plasma in the cellular product prior to transfusion.

   d) It is possible to have a major and minor ABO incompatibility when the donor is blood type A or B and the recipient is the opposite. In this case, an immediate and delayed risk of hemolysis exists, and therefore, the product needs to be depleted of red cells and plasma.

e) Rh incompatibilities do not cause acute or severe complications to the recipient and therefore do not need any additional monitoring.

f) For women whose childbearing potential might be spared, it is important in the future to know if she received Rh+ cellular product if she was Rh−, as the newborn would be at higher risk for hemolysis.

g) If sparing fertility is anticipated, red-cell-depleted products should be used in the case of Rh+ and Rh− recipients.

D. Microangiopathic hemolytic anemia (MAHA) or thrombotic microangiopathy
1. MAHA is a complication that occurs in nearly 15% of patients who undergo allo-HSCT.
2. Conditioning therapies, including TBI and certain medications, can produce generalized endothelial dysfunction in HSCT. This dysfunction results in platelet consumption and microangiopathic hemolysis, creating an environment of excessive thrombosis and fibrin deposition in the microcirculation.
3. The risk factors associated with MAHA are the use of immunosuppression medications such as tacrolimus, cyclosporine, and sirolimus. MAHA usually is reversible by stopping the drug or switching to an alternative.
4. MAHA also can be attributed to the use of HLA-mismatched donor grafts, GVHD, and viral or fungal infections such as aspergillosis and cytomegalovirus (CMV). Diagnostic criteria includes anemia with greater than 2%–4% schistocytes on a peripheral blood smear, as well as an elevated LDH, low haptoglobin, negative Coombs test, falling platelet and RBC counts, renal dysfunction, and sometimes, elevated bilirubin.
5. Treatment of the underlying cause is important. In cases not responding to treatment of underlying GVHD or infection, complications such as renal failure, hypertension, and thrombocytopenia can cause MAHA to become fatal.
6. Plasma exchange has not been very helpful, with only a 35% response noted. Experimental therapies include defibrotide, rituximab, daclizumab, and basiliximab.
7. Close observation of blood counts, LDH, Coombs test, and liver and kidney function is essential to an early diagnosis.

E. Hypercalcemia (Walker-McAdams & Reilly-Burgunder, 2013)
1. Acute or chronic elevation of serum calcium often is not seen in the HSCT setting but may be an additional condition to monitor in patients with residual malignancy.
2. Etiology/risk factors: Patients with lymphoma or multiple myeloma may develop hypercalcemia as a result of uncontrolled malignant disease (called hypercalcemia of malignancy, or HCM) if residual disease is present at the time of HSCT.
3. Pathophysiology
a) Osteoclasts are responsible for bone breakdown. Osteoblasts are responsibility for reabsorbing calcium to build bone.
b) Tumor cells invade the bone and cause increased osteoclast stimulation, which further causes calcium to be released from the bones and into the bloodstream.
c) The kidneys can be overwhelmed by increased cellular calcium, making them unable to excrete calcium ions faster than the bones can reabsorb.
4. Signs and symptoms
a) Fatigue

        b) Anorexia

        c) Constipation

        d) Bone pain

        e) Nausea and vomiting

        f) Confusion

        g) Muscle cramps

        h) Kidney stones

        i) Oliguria

        j) Dysrhythmias

5. Diagnostic studies
   - *a)* Corrected serum calcium (CSC) level greater than 10.5 mg/dl
     - (1) Mild hypercalcemia: CSC level greater than 10.5 mg/dl to 12 mg/dl is treated with hydration; rule out underlying cause.
     - (2) Moderate hypercalcemia: CSC level 12–14 mg/dl is treated with hydration and/or bisphosphonates; rule out underlying cause.
     - (3) Severe hypercalcemia: CSC greater than 14 mg/dl is treated aggressively as it can be life threatening.
   - *b)* Ionized serum calcium level greater than 5.3 mg/dl
   - *c)* Monitoring of additional electrolytes, such as magnesium and potassium, is important, as they are typically low, thus resulting in an increased risk of cardiac dysrhythmias.

6. Medical management
   - *a)* It is vital to treat the underlying cause of malignancy-induced hypercalcemia, as well as to initiate acute strategies to lower serum calcium.
   - *b)* Initial treatment of hypercalcemia with fluid followed by diuresis can accelerate the amount of calcium to be excreted through urine.
   - *c)* Bisphosphonates are effective at slowing disease-related bone destruction, which prevents calcium from spilling into serum circulation. Pamidronate, zoledronic acid, or calcitriol can be administered to treat HCM.
   - *d)* It is important to review the patient's medication list to identify drugs that can contribute to hypercalcemia, such as thiazide diuretics, vitamins A and D, and calcium supplementation.

7. Nursing management: Prevention, early identification, education, and management are essential in caring for patients at risk for hypercalcemia.

F. DIC (Walker-McAdams & Reilly-Burgunder, 2013)

1. Definition
   - *a)* DIC is the simultaneous development of thrombosis and hemorrhage as a result of an overstimulated clotting cascade.
   - *b)* This syndrome can develop suddenly or can be a chronic complication and can progress to severe MAHA.

2. Etiology and risk factors
   - *a)* DIC often is potentiated by septic shock but also is seen in acute leukemia, TLS, liver failure, and vascular injuries.
   - *b)* DIC also can develop as a result of serious hemolytic reactions from ABO-mismatched cellular infusions, massive packed RBC transfusions, or during sepsis.

3. Pathophysiology
   - *a)* Initially, endothelial vascular injury causes activation of clotting cascade and platelet attraction.

    b) Clotting factors and platelets are consumed, causing an excess of circulating thrombin, which separates from fibrinogen and combines with circulating fibrin degradation products (FDPs).

    c) This dysregulation results in insoluble fibrin clot formation, which is responsible for multisystem organ failure from microvascular thrombosis, as well as simultaneous activation of fibrinolysis.

    d) Once clotting factors and platelets have been consumed, hemorrhage occurs.

    e) Excess circulation of thrombin also converts plasminogen to plasmin, resulting in increased fibrinolysis that increases FDPs.

    f) FDPs have anticoagulant properties and cause increased clotting factor and platelet consumption.

4. Signs and symptoms

    a) Hemorrhage, especially from multiple unrelated sites, is the most common and obvious sign of DIC.

    b) Equally important is the development of thrombosis, either through physical examination findings or laboratory evidence of organ damage.

5. Diagnostic studies

    a) Often, platelet counts are low, but this is not sensitive or specific to the DIC diagnosis.

    b) Prothrombin time (PT) and activated partial thromboplastin time (aPTT) can be slow to normal because of interference with the clotting factors.

    c) D-dimer assay is the most reliable test for DIC and is specific for FDPs.

    d) A positive titer for FDPs also is diagnostic of DIC and is more specific than D-dimer.

    e) Assessment of fibrinogen level is essential to decide whether to transfuse fresh frozen plasma and/or cryoprecipitate (if less than 50 mg/dl).

6. Medical management

    a) The cornerstone of treatment of DIC is to treat the underlying cause, such as leukemia or sepsis.

    b) If the cause is unknown or treatment has been unsuccessful, treating the coagulopathy is the next step.

    c) Heparin therapy can be used to inhibit clotting pathways but requires caution in patients with bleeding. The use of heparin in the setting of DIC remains controversial.

    d) Transfusion of blood products such as platelets, fresh frozen plasma, and cryoprecipitate is indicated for patients with active bleeding and DIC. Platelets should be transfused for a platelet count less than $20,000/mm^3$ and cryoprecipitate for a fibrinogen level less than 50 mg/dl. Plasma can be transfused for active bleeding in the setting of prolonged PT or aPTT.

    e) Routine physical examinations to observe for bleeding may assist with earlier diagnosis and treatment.

G. SIADH (Pace, 2016; Walker-McAdams & Reilly-Burgunder, 2013)

1. Definition

    a) SIADH is a potentially life-threatening, endocrine-mediated syndrome causing abnormal production or secretion of antidiuretic hormone (ADH).

    b) The hallmark sign of SIADH is hyponatremia in a euvolemic patient who has not received diuretics, has no edema, and has normal cardiac, renal, thyroid, adrenal, and hepatic function.

2. Etiology and risk factors
   a) The most common cause of SIADH in patients undergoing HSCT is medications. SIADH is mediated through enhanced action of ADH on the renal tubules by various drugs, such as cyclophosphamide, melphalan, vincristine, morphine, nicotine, monoamine oxidase inhibitors, selective serotonin reuptake inhibitors, and tricyclic antidepressants.
   b) Inappropriate secretion of ADH from the hypothalamus (such as with CNS disorders, head trauma or intracranial hemorrhage, brain tumor, stroke, or shock) or increased ADH secretion from another source (such as a tumor cell)
   c) Less common: Nausea, anxiety, stress, trauma, sepsis, uncontrolled headaches, and generalized pain
3. Pathophysiology
   a) Normally, the posterior pituitary gland releases ADH in response to a decreased plasma volume or increased osmolality in the blood (i.e., dehydration). This sends a signal to the collecting ducts in the kidneys to reabsorb water, therefore expanding intravascular osmolality and concentrating urine.
   b) In SIADH, the reabsorption of fluid occurs even if the serum osmolality of the blood is low to normal, causing inappropriate reabsorption of water in the kidneys. This causes increased intravascular volume, reduced urine output, and reduced sodium excretion.
4. Signs and symptoms
   a) Symptoms usually correlate with the rate of onset and severity of hyponatremia. Patients often are asymptomatic when hyponatremia is mild and/or chronic.
   b) When SIADH develops acutely, within one to three days, patients may complain of headache, thirst, anorexia, nausea, vomiting, decreased urine output, and incontinence.
   c) Patients with SIADH and hyponatremia may exhibit hypoactive reflexes, weakness, myoclonus, tremors, and an unsteady gait. When left untreated, patients will eventually develop seizures progressing to coma, which can rapidly become fatal.
5. Diagnostic studies
   a) Serum hyponatremia with sodium less than 135 g/dl on chemistry panel
   b) Serum osmolality less than 270 mOsm/kg
   c) Inappropriately concentrated urine: Urine osmolality greater than 100 mOsm/kg, specific gravity greater than 1.015, urine sodium greater than 20 mEq/L (see Table 4-1)
6. Medical management
   a) SIADH is not a preventable condition but can be successfully treated. It is treated differently than other types of hyponatremia because patients' volume status is euvolemic; therefore, volume expansion with IV fluids should be avoided. Neurologic impairment usually is reversible within two to three weeks.
   b) The first step is to determine the underlying cause and eliminate it if possible.
   c) Mild hyponatremia may respond well to a fluid restriction of 500–1,000 ml/day to promote a negative water balance. It is important to correct sodium slowly to avoid cerebral edema from developing from sudden fluid and electrolyte shifting. Correct serum sodium no faster than 12 mEq in 24 hours or 0.5 mEq/L per hour.
   d) Mild to moderate hyponatremia from SIADH often is treated with fluid restriction and furosemide therapy.

Table 4-1. Syndrome of Inappropriate Antidiuretic Hormone Secretion (SIADH) Diagnostic Tests

Test	Normal	Abnormal Labs in SIADH
Serum osmolality	275–295 mOsm/kg	< 270 mOsm/kg
Serum electrolytes	Na$^+$ 135–145 mmol/L K$^+$ 3.7–5.2 mmol/L Bicarbonate (CO$_2$) 23–29 mmol/L	Na$^+$ 125–134 mmol/L (mild) Na$^+$ 115–124 mmol/L (moderate) Na$^+$ < 115 mmol/L (severe) K$^+$ normal, bicarb normal
Urine osmolality	50–1,200 mOsm/kg	> 100 mOsm/kg Specific gravity > 1.015
Urine electrolytes	Na$^+$ 20 random catch or 20–220 mmol/L	Na$^+$ > 20 mmol/L
Renal function and uric acid	BUN: 6–20 mg/dl Creatinine: 0.7–1.3 mg/dl males; 0.6–1.1 mg/dl females Uric acid: 3.5–7.2 mg/dl	BUN, creatinine, and uric acid may all be reduced.
Chest x-ray	Clear lung fields	Identifies tumor or pulmonary disease
Computed tomography scan of the brain	Absence of abnormal lesions	Identifies anatomic lesions or evidence of cerebral edema

BUN—blood urea nitrogen; K$^+$—potassium; Na$^+$—sodium

Note. Based on information from National Institutes of Health, 2016; Pace, 2016; Walker-McAdams & Reilly-Burgunder, 2013.

      e) If fluid restriction and diuretics are not successful at stabilizing serum sodium levels or if neurologic manifestations are present, pharmacologic therapy with demeclocycline is the typical treatment. Demeclocycline inhibits the action of ADH at the renal tubules, therefore allowing excretion of water. Additionally, administering hypertonic saline (3%) with furosemide on a unit with well-trained staff or in the intensive care setting is appropriate.

   7. Nursing management

      a) Early identification of abnormal serum sodium and assessment of intake, output, and weight are essential in preventing mild SIADH from escalating to a severe and life-threatening condition.

      b) It is important to be aware of medications that may predispose patients to SIADH.

      c) Continued physical and symptom assessments are helpful to identify hyper- or hypovolemia, which excludes the diagnosis of SIADH.

  H. Sepsis and infection (Antin & Raley, 2013; Devine, 2016; O'Leary, 2015; Rovira, Mensa, & Carreras, 2012)

    1. Although great improvement has been made in the understanding and treatment of patients who are immunosuppressed, sepsis and infection remain a major cause of morbidity and mortality in patients undergoing HSCT.

    2. Etiology and risk factors

    a) Increased risk for infection following HSCT is based on the degree and duration of neutropenia following the conditioning regimen.

    b) Additional factors contributing to an increased risk of infection and sepsis include the following:

        (1) Comorbidities (i.e., renal or hepatic insufficiency), which may delay excretion of the chemotherapy drugs

        (2) Donor infectious status

        (3) Disruption of the mucosal barrier from chemoradiotherapy (i.e., mucositis, dermatitis)

        (4) Central venous access

        (5) Decreased production of immunoglobulins

        (6) Development of GVHD

3. Pathophysiology of infectious complications

    a) Early neutropenic phase (days 0–30 post-HSCT): The occurrence of infectious complications is linked to the type of conditioning regimen, with or without radiation therapy. Common pathogenic organisms during this time period include the following:

        (1) Gram-positive bacteria (sinus, respiratory tract)

        (2) Gram-negative bacteria from GI or central catheter origin

        (3) Herpes simplex virus (HSV) reactivation

        (4) Invasive fungal infections, such as aspergillosis or candidemia

        (5) Most common: Bacteremia, pneumonia, cellulitis, proctitis, oropharyngitis, and sinusitis

    b) Intermediate phase (days 30–100 post-HSCT)

        (1) In the intermediate phase, patients have engrafted and neutropenia and mucositis have disappeared, but immunodeficiency and central venous catheters remain.

        (2) The development of acute GVHD and its treatment (e.g., corticosteroids and immunosuppressants) can greatly affect the risk of infection.

        (3) Patients usually are affected by classic opportunistic infections: CMV, adenovirus, BK virus, respiratory viruses, *Pneumocystis jiroveci* pneumonia (PCP, formerly known as *Pneumocystis carinii* pneumonia), toxoplasmosis, nocardiosis, invasive aspergillosis, or mucormycosis.

    c) Late post-transplant phase (greater than 100 days post-HSCT): Chronic and/or frequent infections that occur late post-transplant often can be associated with chronic GVHD, which can prevent normal immune system recovery.

        (1) Encapsulated organisms (*Streptococcus pneumoniae, Haemophilus influenzae*)

        (2) Varicella-zoster virus (VZV)

        (3) PCP

        (4) Invasive aspergillosis or mucormycosis

4. Signs and symptoms

    a) Fever

    b) Hypotension from vasodilation

    c) Dyspnea, or shortness of breath, from capillary leakage or pneumonia

    d) Tachycardia

    e) Dysuria

    f) Diarrhea

    g) Skin rash

   h) New or localized pain

  5. Diagnostic studies

   a) The diagnosis of sepsis is a clinical decision that is based on symptoms (such as fever), laboratory results (positive blood or urine cultures), and radiologic findings (pneumonia or abscess). The most important tests to obtain are blood, urine, sputum, and central venous catheter tip culture and sensitivity tests when clinically indicated.

   b) Blood cultures are the most essential component in diagnosing sepsis. It is vital to draw more than one set at a time, as these can become contaminated with normal bacterial flora or may fail to detect early infestation with bacteria or fungus.

  6. Medical management

   a) During and after transplant and until immune reconstitution occurs, prophylactic antibiotics greatly reduce the risk of infections and sepsis in patients undergoing HSCT (see Table 4-2).

   b) Antibacterial prophylaxis with fluoroquinolones or sulfa, such as ciprofloxacin or trimethoprim-sulfamethoxazole (TMP-SMX), reduces endogenous bacterial flora from the GI tract and prevents infection from exogenous organisms.

   c) TMP-SMX also is indicated to prevent PCP.

   d) Broad-spectrum IV antibiotics are used in the setting of neutropenia and fever.

   e) Gram-negative and gram-positive infections are treated with sensitive narrow antibiotics. Each institution has standards of care concerning which antibiotics to use.

   f) Acyclovir greatly reduces the rates of HSV and VZV reactivation but does not protect against CMV reactivation. Currently, no widely used medication exists to prevent reactivation of CMV. Valganciclovir and IV ganciclovir are used for the treatment of CMV.

   g) Fluconazole, itraconazole, and sometimes voriconazole are used to prevent fungal infections, such as some *Candida* species and *Cryptococcus*.

Table 4-2. Typical Prophylactic Antimicrobial Regimens			
Drug Class	**First Line**	**Second Line**	**Third and Fourth Line**
Antibacterial	Amoxicillin 250 mg PO BID	Azithromycin 250 mg PO daily	Cephalosporins
Anti-PCP	Trimethoprim-sulfamethoxazole double strength PO 3 times per week or single strength daily	Pentamidine aerosolized monthly	Atovaquone or dapsone daily
Antifungal	Fluconazole 400 mg PO daily or itraconazole 200 mg PO daily	Posaconazole 300 mg PO daily	Voriconazole 200 mg PO BID or amphotericin B
Antiviral	Acyclovir 400 mg PO BID	Valacyclovir 500 mg PO BID	Ganciclovir or valganciclovir

PCP—*Pneumocystis jiroveci* pneumonia

Note. Based on information from Antin & Raley, 2013; O'Leary, 2015; Rovira et al., 2012.

    h) Itraconazole is superior to fluconazole in prophylaxis against *Candida glabrata*, *Candida krusei*, and *Aspergillus*.

    i) Currently, voriconazole, posaconazole, micafungin, caspofungin, and amphotericin B preparations are used for treating fungal infections.

    j) Patients undergoing HSCT are known to be deficient of immunoglobulins, a vital part of humoral or innate immunity. IV immunoglobulin (IVIG) can be administered to assist immature immune systems with increased antigen-antibody reactions to infections.

    k) IVIG may prevent encapsulated bacterial infections and also may reduce the rates of viral reactivations such as CMV. Only a small risk of hypersensitivity is present, which usually dissipates if the infusion is slowed and if premedications with diphenhydramine and corticosteroids are given.

    l) The use of colony-stimulating factors, such as filgrastim, can reduce the severity and duration of neutropenia in adult and pediatric patients.

    m) Filgrastim accelerates the maturation of immature neutrophils. It is important to know that filgrastim does not reduce infection-related mortality or overall survival.

    n) It still is unknown if a higher risk of developing acute GVHD exists when filgrastim is administered after allo-HSCT; thus, some centers choose to use it only after AHSCT.

    o) The cornerstone for sepsis treatment in patients undergoing HSCT is early detection and initiation of broad-spectrum IV antibiotics, antifungals, or antivirals. High-rate IV fluids or vasopressor support may be warranted for continued hypotension. Supportive care with acetaminophen and bronchodilators may be helpful as well.

7. Ways to reduce the incidence of sepsis and infections (Estcourt et al., 2015)

    a) Hand washing

    b) Frequent oral care

    c) Screening for ill visitors

    d) HEPA filters in rooms or units

    e) Sterile technique with central line care

    f) Antimicrobial prophylactics

    g) No survival advantage has been linked to a low-bacterial diet over a standard diet, but many institutions still use this diet.

    h) Granulocyte infusions are done occasionally in some institutions; however, low evidence is available that granulocyte infusions are beneficial to improve patients' immune system function.

8. Patient and caregiver education (Walker-McAdams & Reilly-Burgunder, 2013)

    a) Institution-specific education sessions should take place prior to, during, and after transplant with caregivers included.

    b) Information discussed should include the conditioning regimen, medications, side effects, cost, reporting of symptoms, anticipated engraftment time, dietary restrictions, bleeding and infection prevention strategies, central line care, and eligibility criteria for discharge.

    c) Follow-up depends on the type of transplant and institutional protocol. The frequency of outpatient visits should be discussed prior to transplant, and transportation should be arranged by patients and their caregivers.

9. Keep in mind that patients may have reduced concentration abilities as a result of high-dose chemotherapy. Assess patients' ability to retain the vast amount of information required for transplant. Adjust teaching to meet patients' education, reading, and alertness levels. Caregiver attendance at teaching sessions should be mandatory.

IX. Engraftment (Antin & Raley, 2013; Devine, 2016; Walker-McAdams & Reilly-Burgunder, 2013)
   A. Definition
      1. Engraftment in the setting of bone marrow transplant means that patients will experience a steady rise in blood counts following the cellular infusion.
         a) Neutrophil engraftment: Absolute neutrophil count greater than 500/mm^3 for two consecutive days or greater than 1,000/mm^3 in one day
         b) Platelet engraftment: Platelet count greater than 20,000/mm^3 that is unsupported by platelet transfusion
      2. The time to engraftment is dependent on the chemotherapy regimen, stem cell source, and the use of methotrexate for GVHD prophylaxis.
      3. Peripheral autologous stem cells take the shortest time to engraft, while allogeneic UCB takes the longest (see Table 4-3).
   B. Monitoring hematopoietic recovery (Lion, 2012)
      1. Once engraftment has begun, transplant centers typically monitor the serum blood chimerism that identifies the origin of white blood cells as either the donor or recipient.
      2. Monitoring the ratio of recipient versus donor cells allows providers to assess for graft rejections and to identify relapse of malignant disease earlier than when it might be detectable in circulating peripheral blood.
   C. Engraftment syndrome (Carreras, 2012)
      1. Engraftment syndrome is a systemic inflammatory syndrome that can occur during engraftment after AHSCT, as well as during allogeneic engraftment, and can

Table 4-3. Timing of Engraftment	
Type of HSCT	**Days From Chemotherapy to Engraftment**
Autologous peripheral blood HSCT	7–10
Autologous bone marrow HSCT	14–20
Allogeneic bone marrow HSCT	22–24
Allogeneic multiple cord HSCT	12–24
Allogeneic peripheral blood HSCT	10–14
Allogeneic reduced-intensity conditioning	7–30 (on average)

HSCT—hematopoietic stem cell transplantation

Note. Based on information from Antin & Raley, 2013; Lion, 2012; Tierney, 2013; Walker-McAdams & Reilly-Burgunder, 2013.

occur in 5%–25% of patients. Rapid engraftment increases the risk of developing engraftment syndrome.

2. Etiology and risk factors: It is mostly observed in patients receiving autologous transplant who may not have encountered intensive chemotherapy before, such as patients with myeloma, amyloid, or solid tumors.
3. Pathophysiology: Patients experience a massive release of proinflammatory cytokines, resulting in capillary leak syndrome and systemic endothelial damage, which can lead to systemic, multisystem organ failure.
4. Signs and symptoms
    a) Fever
    b) Rash
    c) Hypoxemia
    d) Pulmonary edema
    e) Weight gain
    f) Hepatic or renal dysfunction
    g) Encephalopathy
5. Diagnostic studies
    a) No specific diagnostic studies currently exist, as engraftment syndrome is a clinical diagnosis. The diagnosis is made by requiring three major criteria or two minor and one major criteria, according to Spitzer's criteria.
    b) Major criteria: Noninfectious fever, rash, pulmonary edema, or hypoxia
    c) Minor criteria: Weight gain, hepatic or renal dysfunction, or encephalopathy
6. Medical management: Methylprednisolone 1 mg/kg BID for three days, then taper the dose of the medication over one week. Resolution is expected within five days in the majority of cases.
7. Nursing management
    a) It is important that an infectious workup is completed before the initiation of high-dose methylprednisolone.
    b) Also important is for patients to be at baseline weight during engraftment. Retained fluids, especially pulmonary, can escalate engraftment syndrome.

X. UCB transplant (Antin & Raley, 2013; Gluckman, 2012; van Besien, 2014; Walker-McAdams & Reilly-Burgunder, 2013)
    A. UCB is most often used in unrelated allo-HSCTs. Although traditionally given in the pediatric setting, it has been especially useful for older patients who may not have a healthy, living relative or suitable donors within the registry.
    B. UCB can be used for sibling transplants in children and has been most successful in the pediatric population, using a single cord unit.
    C. Adults require multiple UCB units, as administering a single unit in adults is associated with increased rate of graft failure because of limited cell dose.
    D. The cells are cryopreserved immediately after birth and are readily available at donation centers that work closely with transplant centers, with no risk to the mother or child.
    E. Cord blood transplants offer a more immature and therefore more tolerant immune system that allows for a greater degree of HLA mismatch.
    F. It is vital to pick the correct donor cord blood by assessing the cell dose and HLA-match grade, as low cell dose and HLA mismatches can potentially cause graft failure.
    G. Although multiple units are given, patients will eventually only engraft stem cells from one of the donor units.

H. Cord blood transplants offer lower rates of chronic GVHD than marrow or peripheral stem cell donor transplants, as well as reduced rates of transmission of CMV to the recipient.

I. One concern regarding cord blood transplantation is delayed engraftment compared with marrow or peripheral stem cells, which can lead to more infectious complications and higher mortality rates.

J. Effort has been made to reduce the time to engraftment by studying RIC regimens and expanding the cord blood units, which would in theory expand the cells' homing.

Key Points

- The conditioning regimen is based on the disease, goal of treatment, cell source, and patient factors.
- Reduced-intensity treatments have provided opportunities for patients to receive a transplant who might not otherwise be eligible because of comorbidities.
- Although total body irradiation remains the standard for allogeneic transplant conditioning regimens, it has significant side effects.
- Conditioning regimens combine chemotherapies with different toxicities to protect healthy organs.
- Hematopoietic stem cells are cryopreserved using dimethyl sulfoxide (DMSO) but also can be infused fresh.
- The most common reaction associated with autologous stem cells is DMSO toxicity.
- Acute complications after hematopoietic stem cell transplantation can result from the conditioning regimen, cellular product infusion, or engraftment process.
- ABO incompatibilities can be overcome by depletion of red blood cells or plasma but still require monitoring after cellular infusion.
- Slow engraftment in cord blood transplantation remains a challenge.

References

Antin, J.H., & Raley, D.Y. (Eds.). (2013). *Manual of stem cell and bone marrow transplantation* (2nd ed.). New York, NY: Cambridge University Press.

Bubalo, J. (2011). Conditioning regimens. In R.T. Maziarz & S. Slater (Eds.), *Blood and marrow transplant handbook: Comprehensive guide for patient care* (pp. 39–49). New York, NY: Springer.

Carreras, E. (2012). Early complications after HSCT. In J. Apperley, E. Carreras, E. Gluckman, & T. Masszi (Eds.), *The EBMT handbook: Haematopoietic stem cell transplantation* (6th ed., pp. 176–195). Paris, France: European School of Haematology.

Cheuk, D.K.L. (2013). Optimal stem cell source for allogeneic stem cell transplantation for hematological malignancies. *World Journal of Transplantation, 3,* 99–112.

Cope, D.G. (2016). Metabolic emergencies. In B.H. Gobel, S. Triest-Robertson, & W.H. Vogel (Eds.), *Advanced oncology nursing certification review and resource manual* (2nd ed., pp. 643–692). Pittsburgh, PA: Oncology Nursing Society.

Devine, H. (2016). Blood and marrow stem cell transplantation. In B.H. Gobel, S. Triest-Robertson, & W.H. Vogel (Eds.), *Advanced oncology nursing certification review and resource manual* (2nd ed., pp. 293–344). Pittsburgh, PA: Oncology Nursing Society.

Estcourt, L.J., Stanworth, S., Doree, C., Blanco, P., Hopewell, S., Trivella, M., & Massey, E. (2015). Granulocyte transfusions for preventing infections in people with neutropenia or neutrophil dysfunction. *Cochrane Database of Systematic Reviews, 2015*(6). doi:10.1002/14651858.CD005341.pub3

Giralt, S., & Bensinger, W. (2013). Stem cell transplantation for multiple myeloma: Current and future status. *Leukemia Supplements, 2,* S10–S14. doi:10.1038/leusup.2013.3

Gluckman, E. (2012). Choice of donor according to HLA typing and stem cell source. In J. Apperley, E. Carreras, E. Gluckman, & T. Masszi (Eds.), *The EBMT handbook: Haematopoietic stem cell transplantation* (6th ed., pp. 90–107). Paris, France: European School of Haematology.

Gratwohl, A., & Carreras, E. (2012). Principles of conditioning. In J. Apperley, E. Carreras, E. Gluckman, & T. Masszi (Eds.), *The EBMT handbook: Haematopoietic stem cell transplantation* (6th ed., pp. 124–137). Paris, France: European School of Haematology.

Gyurkocza, B., & Sandmaier, B.M. (2014). Conditioning regimens for hematopoietic cell transplantation: One size does not fit all. *Blood, 124,* 344–353. doi:10.1182/blood-2014-02-514778

Lally, R.M. (2008). From then to now: An update on blood and marrow transplantation. *ONS Connect, 23*(3), 10–14.

Lexicomp Online. (2014a). Antithymocyte globulin (equine). Retrieved from http://online.lexi.com/lco/action/doc/retrieve/docid/ccf_f/221846

Lexicomp Online. (2014b). Carboplatin. Retrieved from http://online.lexi.com/lco/action/doc/retrieve/docid/ccf_f/221476

Lexicomp Online. (2014c). Cytarabine. Retrieved from http://online.lexi.com/lco/action/doc/retrieve/docid/ccf_f/221559

Lexicomp Online. (2014d). Ifosfamide. Retrieved from http://online.lexi.com/lco/action/doc/retrieve/docid/ccf_f/221771

Lexicomp Online. (2014e). Thiotepa. Retrieved from http://online.lexi.com/lco/action/doc/retrieve/docid/ccf_f/222160

Lion, T. (2012). Molecular monitoring after HSCT. In J. Apperley, E. Carreras, E. Gluckman, & T. Masszi (Eds.), *The EBMT handbook: Haematopoietic stem cell transplantation* (6th ed., pp. 280–287). Paris, France: European School of Haematology.

National Institutes of Health. (2016). Ectopic ADH secretion. Retrieved from https://www.nlm.nih.gov/medlineplus/ency/article/000314.htm

O'Leary, C. (2015). Neutropenia and infection. In C.G. Brown (Ed.), *A guide to oncology symptom management* (2nd ed., pp. 483–504). Pittsburgh, PA: Oncology Nursing Society.

Pace, A.F. (2015). Electrolyte imbalances, tumor lysis syndrome, and syndrome of inappropriate antidiuretic hormone. In C.G. Brown (Ed.), *A guide to oncology symptom management* (pp. 319–368). Pittsburgh, PA: Oncology Nursing Society.

Poliquin, C.M. (2007). Conditioning regimens in hematopoietic stem cell transplantation. In S. Ezzone & K. Schmit-Pokorny (Eds.), *Blood and marrow stem cell transplantation: Principles, practice, and nursing insights* (3rd ed., pp. 109–143). Burlington, MA: Jones & Bartlett Learning.

Rovira, M., Mensa, J., & Carreras, E. (2012). Infections after HSCT. In J. Apperley, E. Carreras, E. Gluckman, & T. Masszi (Eds.), *The EBMT handbook: Haematopoietic stem cell transplantation* (6th ed., pp. 196–215). Paris, France: European School of Haematology.

Schmit-Pokorny, K. (2007). Blood and marrow transplant: Indications, procedure, process. In S. Ezzone & K. Schmit-Pokorny (Eds.), *Blood and marrow stem cell transplantation: Principles, practice, and nursing insights* (3rd ed., pp. 75–108). Burlington, MA: Jones & Bartlett Learning.

Tierney, D.K. (2013). Hematopoietic cell transplantation. In M. Olsen & L.J. Zitella (Eds.), *Hematologic malignancies in adults* (pp. 499–536). Pittsburgh, PA: Oncology Nursing Society.

van Besien, K. (2014). Advances in umbilical cord blood transplant: An overview of the 12th International Cord Blood Symposium, San Francisco, 5–7 June, 2014. *Leukemia and Lymphoma, 56,* 877–881. doi:10.3109/10428194.2014.947980

Walker-McAdams, F., & Reilly-Burgunder, M. (2013). Transplant treatment course and acute complications. In S.A. Ezzone (Ed.), *Hematopoietic stem cell transplantation: A manual for nursing practice* (2nd ed., pp. 47–66). Pittsburgh, PA: Oncology Nursing Society.

Wilson, F.P., & Berns, J.S. (2014). Tumor lysis syndrome: New challenges and recent advances. *Advances in Chronic Kidney Disease, 21,* 18–26. doi:10.1053/j.ackd.2013.07.001

Study Questions

1. What is the most important rationale for giving total body irradiation in multiple fractions?
   A. It is easier for patients.
   B. It decreases short-term side effects.
   C. It decreases long-term side effects.
   D. It is easier for radiation staff.

2. What change can decrease side effects of busulfan?
   A. Using oral busulfan
   B. Basing the busulfan dose on blood levels
   C. Giving busulfan intravenously
   D. B and C

3. Which regimen is the most appropriate for a 70-year-old patient with multiple myeloma undergoing autologous stem cell transplantation?
   A. Myeloablative busulfan and cyclophosphamide
   B. Reduced-intensity melphalan
   C. Reduced-intensity total body irradiation and fludarabine
   D. Myeloablative melphalan

4. Why would a reduced-intensity conditioning regimen be chosen for a patient with low-risk disease and multiple comorbidities who has been determined to be a high-risk transplant patient?
   A. Transplant-related mortality would decrease with lower-intensity conditioning regimens.
   B. Relapse rate would decrease with lower-intensity conditioning regimens.
   C. Conditioning regimens are easier to administer.
   D. Organ toxicities would increase with lower-intensity conditioning regimens.

5. What is NOT a rationale for using a myeloablative transplant conditioning regimen?
   A. Increased tumor kill
   B. Decreased risk of graft rejection
   C. Increased graft-versus-tumor effect
   D. Increased immunosuppression

6. P.J. is a 58-year-old woman who is receiving a reduced-intensity allogeneic stem cell transplant for acute myeloid leukemia. During allogeneic stem cell infusion, P.J. begins to feel short of breath and appears pale and diaphoretic. The nurse notes bronchospasms and wheezing upon auscultation of the lungs. P.J. is most likely experiencing what type of reaction?
   A. Acute hemolytic reaction
   B. Anaphylactic reaction
   C. Urticarial reaction
   D. Dimethyl sulfoxide toxicity

7. Acute tumor lysis syndrome is characterized by all of the following electrolyte abnormalities EXCEPT:
   A. Hyperkalemia
   B. Hyperuricemia
   C. Hypophosphatemia
   D. Hypocalcemia

8. C.T.'s blood type and his donor blood type have a minor ABO incompatibility. Which statement about minor ABO incompatibility is incorrect?
   A. It is noted when the recipient is type O and the donor is type A, B, or AB.
   B. The recipient is at risk for acute and delayed hemolytic reactions after the product is transfused.
   C. The type O donor has natural antibodies to A or B blood types, giving the recipient a risk of acute hemolysis.
   D. Delayed hemolysis can occur once the graft produces anti-A and anti-B antibodies to the recipient's current blood type of A, B, or AB. The recipient usually will have a mixed blood type for a time.

9. What is the correct method for preventing the side effect of syndrome of inappropriate antidiuretic hormone secretion (SIADH)?
   A. SIADH is not a preventable condition.
   B. Give high-rate IV fluids throughout the conditioning chemotherapy regimen.
   C. Keep patients on fluid restriction throughout the conditioning chemotherapy regimen.
   D. Give furosemide throughout the chemotherapy regimen.

10. What is the first-line medication used to prevent *Pneumocystis jiroveci* pneumonia?
    A. Ciprofloxacin
    B. Acyclovir
    C. Voriconazole
    D. Trimethoprim-sulfamethoxazole

11. Which is NOT a symptom of engraftment syndrome?
    A. Fever
    B. Mouth sores
    C. Rash
    D. Hypoxemia

12. The major cause of mortality in cord blood transplant is which of the following?
    A. Bleeding
    B. Malnutrition
    C. Infection
    D. Renal failure

CHAPTER 5

Graft-Versus-Host Disease

Rita M. Jakubowski, MSN, RN, OCN®, ANP-BC, BMTCN®

I. Introduction
   A. Hematopoietic stem cell transplantation (HSCT) is a lifesaving measure for hematologic disorders—both malignant and nonmalignant—as well as for immune disorders. Despite advances in stem cell sources (umbilical cord blood [UCB], haploidentical grafts, bone marrow, and peripheral blood stem cells [PBSCs]), conditioning regimens (nonmyeloablative and reduced intensity), and treatment of infectious complications, graft-versus-host disease (GVHD) remains one of the most common complications of allogeneic HSCT (allo-HSCT) and is a major cause of morbidity and mortality following transplant. It also significantly affects the quality of life for patients and caregivers. GVHD is an immunologic response that occurs when donor lymphocytes are infused into the recipient and identified as foreign. This process essentially is an exaggerated response of a normal physiologic inflammatory mechanism of the donor lymphocytes. Despite routine prophylactic immunosuppression, the overall incidence rate of acute GVHD is reported as 20%–80%, depending on the recipient's risk factors and stem cell source (Martin et al., 2012).
   B. According to the Center for International Blood and Marrow Transplant Research, mortality due to GVHD was 18% for matched sibling transplants in 2011–2012 and 20% for transplants with unrelated donors (Pasquini & Zhu, 2015). GVHD significantly affects overall survival rates and quality of life for patients. Strategies to reduce GVHD can affect morbidity and mortality rates by increasing not only the incidence of relapse, but also the likelihood that fatal infectious complications will occur. Finding a balance between the newly transplanted cells by creating an immunologic effect against any remaining diseases (e.g., graft-versus-leukemia effect) and new cells fighting the host's normal cells (GVHD) is one of the biggest challenges in HSCT.

II. GVHD (Ferrara, Levine, Reddy, & Holler, 2009; Jacobsohn & Vogelsang, 2007; Mitchell, 2013)
   A. Definition
      1. GVHD occurs when immunologically competent donor T lymphocytes (in the transplanted graft) recognize antigens on cells in the recipient's organs as foreign and mount an immunologic response.
      2. The cells attack or injure the immunocompromised host's tissues either directly or through the secretion of inflammatory cytokines.

3. This immunologic response of donor lymphocytes (graft) causes varying degrees of damage to the host's tissues (disease).

   a) The revised National Institutes of Health criteria describe two main categories of GVHD: acute and chronic (Alousi, Bullinger, Couriel, Massaro, & Neumann, 2007; Deeg & Antin, 2006; Filipovich et al., 2005; Jagasia et al., 2015).

   b) Historically, the distinction between the two was arbitrarily made based on the time of onset following transplant (fewer than 100 days was termed *acute*, and more than 100 days following transplant was called *chronic*). However, with donor lymphocyte infusion (DLI) and reduced-intensity conditioning (RIC), time from transplant is no longer the standard determining factor. Acute GVHD can occur post-DLI and there can be an overlap syndrome, where acute and chronic GVHD exist concomitantly. Therefore, clinical manifestations now play a major role in diagnosing GVHD.

B. Classifications of GVHD (Jagasia et al., 2015)

   1. Acute GVHD

      a) Classic acute GVHD presents as erythematous, maculopapular rash, nausea, vomiting, anorexia, profuse diarrhea, ileus, or cholestatic liver disease that occurs within 100 days after transplant or DLI in patients not meeting criteria for chronic GVHD.

      b) Persistent, recurrent, or late-onset acute GVHD includes features of acute GVHD and occurs beyond 100 days post-transplant or DLI and without criteria for a diagnosis of chronic GVHD.

      c) Classic acute GVHD often is seen during taper or withdrawal of immunosuppressants.

   2. Chronic GVHD (Jagasia et al., 2015; Mitchell, 2013)

      a) Classic chronic GVHD has manifestations of autoimmune diseases and no features characteristic of acute GVHD. It is a syndrome that involves multiple organs including skin, eyes, oral mucosa, lung, gastrointestinal (GI) tract, and liver.

      b) Most cases are diagnosed within the first year at a median of four to six months after HSCT, but 5%–10% of cases are initially diagnosed beyond the first post-transplant year.

   3. A subcategory of chronic GVHD is termed *overlap syndrome* and occurs when features of both chronic and acute appear together. Symptoms can be transient and often are dependent on the degree of immunosuppression.

      a) Patients who present with overlap chronic GVHD can resolve the acute features, but chronic GVHD features persist. Patients with classic chronic GVHD may develop acute GVHD symptoms when immunosuppression is tapered.

      b) Hyperacute GVHD is a severe form of acute GVHD that can be fatal (Kim et al., 2004; Mitchell, 2013).

      c) Diagnosis is based upon the following criteria.

         (1) Fever of greater than 38.3°C (100.4°F) on two occasions for more than three days prior to engraftment, with a lack of resolution after a minimum of three days of treatment with antibiotics and antifungal agents (including amphotericin B)

(2) Rapid development of skin rash before engraftment, which can start as generalized erythroderma and progress to desquamation

(3) Hepatic dysfunction, especially alkaline phosphatase and bilirubin before engraftment (excluding causes such as veno-occlusive disease, drug-induced hepatitis, or right-sided heart failure)

(4) Development of mucoid, greenish diarrhea, with more than five stools per day (excluding etiology of mucositis)

    d) Treatment is high-dose steroids.

    e) It may be difficult to differentiate from engraftment syndrome, which presents as fever in addition to one of the following: skin rash, pulmonary infiltrates, or diarrhea.

C. Incidence (Martin et al., 2012; Pasquini & Zhu, 2015; Slater, 2011)

  1. The incidence rates of grades 2–4 acute GVHD are reported as being 20%–85%, depending on the recipient's risk factors and stem cell source.

  2. The same degree of human leukocyte antigen (HLA) mismatch results in lower risk of acute GVHD using UCB grafts.

D. Risk factors (Lee et al., 2013; Mitchell, 2013; Slater, 2011)

  1. Degree of HLA mismatch (most important risk factor); essential to match HLA-A, HLA-B, HLA-C, and HLA-DRB1 antigens

  2. PBSCs as the graft source

  3. Sex mismatch: Greatest risk with a parous female donor and a male recipient

  4. Recipients and donors older than 40 years of age

  5. High doses of total body irradiation (TBI) in the preparative regimen

  6. Conditioning intensity: Higher risk with myeloablative conditioning regimens than nonmyeloablative regimens

  7. Higher CD34+ cell dose

  8. GVHD prophylaxis (single agent or reduced dose)

  9. Unmanipulated graft (not depleted of T cells)

  10. Donor transfusion status (previously transfused)

  11. Related versus unrelated: Most severe GVHD occurs with HLA-mismatched or unrelated donors, compared with HLA-matched sibling.

E. Requirements for GVHD: Billingham criteria (Ferrara et al., 2009)

  1. Graft must contain immunocompetent cells.

  2. Histoincompatibility must exist between the donor and recipient. The recipient must possess tissue antigens that are not present in the donor; when this occurs, the recipient appears foreign to the graft.

  3. The recipient must be incapable of mounting an effective immunologic reaction against the graft; this would eliminate the foreign transplanted cells.

F. Pathophysiology (Alousi et al., 2007; Apperley & Masszi, 2012; Ferrara & Reddy, 2006; Mitchell, 2013; Slater, 2011): Three phases of GVHD

  1. Phase 1: Occurs prior to the transplant when the preparative, or conditioning, regimen of chemotherapy (with or without radiation) may damage host tissues, including intestinal mucosa, skin, and liver, and the mucosa becomes permeable

    a) The permeable mucosa leads to secretion of large amounts of inflammatory cytokines, such as tumor necrosis factor-alpha (TNF-α) and interleukin-1 (IL-1).

    b) These cytokines also upregulate major histocompatibility complexes and minor histocompatibility antigens present on the host tissues.

      c) This upregulation makes it easy for mature donor T cells within the graft to recognize the host tissues as foreign and mount an inflammatory response.

  2. Phase 2: Donor T-cell activation

      a) Transplanted naïve donor T lymphocytes circulate in the recipient's bloodstream and come into contact with minor antigens expressed on the surface of the recipient's cells. These are called *antigen-presenting cells* (APCs).

      b) Even when major histocompatible antigens are matched, some donor T cells recognize the recipient's minor antigens as foreign and bind to the antigen.

      c) Host APCs present alloantigens to the resting T cells and activate them.

      d) Once the T cells are bound to APCs, signals direct a subset of T lymphocytes (helper T or Th-1 lymphocytes) to begin producing proinflammatory cytokines (IL-12, IL-2, and interferon) and increase the expression of receptors for these cytokines on the surface of the T cell.

      e) These activated T cells expand and differentiate, producing specific cytokines that recruit cytotoxic T lymphocytes and natural killer cells to cause cell and tissue destruction of target organs.

  3. Phase 3: Cellular and inflammatory effector phase (target tissue destruction)

      a) An inflammatory cascade initiates a number of cytotoxic pathways, targeting and attacking host cells in multiple organ systems (much like a cytokine storm).

      b) Once the T cells have been stimulated against the host, they are either directly or indirectly responsible for tissue damage.

      c) Inflammation recruits effector cells into target organs, amplifying local tissue injury with further secretion of inflammatory cytokines, which, when combined with cytotoxic T lymphocytes, leads to tissue destruction.

      d) The entire process becomes cyclical: More tissue damage leads to more cytokine production, which causes a greater risk of GVHD.

G. Organs most commonly affected by acute GVHD (Alousi et al., 2007; Jacobsohn & Vogelsang, 2007; Mitchell, 2013; Slater, 2011)

  1. Skin

  2. Liver

  3. GI tract

H. Biomarkers and diagnostic evaluation (Levine, Paczesny, & Sarantopoulos, 2012)

  1. Currently, ongoing research is being devoted to identifying organ-specific acute and chronic GVHD serum biomarkers. A biomarker is a characteristic that can be measured to diagnose disease.

      a) Regenerating islet-derived 3-alpha for lower GI

      b) Elafin for skin

      c) B-cell activating factor (known as BAFF) for chronic GVHD

  2. The ability to measure these biomarkers can prove useful in predicting, diagnosing, and developing management strategies for GVHD, as well as monitoring response to treatment.

I. Prevention (Antin & Raley, 2013; Apperley & Masszi, 2012; Corella, 2011; Cutler et al., 2005; Mitchell, 2013)

  1. Depletion of T cells in the graft (used in some centers)

  2. Immunosuppressant therapy

      a) This therapy is given prophylactically prior to transplant.

b) Immunosuppressive drugs have different mechanisms of action or specific pathways (e.g., blocking TNF, IL-2 pathways) and therefore often are used in combination.

c) A two-drug combination of calcineurin inhibitors (CNIs) (cyclosporine or tacrolimus) and a short course of methotrexate (MTX) is standard for acute GVHD prophylaxis.

d) A newer combination of sirolimus and tacrolimus can be used as preventive GVHD therapy. However, increased incidence of transplant-associated microangiopathy has occurred when sirolimus is combined with a CNI.

3. GVHD prophylaxis (Antin & Raley, 2013; Ippoliti & Massaro, 2007)

   a) CNIs

   (1) Both cyclosporine and tacrolimus have a similar mechanism of action. Cyclosporine binds to cyclophilin and tacrolimus binds to FKBP12, both of which are proteins.

   (2) These complexes inhibit calcineurin phosphatase, which is a protein necessary for cellular processes, and signal transduction pathways.

   (3) They serve to inhibit activation and proliferation of T lymphocytes by interfering with IL-2 production and expression of IL-2 receptor. IL-2 is one of the major cytokines responsible in the activation and proliferation of T cells.

   (4) CNIs carry a risk of the development of transplant-associated thrombotic microangiopathy (TA-TMA) (Chapin et al., 2014).

   (a) TA-TMA refers to inflammatory and thrombotic diseases of the microvasculature. It is manifested by thrombocytopenia, microangiopathic hemolytic anemia, and organ dysfunction. Acute renal dysfunction is not uncommon.

   (b) Occurs in 10%–20% of allogeneic HSCT recipients

   (c) Carries a high mortality rate

   (d) May be difficult to diagnose, as clinical symptoms of TA-TMA are similar to atypical hemolytic uremic syndrome and thrombotic thrombocytopenic purpura

   (e) Pathophysiology is not well understood. Diagnosis is made by the presence of schistocytes on peripheral blood smear, high lactate dehydrogenase, low hemoglobin and platelet counts, increased unconjugated bilirubin, Coombs-negative hemolysis, increased serum creatinine, or changes in mental status.

   (f) Treatment is removal of CNIs. Other modalities of treatment have included plasma exchange, high-dose steroids, and rituximab; however, limited data exist that these are of benefit.

   b) Cyclosporine

   (1) Mechanism of action: Prevents IL-2 gene expression, therefore impairing IL-2 synthesis and activation of T lymphocytes

   (2) Available in capsule and IV formulation

   (3) IV dose: 1.5 mg/kg every 12 hours

   (4) Conversion factor of IV to PO: Approximately 1:3

   (5) Begin cyclosporine at least two days prior to stem cell infusion to ensure therapeutic serum levels when the graft is infused.

   (6) Side effects

    (a) Metabolic

        i. Hyperglycemia (diabetes mellitus)

        ii. Hypomagnesemia

        iii. Hyperlipidemia

        iv. Osteoporosis

        v. Hyperkalemia

    (b) Neurologic (Bechstein, 2000)

        i. Posterior reversible encephalopathy syndrome: A clinico-radiologic process characterized by varying degrees of tremors, neuralgia, peripheral neuropathy, psychoses, hallucinations, blindness, cerebellar ataxia or leukoencephalopathy, vomiting, visual disturbance, and focal neurologic signs

        ii. Headaches

        iii. Tremors

        iv. Seizures

        v. Paresthesias

        vi. Ataxia

        vii. Dizziness

        viii. Insomnia

    (c) GI

        i. Nausea and vomiting

        ii. Constipation

        iii. Anorexia

        iv. Abnormal liver function tests (LFTs) (hyperbilirubinemia)

        v. Gingival hyperplasia

        vi. Dysphagia

        vii. Gastritis

        viii. Pancreatitis

    (d) Cardiovascular

        i. Hypertension: Treat with calcium channel blocker (i.e., nifedipine extended release [ER], amlodipine).

        ii. Peripheral edema

    (e) Renal: Nephrotoxicity (elevated serum creatinine)

    (f) Hematologic: TA-TMA

    (g) Dermatologic

        i. Acneform rash

        ii. Hirsutism

    (h) Other

        i. Infection

        ii. Impaired wound healing

        iii. Flushing

        iv. Night sweats

(7) Administration

    (a) Designate an IV lumen for cyclosporine administration to prevent erroneous blood level results.

    (b) Instruct patients not to change oral formulation. Bioavailability differs between capsule formulations.

    (c) Instruct patients to take oral formulation with food.

(d) Emphasize the importance of strict adherence to the schedule of every 12 hours.

(e) Monitor serum creatinine, blood urea nitrogen (BUN), potassium, and magnesium levels.

(f) Coadministration of grapefruit juice may increase levels.

(g) Drug–drug combinations, especially cytochrome P450 inhibitors or inducers, can induce toxic or subtherapeutic levels.

(h) Many drug–drug interactions exist. Reduce initial dose by 50% when beginning voriconazole therapy. When discontinuing voriconazole, monitor and adjust cyclosporine dose according to levels.

(i) Therapeutic range varies in institutions and with assay (approximately 200–400 ng/ml).

(j) Routine monitoring is recommended at least twice per week early in transplant course. Aim for therapeutic level just prior to engraftment in an attempt to reduce the chance of developing GVHD.

(k) Dose adjust for renal dysfunction (see Table 5-1).

c) Tacrolimus (Alousi et al., 2007; Antin & Raley, 2013; Corella, 2011; Ippoliti & Massaro, 2007; Mitchell, 2013)

(1) A macrolide antibiotic that inhibits the factor that turns on the genes for cytokines essential to early T-cell activation (IL-2, interferon, and TNF)

(2) Available in PO and IV formulation

(3) Initial IV dose: 0.02–0.03 mg/kg continuous infusion (doses adjusted to achieve therapeutic levels)

(4) Initiate at least two days prior to stem cell infusion to ensure adequate level.

(5) Conversion factor of IV to PO: Approximately 1:4

(6) Monitor serum levels drawn from uncontaminated lumen.

(7) Side effects

(a) Metabolic

i. Hyperkalemia

ii. Hyperglycemia

iii. Hypomagnesemia

iv. Hypophosphatemia

Table 5-1. Sample Dose Adjustments of Tacrolimus and Cyclosporine in Patients With Renal Dysfunction

Creatinine (mg/dl)	Tacrolimus/Cyclosporine Dosage
< 1.5	100%
1.5–1.7	75%
1.8–2	50%
> 2	Hold dose until creatinine is < 2 and resume at 50%–75% prior dose.

Note. Based on information from Evans, 2009; Goker et al., 2001.

From "Acute and Chronic Graft-Versus-Host Disease" (p. 126), by S.A. Mitchell in S.A. Ezzone (Ed.), *Hematopoietic Stem Cell Transplantation: A Manual for Nursing Practice* (2nd ed.), 2013, Pittsburgh, PA: Oncology Nursing Society. Copyright 2013 by Oncology Nursing Society. Adapted with permission.

       v. Hyperlipidemia
- (b) Neurologic
  - i. Headache
  - ii. Tremors
  - iii. Dizziness
  - iv. Seizures
- (c) GI
  - i. Diarrhea
  - ii. Nausea and vomiting
  - iii. Anorexia
  - iv. Constipation
  - v. Abdominal pain
  - vi. Dysphagia
  - vii. Elevated LFTs (hyperbilirubinemia)
- (d) Renal
  - i. Elevated serum creatinine
  - ii. Nephrotoxicity
- (e) Cardiovascular
  - i. Hypertension (requires treatment with calcium channel blocker [nifedipine ER or amlodipine])
  - ii. Peripheral edema
- (f) Hematologic: TA-TMA
- (g) Dermatologic
  - i. Pruritus
  - ii. Skin rash
- (h) Other
  - i. Peripheral edema
  - ii. Infection
  - iii. Impaired wound healing

(8) Administration
- (a) Instruct the patient to take PO formulations on an empty stomach.
- (b) Emphasize the importance of strict adherence to the schedule of every 12 hours.
- (c) Bioavailability may vary with different formulations.
- (d) Coadministration of grapefruit juice may increase levels.
- (e) Drug–drug interactions with cytochrome P450 inhibitors or inducers can cause subtherapeutic or toxic levels.
- (f) Major interaction in HSCT setting is with voriconazole. Consider decreasing tacrolimus to one-half to one-third dose with voriconazole initiation.
- (g) Do not administer simultaneously with cyclosporine.
- (h) Discontinue tacrolimus 24 hours prior to starting cyclosporine.
- (i) Dose adjust for renal dysfunction (see Table 5-1).

d) Other considerations: Generic CNIs
- (1) Patients should be educated on the possibility that their immunosuppressant medications may change in shape, size, or color.
- (2) There should be consistent use of one drug formulation, as drug levels may vary with different formulations.

(3) Dose adjustments of supratherapeutic or subtherapeutic levels are made considering renal function. Adjustments of 25%–50% reduction or increase in levels are common. For supratherapeutic levels above institutional range, the CNI may be held and repeat levels followed and redose based on levels.

e) Sirolimus (Alousi et al., 2007; Corella, 2011; Cutler et al., 2008; Ippoliti & Massaro, 2007; Mitchell, 2013; Slater, 2011)

(1) Immunosuppressant used in both prevention and treatment

(2) Macrolide antibiotic that inhibits the response of B and T lymphocytes to cytokine stimulation by IL-2. It also inhibits antibody production by B cells.

(3) Available only as PO formulation

(4) Has a long half-life and requires once-daily dosing

(5) Standard dose: 12 mg PO loading (6 mg BID) then 4 mg PO daily

(6) Monitor serum concentrations. Varies with institutions, but therapeutic levels range from 5–15 ng/ml.

(7) Metabolized through the cytochrome P450 3A system and therefore has many drug–drug interactions

(8) Needs to be monitored closely with voriconazole

(9) Side effects: Hyperlipidemia, headache, nausea, dizziness, thrombocytopenia, leukopenia, peripheral edema, hypertension, hypokalemia, increased serum creatinine, pneumonitis, and pulmonary toxicity. Sirolimus has a lower risk of transplant-related microangiopathy, but this risk is increased when used in combination with tacrolimus.

(10) Sirolimus may suppress hematopoietic recovery if used after recent high-dose therapy.

(11) Oral bioavailability is variable and improved with high-fat meals.

III. Antibodies (Alousi et al., 2007; Antin & Raley, 2013; Corella, 2011; Mitchell, 2013; Slater, 2011)

A. Antithymocyte globulin (ATG)

1. Either horse-derived or rabbit-derived. Both affect cell-mediated immunity. Each product contains antibodies against T lymphocytes and selectively destroys T lymphocytes.

2. Dose ranges: No consensus exists, and the dose may vary with institutional guidelines and conditioning regimens (myeloablative versus RIC).

a) Rabbit ATG usually is administered for three days prior to infusion of cells (i.e., days –3, –2, –1). Doses vary with institutional protocols, but common dosing is 2.5 mg/kg per day. Doses also can be escalated (e.g., 0.5 mg/kg day –3 , 1 mg/kg day –2, 2 mg/kg day –1).

b) Horse ATG: Doses vary with institutional protocols, ranging from 10 mg/kg per day to 40 mg/kg per day. Administer prior to transplant (days –3, –2, –1).

3. Used as an immunosuppressant before transplant to prevent graft rejection and GVHD. Also used as treatment for GVHD after transplant.

4. Administration

a) Horse ATG requires a test dose prior to the first dose. No test dose is required for rabbit ATG. A conservative approach recommended by manufacturer is a "prick test" (epicutaneous) with undiluted ATGAM.

    (1) If there is no wheal 10 minutes after pricking, proceed to intradermal testing with 0.02 ml of a 1:1,000 volume/volume saline dilution of horse ATG, with a separate saline control injection of similar volume.

    (2) Result is read at 10 minutes: A wheal at the horse ATG site of 3 mm or larger in diameter than the saline control site suggests a sensitivity and increased possibility of allergic reaction to infusion.

   b) ATG is infused over four to six hours (based on concentration) because of the potential for adverse side effects or reaction (e.g., rigors, fevers, hypotension, shortness of breath [SOB], laryngospasm, anaphylaxis, pulmonary edema, cytokine release syndrome).

   c) Administering steroids and antihistamine prior to initiating the infusion as well as halfway through the infusion can help reduce the incidence of serious reactions. Standard premedications of diphenhydramine 50 mg IV and steroids. (Methylprednisolone 0.5 mg/kg pre-infusion and 0.5 mg/kg halfway through the infusion often are used.)

    (1) Monitor the patient closely during and following infusion.

    (2) Anaphylaxis kit must be at bedside during infusion.

    (3) Meperidine: 12.5–25 mg IV can be used for rigors if hemodynamically stable.

    (4) Adverse effects: Tachycardia, hypertension, hyperkalemia, diarrhea, nausea, vomiting, fever, chills

    (5) Side effects: Dyspnea, pulmonary edema, chest pain, anaphylaxis, sepsis, fever, rigors, rash, nausea and vomiting

    (6) Serum sickness may develop after infusion: myalgias, arthralgias, fever, rash, and hand and facial edema. Serum sickness is treated with steroids.

    (7) ATG's immunosuppressive effect causes high risk of morbidity and mortality due to infectious complications.

B. Mycophenolate mofetil (Alousi et al., 2007; Antin & Raley, 2013; Apperley & Masszi, 2012; Corella, 2011; Ippoliti & Massaro, 2007; Mitchell, 2013; Slater, 2011): Interferes with purine nucleotide synthesis and selectively inhibits proliferation of T and B lymphocytes

  1. Dose: 15 mg/kg IV or PO every 8 or 12 hours (institutional guidelines vary). IV and PO doses are equivalent. Maximum of 1,000–1,500 mg per dose.

  2. Side effects

   a) Metabolic

    (1) Hyperkalemia

    (2) Hypokalemia

    (3) Hyperlipidemia

    (4) Hyperglycemia

    (5) Hypocalcemia

    (6) Hypomagnesemia

   b) Neurologic

    (1) Headache

    (2) Insomnia

    (3) Dizziness

    (4) Tremors

    (5) Paresthesias

    c) GI
        (1) Diarrhea
        (2) Nausea and vomiting
        (3) Constipation
        (4) Anorexia
        (5) Abdominal pain
        (6) Hepatotoxicity
        (7) Ascites
        (8) Abnormal LFTs
    d) Cardiovascular
        (1) Hypertension
        (2) Peripheral edema
    e) Hematologic
        (1) Anemia
        (2) Leukocytosis or leukopenia
        (3) Thrombocytopenia
    f) Renal: Elevated serum BUN and creatinine
    g) Respiratory
        (1) SOB
        (2) Pleural effusion
        (3) Cough
    h) Dermatologic: Acneform rash
    i) Other
  3. Administration
    a) Instruct patient to take on an empty stomach.
    b) Monitor LFTs and complete blood counts.
    c) Mycophenolate mofetil may have decreased absorption when administered with magnesium oxide-, aluminum-, or magnesium-containing antacids or cholestyramine. There should be a gap of at least two hours between antacids and mycophenolate because of decreased absorption secondary to antacids.
    d) GI pathology of mycophenolate mofetil may mimic that of GVHD (Selbst et al., 2009).
C. MTX (Alousi et al., 2007; Antin & Raley, 2013; Apperley & Masszi, 2012; Corella, 2011; Ippoliti & Massaro, 2007; Mitchell, 2013; Slater, 2011): An antimetabolite that affects DNA synthesis and cell reproduction and inhibits lymphocyte proliferation
  1. Dose
    a) Standard regimen: 15 mg/m^2 IV on day +1, followed by 10 mg/m^2 on days +3, +6, and +11
    b) Mini-dosing regimen: 5 mg/m^2 IV on days +1, +3, +6, and +11
  2. Side effects: Myelosuppression, mucositis, interstitial pneumonitis, hepatotoxicity, and nephrotoxicity
  3. Administration
    a) Doses may be adjusted or held for severe mucositis and renal or liver insufficiency, significant ascites, weight gain, or fluid retention.
    b) First dose should be given at least 24 hours following stem cell infusion.
    c) Leucovorin rescue for side effects or toxicities (mucositis) of MTX can begin 12–24 hours after administration of MTX. Dose is the same as the MTX dose and is given for two to eight doses.

D. Cyclophosphamide (Luznik et al., 2008, 2010): An alkylating agent that targets pro-
   liferating alloreactive T cells
   1. Used most often in haploidentical transplants but can be used in other protocols
   2. Dose: 50 mg/kg per day on days +3 and +4 after stem cell infusion

IV. Acute GVHD (Alousi et al., 2007; Jacobsohn & Vogelsang, 2007; Mitchell, 2013; Slater,
    2011; Vargas-Díez, Garcia-Díez, Marin, & Fernández-Herrera, 2005)
   A. Diagnosis: Biopsy of the involved tissues is the gold standard for diagnosing GVHD,
      but biopsies often are not definitive. Thus, GVHD diagnosis is made based on sug-
      gestive pathology and clinical correlation (laboratory values, symptoms). Biopsies can
      confirm the diagnosis when other diagnoses are included in the differential, such as
      infection or drug reaction.
   B. Clinical presentation
      1. Clinical manifestations of acute GVHD can present as dermatitis, enteritis, or
         hepatitis, representing skin, GI, and liver.
      2. Patients may have disease in one or multiple organs.
   C. Organs involved
      1. Skin (Alousi et al., 2007; Antin & Raley, 2013; Apperley & Masszi, 2012; Ferr-
         ara et al., 2009; Garnett, Apperley, & Pavlů, 2013; Jacobsohn & Vogelsang, 2007;
         Mitchell, 2013; Slater, 2011)
         a) Clinical characteristics
            (1) The skin usually is the first organ to be involved.
            (2) An erythematous, maculopapular rash (painful or pruritic) can occur
                at or near time of engraftment. It involves the palms of hands, soles of
                feet, and neck, spreading to trunk and extremities.
            (3) Distribution progresses and becomes more confluent.
            (4) Severity is determined by percentage of body surface area involved using
                the Rule of Nines (see Figure 5-1).
            (5) Appearance is similar to sunburn with blanching.
            (6) In more severe cases, skin is erythrodermic and can have bullous lesions
                or desquamation.
            (7) Manifestations usually develop two to three weeks after stem cell trans-
                plant.
         b) Pathologic features (Apperley & Masszi, 2012): Lichenoid infiltration of
            the upper dermis and lower epidermis with vacuolation, degeneration, and
            individual cell necrosis of the basal layer of the epidermis. Pathologic fea-
            tures also include apoptosis at dermal–epidermal junction.
            (1) Grade 1: Vacuolation of epidermal basal cells
            (2) Grade 2: Presence of individually necrotic keratinocytes
            (3) Grade 3: Formation of bullae on confluent areas of keratinocyte necrosis
            (4) Grade 4: Sloughing of the epidermis
         c) Differential diagnosis
            (1) Chemotherapy and radiation effects
            (2) Drug allergy
            (3) Viral infection
         d) Nursing implications (Alousi et al., 2007; Slater, 2011): Ancillary skin care
            (1) Monitor progression of rash.
            (2) Monitor pruritus.

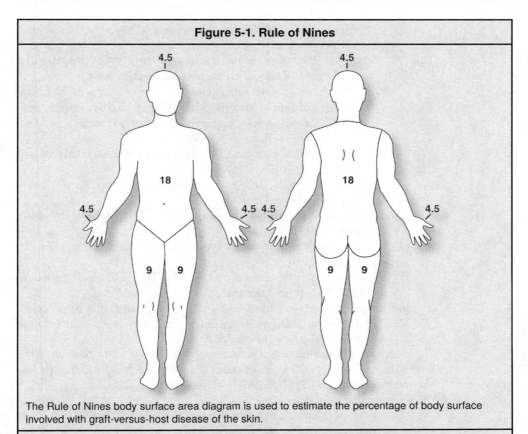

Figure 5-1. Rule of Nines

The Rule of Nines body surface area diagram is used to estimate the percentage of body surface involved with graft-versus-host disease of the skin.

Note. From "Acute and Chronic Graft-Versus-Host Disease" (p. 110), by S.A. Mitchell in S.A. Ezzone (Ed.), *Hematopoietic Stem Cell Transplantation: A Manual for Nursing Practice* (2nd ed.), 2013, Pittsburgh, PA: Oncology Nursing Society. Copyright 2013 by Oncology Nursing Society. Reprinted with permission.

(3) Cleanse the skin using a mild hypoallergenic nondrying soap on intact skin and warm normal saline on areas of desquamation.

(4) Avoid perfumed lotions.

(5) Use sunscreen and avoid exposure to sunlight.

 e) Pharmacologic treatment of cutaneous acute GVHD

  (1) CNI levels should be therapeutic at all times.

  (2) Topical steroids

   (a) Stage 1 and 2 skin GVHD often can be successfully treated with topical steroid creams and should be tried to avoid further systemic immunosuppressant therapy.

   (b) Institutional protocols vary from beginning with high-dose topical steroids to trying a lower dose first for stages 1 and 2.

   (c) Physician preference determines if moderate- or high-dose topical steroid cream or ointment will be initiated.

   (d) Triamcinolone (0.1%) or betamethasone (0.1%) are considered moderate-dose topical steroids, which should be used on only

trunk and extremities. Hydrocortisone (1%) cream can be used on face, neck, and groin.

(e) If possible, wrap affected areas with warm moist dressing after application of steroid cream to increase absorption.

(f) High-potency steroids (e.g., clobetasol dipropionate [0.05%], betamethasone dipropionate [0.05%]) can be applied two to three times daily. To avoid atrophy, higher-potency steroid creams should not be used longer than two weeks.

(g) If still needed, change to a lower-potency steroid cream (e.g., triamcinolone [0.1%]).

(h) The face, axilla, and groin require low-potency steroid cream (hydrocortisone [1%]).

(3) Tacrolimus ointments have been used with, or in place of, steroids for cutaneous GVHD.

(4) Systemic antihistamines can be symptomatically helpful if topical treatment is inadequate.

(5) Wound care may be necessary: Stage 4 GVHD with blistering exfoliation usually requires burn care.

(6) Frequent dressing changes with warm normal saline may be necessary.

(7) Application of antibiotic ointment (e.g., mupirocin ointment) and nonadherent dressings may be helpful.

2. The GI tract is the second most common organ affected (Antin & Raley, 2013; Jacobsohn & Vogelsang, 2007; Kalantari et al., 2003; Mitchell, 2013; Parfitt, Jayakumar, & Driman, 2008; Slater, 2011; Vargas-Díez et al., 2005).

a) Clinical characteristics

(1) Lower GI (involving distal small bowel and colon): Diarrhea is the main symptom. It may be voluminous and often is green, mucoid, watery, and mixed with exfoliated cells and tissue shreds. It often is accompanied by crampy abdominal pain and distension. Diarrhea may become bloody with progression of GVHD.

(2) Upper GI: Persistent nausea, vomiting, bloating, or anorexia

(3) Hypoalbuminemia occurs secondary to GVHD-associated intestinal protein leak and negative nitrogen balance.

(4) Stage 4 GI GVHD involves painful cramping, bloody diarrhea, and, ultimately, ileus.

(5) Severity of GI GVHD is measured by volume of diarrhea (see Table 5-2).

b) Differential diagnosis: Must rule out other causes of diarrhea.

(1) Food poisoning

(2) Infection

(3) Mucositis from preparative regimen

(4) Bacterial or viral infection (e.g., cytomegalovirus [CMV], *Clostridium difficile* [*C. difficile*], norovirus, adenovirus)

(5) Drug side effect

c) Diagnosis: Lower or upper endoscopy

(1) Endoscopy findings: Mucosal erythema, edema, mucosal sloughing and, possibly, bleeding. This may involve the cecum, ileum, and colon, as well as the upper GI tract.

(2) Areas may be denuded.

Table 5-2. Staging and Grading for Acute Graft-Versus-Host Disease (GVHD)		
Consensus Criteria for Clinical Staging and Grading of Acute GVHD		
Organ	**Grade**	**Description**
Skin	+1	Maculopapular eruption over < 25% of body area
	+2	Maculopapular eruption over 25%–50% of body area
	+3	Generalized erythroderma
	+4	Generalized erythroderma with bullous formation and often with desquamation
Liver	+1	Bilirubin 2–3 mg/dl
	+2	Bilirubin 3.1–6 mg/dl
	+3	Bilirubin 6.1–15 mg/dl
	+4	Bilirubin > 15 mg/dl
Gut	+1	Diarrhea > 500 ml/day or > 30 ml/kg
	+2	Diarrhea > 1,000 ml/day or > 60 ml/kg
	+3	Diarrhea > 1,500 ml/day or > 90 ml/kg
	+4	Diarrhea > 2,000 ml/day or > 120 ml/kg

Overall Stage				
Stage	**Skin***	**Liver**	**Gut**	**Performance Status**
I	+1 to +2	0	0	No decrease
II	+1 to +3	+1	and/or +1	Mild decrease
III	+2 to +3	+2 to +3	and/or +2 to +3	Marked decrease
IV	+2 to +4	+2 to +4	and/or +2 to +4	Extreme decrease

*If no skin disease is present, the overall grade is the higher, single organ stage.

Note. Based on information from Chao, 2015; Glucksberg et al., 1974; Przepiorka et al., 1995.

From "Graft Versus Host Disease" (p. 92), by S.A. Mitchell in S.A. Ezzone (Ed.), *Hematopoietic Stem Cell Transplantation: A Resource Book for Nurses*, 2004, Pittsburgh, PA: Oncology Nursing Society. Copyright 2004 by Oncology Nursing Society. Adapted with permission.

      d) Diagnostic imaging of bowel
          (1) X-ray: Plain films may show bowel dilatation, bowel wall thickening, air fluid levels, and paucity of gas; this, however, may not be diagnostic of GVHD. Infectious and neutropenic colitis are among the differential diagnosis in plain film imaging.
          (2) Computed tomography (CT) scan will show bowel wall thickening with or without proximal dilatation, engorgement of the vasa recta, mesenteric fat stranding, mucosal enhancement, gallbladder–biliary tract abnormalities, and ascites. CT findings associated with high-grade GVHD include thickening of the distal esophagus, ileum, or ascending colon and increasing number of thickened bowel wall segments.
      e) Pathology
          (1) Crypt cell apoptosis
          (2) May be difficult to distinguish GVHD from effects of chemotherapy or radiation

        (a) Grade 1: Individual cell necrosis

        (b) Grade 2: Loss of individual crypts

        (c) Grade 3: Loss of two or more adjacent crypts with ulceration

        (d) Grade 4: Denudation of epithelium

    f) Nursing implications and supportive care for GI GVHD

       (1) Strict intake and output

       (2) Daily weights

       (3) Rectal skin care

       (4) Bowel rest: Primary first-treatment strategy for acute GI GVHD

       (5) Aggressive hydration and electrolyte repletion if large-volume diarrhea

       (6) Total parenteral nutrition (TPN) (often required)

       (7) May require IV narcotics but must be used cautiously and with close monitoring. Paralytic ileus is grade 4 of GVHD, and use of narcotics may contribute.

    g) Once the patient begins to show signs of improvement, diet should be advanced slowly with the GVHD Progressive Diet (see Table 5-3).

Table 5-3. Graft-Versus-Host Disease Progressive Diet Regimen		
Stage	**Diet Principles**	**Suggested Foods**
1	Bowel rest	NPO (nothing by mouth); consider need for total parenteral nutrition (TPN).
2	Liquids, isotonic, lactose-free, low residue, no caffeine, allow 60 ml every two to three hours. If diarrhea or cramps recur or persist, return to bowel rest. Continue TPN.	Water, decaffeinated tea, decaffeinated coffee, caffeine-free diet soft drinks, caffeine-free and sugar-free imitation fruit drinks (e.g., Crystal Light®), sugar-free Jell-O®, sugar-free Popsicles®, clear broth, consommé, bouillon, sugar-free or dietetic hard candy that does not contain sorbitol or xylitol
3	Introduce solid foods, choosing low-fiber, lactose-free, fat-free, starchy foods. Sugar is introduced during this phase. Small portions only. No meat or meat products are allowed. Low total acidity; no gastric irritants such as caffeine. Introduce one food at a time. Each new food may be tried with foods taken previously. Discontinue the most recently added food if diarrhea or abdominal pain increases. If symptoms persist, return to bowel rest. Continue TPN until calorie and protein counts and fluid intake are adequate. May drink water, decaffeinated tea, decaffeinated coffee, caffeine-free diet soft drinks, and caffeine-free and sugar-free imitation fruit drinks (e.g., Crystal Light), in addition to foods chosen from list.	Plain white bread/toast, bagel, English muffin Soda crackers, melba toast, matzo, graham crackers Cream of Wheat®, crisped rice, cornflakes, Cheerios® White rice, plain noodles Arrowroot cookies, social tea cookies Fruit juices (less than 60 ml serving/may try half strength): apple, cranberry, grape, pineapple, orange, grapefruit, or tomato juice (no more than two servings/day) Mashed or boiled potato without skin or butter Clear chicken, meat, or vegetable broth; consommé; broth containing noodles or rice Jell-O, Popsicles
		(Continued on next page)

Table 5-3. Graft-Versus-Host Disease Progressive Diet Regimen *(Continued)*		
Stage	**Diet Principles**	**Suggested Foods**
4	Solid foods as in stage 3 but with fat intake slowly increased	Lactose-free milk Plain white bread/toast, bagel, English muffin, soda crackers, melba toast, matzo, graham crackers Cream of Wheat, crisped rice, cornflakes, Cheerios White rice, plain noodles Arrowroot cookies, social tea cookies Fruit juices (half strength or less than 60 ml serving): apple, cranberry, grape, pineapple, orange, grapefruit, or tomato juice (may increase to four servings/day) Mashed or boiled potato without skin or butter Trimmed lean meats, fish, and poultry baked, broiled, boiled, poached, roasted, or stewed Maximum one egg per day, boiled or poached Tuna or salmon packed in water or broth Cooked vegetables one to two servings/day (asparagus, carrots) Clear chicken, beef, or vegetable broth; consommé; broth containing noodles or rice Cream soups prepared with lactose-free milk Natural hard, low-fat cheese (skim-milk mozzarella, parmesan) Jell-O, Popsicles, peaches or pears canned in juice or water (maximum of half cup or two halves)
5	Advance to regular diet by adding restricted foods, one per day, to assess tolerance.	Last foods to be tried include high-fiber foods, food or drinks that contain caffeine (e.g., coffee, chocolate, soft drinks with caffeine), and lactose-containing foods, including ice cream, custard, milk, and cottage cheese.

Note. Based on information from Charuhas, 2006; Gauvreau et al., 1981; Henry & Loader, 2009; McCrudden et al., 2004.

From "Acute and Chronic Graft-Versus-Host Disease" (p. 135), by S.A. Mitchell in S.A. Ezzone (Ed.), *Hematopoietic Stem Cell Transplantation: A Manual for Nursing Practice* (2nd ed.), 2013, Pittsburgh, PA: Oncology Nursing Society. Copyright 2013 by Oncology Nursing Society. Reprinted with permission.

h) Once infectious etiology is ruled out as the cause of diarrhea, management strategies include antimotility agents.
   (1) Loperamide
   (2) Diluted tincture of opium: 0.3–1 ml PO every two to six hours PRN (maximum daily dose of 6 ml)

(3) Octreotide: 100–150 mcg IV TID

(4) Oral beclomethasone dipropionate: 2 mg PO every six hours

(5) Budesonide: 3 mg PO TID or 9 mg PO every day

3. The liver is the third most commonly affected organ (Jacobsohn & Vogelsang, 2007; Mitchell, 2013).

   a) Clinical characteristics (hepatic): Specific laboratory values may suggest liver involvement of GVHD, also called a *cholestatic picture.*

     (1) Hyperbilirubinemia

     (2) Increased alkaline phosphatase

     (3) Lesser-degree elevated transaminases (alanine transaminase, aspartate transaminase)

   b) Differential diagnosis

     (1) Hepatic veno-occlusive disease

     (2) Effects of preparatory regimen

     (3) Effects of TPN

     (4) Viral infection

     (5) Sepsis

     (6) Drug toxicity, including drugs used for prophylaxis of GVHD (e.g., cyclosporine, tacrolimus, MTX)

   c) Diagnosis of liver GVHD

     (1) Transjugular liver biopsy

     (2) Pathology

       (a) Bile duct apoptosis, lymphocytic attack on bile ducts, and bizarre irregular bile ducts

       (b) Loss of bile duct integrity leads to jaundice.

   d) Nursing implications

     (1) Avoid all hepatotoxic medications. Dose adjust those medications that cannot be discontinued and are potentially hepatotoxic.

     (2) Monitor LFTs and coagulation studies.

     (3) Consider adding ursodiol 300 mg PO BID or TID to protect liver cells from damaging activity of toxic bile salts.

4. Other manifestations of acute GVHD (Mitchell, 2013)

   a) Leukopenia, anemia, and thrombocytopenia

   b) Hypogammaglobulinemia

   c) Increased risk of infections, especially CMV

   d) Hemolysis

5. Grading and staging of acute GVHD (Alousi et al., 2007; Apperley & Masszi, 2012; Mitchell, 2013; Slater, 2011)

   a) Severity of GVHD is based on histology and clinical factors.

   b) Glucksberg grading and staging of acute GVHD involves the degree of skin, liver, and GI involvement.

     (1) Each organ is graded from 0–4.

       (a) GI: Daily volume of diarrhea

       (b) Liver: Bilirubin level

       (c) Skin: Rule of Nines

     (2) To determine the overall stage of GVHD, these grades are combined, taking into consideration the grade of each organ and its effect on performance status to provide an overall stage (see Table 5-2).

(3) In 1994, the Consensus Workshop attempted to improve the scoring system. They retained much of the Glucksberg scoring system but dropped the clinical performance score status.

D. Treatment of acute GVHD (Alousi et al., 2007; Antin & Raley, 2013; Apperley & Masszi, 2012; Garnett et al., 2013; Martin et al., 2012; Mitchell, 2013)

   1. Key concepts
      a) Patients receive prophylactic immunosuppressive therapy prior to transplant or depletion of T cells in grafts to minimize the risk of acute GVHD.
      b) GVHD often occurs while patients are still on CNI prophylaxis.
      c) Despite measures to prevent it, 20%–80% patients still develop acute GVHD.
      d) Symptoms usually develop two to three weeks after transplant.
      e) Management of acute GVHD is challenging and requires a multidisciplinary team of experts and clinicians who are knowledgeable in HSCT, as well as social workers and psychiatrists for emotional and psychological support.
      f) Survival correlates directly with response to initial therapy.
      g) Decision to begin systemic treatment depends on the severity of GVHD and the rate of progression.
      h) Rapid progression of GI or liver GVHD requires prompt systemic treatment.
      i) Immunosuppression is the main treatment strategy for acute GVHD.
      j) If the patient is on a CNI, therapeutic levels should be maintained.
      k) Grade 1 acute GVHD may respond to topical agents (e.g., cream or ointment for skin GVHD, oral budesonide or beclomethasone for upper GI GVHD). This will limit the toxicities of systemic steroids.
      l) Cases of indolent progression of rash without intestinal or liver involvement need assessment of risk-benefit ratio of adding additional high-dose systemic immunosuppressants (Martin et al., 2012).
      m) Cases that do not resolve with topical treatment may require systemic treatment or additional immunosuppression.
      n) Generally, systemic therapy is required for grades 2–4.

   2. Primary therapy for GVHD (immunosuppressive agents) (Alousi et al., 2007; Antin & Raley, 2013; Apperley & Masszi, 2012; Garnett et al., 2013; Ippoliti & Massaro, 2007; Martin et al., 2012; Mitchell, 2013)
      a) The goal is to disrupt the immune pathways and interactions that initiate and perpetuate the destructive behavior of donor T cells.
      b) Risk of infection can be caused by severe immunosuppression.
      c) Risk of relapse of underlying malignancy occurs from the inhibition of the graft-versus-tumor effect of lymphocytes.
      d) Systemic corticosteroids remain the mainstay of first-line treatment in grades 2–4 acute GVHD.
         (1) Methylprednisolone has direct lymphocyte activity that serves to decrease cytotoxic T-cell proliferation and inhibit production of IL-1, IL-2, and interferon alpha.
         (2) Approximately 50% of patients with acute GVHD will have a partial or complete response to high-dose steroids.
         (3) Patients with steroid-resistant acute GVHD have a poor prognosis, with mortality rates in excess of 90%.
         (4) In most centers, the starting dose of methylprednisolone is 1–2 mg/kg per day, depending on the severity of GVHD.

(5) Steroids are added to the CNI that the patient may already be receiving. CNI levels should be therapeutic.

(6) Side effects of corticosteroids

    (a) Metabolic

        i. Fluid and electrolyte imbalance

        ii. Diabetes mellitus

        iii. Hyperlipidemia

        iv. Osteopenia, osteoporosis

        v. Hyperglycemia

    (b) Neurologic

        i. Tremors

        ii. Headache

        iii. Insomnia

        iv. Difficulty concentrating

    (c) Cardiovascular: Hypertension

    (d) GI

        i. Gastritis

        ii. Bleeding

    (e) Dermatologic

        i. Bruising

        ii. Fragile skin

    (f) Ophthalmic

        i. Cataract

        ii. Glaucoma

    (g) GI: Irritation

    (h) Other

        i. Peripheral edema

        ii. Infection

        iii. Impaired wound healing

        iv. Hirsutism

        v. Cushingoid changes

        vi. Muscle wasting

        vii. Avascular necrosis (AVN)

        viii. Gastritis

        ix. Increased risk of infections

        x. Weight gain

        xi. Steroid myopathy

    (i) Psychiatric

        i. Psychosis

        ii. Mood changes

        iii. Confusion

        iv. Insomnia

e) Administration of corticosteroids

(1) Corticosteroids often are used in combination with cyclosporine or tacrolimus.

(2) Prolonged high-dose steroids can cause proximal muscle weakness. Physical therapy consult should be recommended.

(3) Administer with food or milk to minimize GI upset.

(4) Administer with H_2 blocker.

(5) Once clinical improvement is noted, steroids should be tapered. No consensus exists regarding tapering. A more rapid taper reduces the risk of infectious complications but may precipitate a GVHD flare. A possible approach is a 10% reduction every week in the absence of GVHD symptoms and after GVHD has been controlled for about one month.

(6) Prolonged steroids render the patient at risk for relapse caused by suppression of immunologic graft-versus-disease effect.

(7) Prolonged steroids pose a high risk of fungal, viral, and bacterial infections. Administration of concomitant antimicrobials, including antibacterial, antiviral, and antifungal agents, should be considered.

(8) All CNIs used in combination with steroids should be maximized, and therapeutic levels should be achieved and monitored.

(9) The most important predictor of long-term survival is patient response to high-dose steroids.

3. Second- and third-line therapy (Alousi et al., 2007; Antin & Raley, 2013; Apperley & Masszi, 2012; Deeg, 2007; Garnett et al., 2013; Ippoliti & Massaro, 2007; Martin et al., 2012; Mitchell, 2013; Slater, 2011)

   a) Failed initial therapy with high-dose steroids is defined as progression of GVHD after three days, no change after seven days, or incomplete response after 14 days of steroids. Failed initial therapy requires further treatment.

   (1) No individual secondary therapy is preferred or considered standard of care.

   (2) Often, second- and third-line treatment is physician preference.

   (3) The higher the grade of acute GVHD, the poorer the outcome.

   (4) Second-line treatment is characterized by high failure rates, significant toxicities, and poor survival.

   (5) Response to treatment is a predictor of outcome, with mortality and morbidity rates highest in patients who do not achieve a complete response to initial strategy.

   (6) Patients who receive additional immunosuppressive therapy are at risk for opportunistic infections, CMV, and invasive fungal infections.

   b) Options for secondary therapy for GVHD (Antin & Raley, 2013; Deeg, 2007; Garnett et al., 2013; Hsu, May, Carrum, Krance, & Przepiorka, 2001; Mitchell, 2013; Slater, 2011)

   (1) If the patient is not on a CNI, tacrolimus, cyclosporine, or sirolimus can be added if not already used as GVHD prophylaxis.

   (2) Mycophenolate mofetil (Alousi et al., 2007; Antin & Raley, 2013; Apperley & Masszi, 2012; Corella, 2011; Ippoliti & Massaro, 2007; Mitchell, 2013; Slater, 2011): Interferes with purine nucleotide synthesis and selectively inhibits proliferation of T and B lymphocytes

      (a) Dose: 15 mg/kg IV or PO every 8 or 12 hours (institutional guidelines vary). IV and PO doses are equivalent. Maximum of 1,000–1,500 mg per dose.

      (b) Side effects

         i. Metabolic: Hyperkalemia, hypokalemia, hyperlipidemia, hyperglycemia, hypocalcemia, hypomagnesemia

      ii. Neurologic: Headache, insomnia, dizziness, tremors, paresthesias

     iii. GI: Diarrhea, nausea and vomiting, constipation, anorexia, abdominal pain, hepatotoxicity, ascites, abnormal LFTs

     iv. Cardiovascular: Hypertension, peripheral edema

     v. Hematologic: Anemia, leukocytosis, leukopenia, thrombocytopenia

     vi. Renal: Elevated serum BUN and creatinine

    vii. Respiratory: SOB, pleural effusion, cough

   viii. Dermatologic: Acneform rash

  (c) Administration

      i. Instruct patient to take on an empty stomach.

     ii. Monitor LFTs and complete blood counts.

    iii. Mycophenolate mofetil may have decreased absorption when administered with magnesium oxide-, aluminum-, or magnesium-containing antacids or cholestyramine. There should be a gap of at least two hours between antacids and mycophenolate because of decreased absorption secondary to antacids.

    iv. GI pathology of mycophenolate mofetil may mimic that of GVHD (Selbst et al., 2009).

(3) Sirolimus (Alousi et al., 2007; Corella, 2011; Cutler et al., 2008; Ippoliti & Massaro, 2007; Mitchell, 2013; Slater, 2011)

  (a) Immunosuppressant used in both prevention and treatment

  (b) Macrolide antibiotic that inhibits the response of B and T lymphocytes to cytokine stimulation by IL-2. It also inhibits antibody production by B cells.

  (c) Available only as PO formulation

  (d) Has a long half-life and requires once-daily dosing

  (e) Standard dose: 12 mg PO loading (6 mg BID) then 4 mg PO daily

  (f) Monitor serum concentrations. Varies with institutions, but therapeutic levels range from 5–15 ng/ml.

  (g) Metabolized through the cytochrome P450 3A system and therefore has many drug–drug interactions.

  (h) Needs to be monitored closely with voriconazole

  (i) Side effects: Hyperlipidemia, headache, nausea, dizziness, thrombocytopenia, leukopenia, peripheral edema, hypertension, hypokalemia, increased serum creatinine, pneumonitis, and pulmonary toxicity. Sirolimus has a lower risk of transplant-related microangiopathy, but this risk is increased when used in combination with tacrolimus.

  (j) Sirolimus may suppress hematopoietic recovery if used after recent high-dose therapy.

  (k) Oral bioavailability is variable and improved with high-fat meals.

(4) ATG: Horse or rabbit serum that consists of antibodies to human T cells. ATG is capable of destroying lymphocytes.

      (a) Dose ranges: No single consensus exists. Examples of dosing include the following (Hsu et al., 2001):
          i. Horse ATG: 5 mg/kg (40 mg/kg infused daily, BID, or every other day for 1–10 days)
          ii. Rabbit ATG: 1 mg/kg (10 mg/kg infused daily or every other day for 2–10 days)
      (b) Horse and rabbit ATG should not be used interchangeably, as their potency differs. Horse ATG requires a test dose prior to the first dose. No test dose is required for rabbit ATG.
      (c) ATG and ATGAM are administered with premedications of diphenhydramine and corticosteroids.
      (d) Improvements with ATG are noted in 20%–50% of patients.
      (e) Responses of 60%–75% have been observed for skin GVHD.
c) Other monoclonal antibodies (mAbs) (Alousi et al., 2007; Antin & Raley, 2013; Garnett et al., 2013; Mitchell, 2013; Przepiorka et al., 2000; Slater, 2011)
  (1) Infliximab
      (a) Mechanism of action: Chimeric mAb that binds to TNF-α, neutralizing its activity and causing cell lysis. TNF-α is present in high levels in patients with GVHD.
      (b) Dose: Standard dose is 10 mg/kg IV over two hours for one to four weeks.
      (c) Infliximab must be given with low protein-binding filter of 1.2 microns or less.
      (d) Infusion reactions (i.e., hypersensitivity reactions) can occur and include fever, chills, chest pain, hypotension, headache, and urticaria.
      (e) Other side effects include nausea, abdominal pain, fatigue, and coughing.
      (f) Delayed serum sickness–like symptoms include myalgias, arthralgias, fever, rash, sore throat, and hand and facial edema and can be seen 3–12 days after infusion.
      (g) Premedications of acetaminophen and diphenhydramine may be administered.
      (h) Increased risk of serious infections is present with infliximab.
  (2) Basiliximab
      (a) Mechanism of action: IL-2 receptor antagonist that blocks IL-2 receptor alpha chain on surface of activated T lymphocytes (off-label use) (Massenkeil et al., 2002)
      (b) Dose: 20 mg IV on days 1 and 4. May repeat for recurrent acute GVHD.
      (c) Side effects: Anaphylactic or hypersensitivity reactions, hypertension, edema, fever, and headache
          i. Metabolic: Hypercholesterolemia, hyperglycemia, hyperkalemia, hypokalemia, hypophosphatemia, and hyperuricemia
          ii. GI: Constipation, diarrhea, nausea and vomiting, dyspepsia
          iii. Neurologic: Tremor, headache

      iv. Pulmonary: Dyspnea

      v. Cardiac: Hypotension

      vi. Other: Infection and lymphoproliferative disorder, peripheral edema, fever, viral infections

(3) Alemtuzumab

  (a) Mechanism of action: Binds to cell surface CD52, which is present on all B and T lymphocytes, resulting in cell lysis

  (b) Dose: 10 mg per day IV for five doses

  (c) Adverse effects: Infusional reactions may be severe and include fever and rigors. Premedicate with acetaminophen and diphenhydramine.

  (d) Rare side effects include fatal pancytopenia with bone marrow hypoplasia, autoimmune idiopathic thrombocytopenia, and autoimmune hemolytic anemia.

  (e) Other side effects

      i. Nausea and vomiting

      ii. Rash

      iii. Fatigue

      iv. Hypotension

      v. Flu-like syndrome

      vi. Fever

      vii. Hypovolemia

      viii. Arrhythmias (ventricular, atrial)

      ix. Esophagitis, gastroenteritis, pancreatitis, colitis

      x. Acute coronary syndrome

      xi. Abnormal renal function

      xii. Muscle weakness

      xiii. Severe lymphopenia (increases risk of infection, especially opportunistic infections)

      xiv. Myelosuppression

(4) Pentostatin

  (a) Mechanism of action: Nucleoside analog that potentially inhibits adenosine deaminase, thus inducing lymphocyte apoptosis

  (b) Dose: 1.5 mg/m^2 IV daily on days 1–3 and 15–17

  (c) Requires dose adjustment by 50% for absolute neutrophil count less than 1,000/mm^3 or creatinine clearance of 30–50 ml/min

  (d) Side effects

      i. Increased risk of infection

      ii. Cytopenia

      iii. Abdominal pain, nausea, vomiting

      iv. Flu-like symptoms

      v. Transaminitis

      vi. Hypotension

      vii. Arthralgias

      viii. Hypercalcemia

      ix. Hyponatremia

(5) Etanercept

  (a) TNF receptor that inactivates TNF-α and TNF-beta

      (b) Dose: 0.4 mg/kg per dose (25 mg maximum) subcutaneous twice weekly for four to eight weeks (must be at least 72 hours apart)

      (c) Adverse reactions

        i. Increased risk for serious infection, including bacterial, fungal, and opportunistic infections

        ii. Headache

        iii. Injection site reaction

        iv. Rhinitis, upper respiratory infection

        v. Rare complications: Cytopenias, aplastic anemia, Stevens-Johnson syndrome

        vi. Autoimmune hepatitis and malignant lymphoma

        vii. Hepatitis B reactivation

        viii. New onset or exacerbation of central nervous system demyelinating disorder

d) Nonabsorbable enteral steroids: Budesonide and beclomethasone

  (1) Budesonide

      (a) Mechanism of action: Anti-inflammatory corticosteroid with low systemic bioavailability because of rapid first-pass metabolism in the liver

      (b) Dose: 3 mg PO TID

      (c) Fewer corticosteroid-related side effects because of low absorption

  (2) Beclomethasone (off-label use)

      (a) Mechanism of action: Synthetic corticosteroid with potent glucocorticoid activity but weak mineralocorticoid activity; mechanism of action not clearly understood

      (b) May be given in addition to IV steroids

      (c) Dose: 2 mg PO every six hours

e) Phototherapy (Peritt, 2006; Slater, 2011)

  (1) Often used as an adjunct to systemic therapy

  (2) Extracorporeal photopheresis (ECP) used for acute and chronic GVHD

  (3) Mechanism of action is not clearly understood, but it induces apoptosis of lymphocytes.

  (4) Infusions of apoptotic cells are taken up by APCs. These APCs decrease production of proinflammatory cytokines, increase production of anti-inflammatory cytokines, lower ability to stimulate T-cell responses, and induce regulatory T cells.

  (5) Performed by standard apheresis process

      (a) 8-Methoxypsoralen: 200 mcg is injected into the buffy coat/plasma.

      (b) This cell solution then is exposed to ultraviolet light and reinfused into the patient.

      (c) Patients are treated for two consecutive days at two- to four-week intervals.

      (d) Responding patients continue every two weeks for an extended period of time.

      (e) Abrupt termination of ECP is avoided, as symptoms may worsen or rebound.

      (f) Used for both acute and chronic GVHD

(6) Adverse effects include hypotension, anemia and thrombocytopenia, bleeding caused by procedure-related anticoagulant, and central venous catheter–associated bacterial infection or sepsis.

    4. Mesenchymal cells (Le Blanc & Ringdén, 2006)

      a) Mesenchymal cells have immunosuppressant properties.

      b) Cells are isolated from bone marrow, adipose tissue, and UCB and have the ability to differentiate into several tissues and produce growth factors and cytokines that promote hematopoietic cell expansion and differentiation.

      c) Mesenchymal cells also have antiproliferative, immunomodulatory, and anti-inflammatory properties but only evoke little immune reactivity.

E. Key points to acute GVHD treatment (Alousi et al., 2007; Antin & Raley, 2013; Apperley & Masszi, 2012; Deeg, 2007; Martin et al., 2012; Slater, 2011)

    1. Skin: ATG (either rabbit or horse), alemtuzumab, basiliximab, phototherapy, ECP, pentostatin, sirolimus, and mycophenolate

    2. Liver: ATG, alemtuzumab, ECP, mycophenolate, pentostatin, and sirolimus

    3. GI: ATG, beclomethasone, budesonide, etanercept, infliximab, pentostatin, and sirolimus

    4. First-line therapy: Steroids, CNIs

    5. Second- and third-line therapy

      a) Anti-TNF antibodies (infliximab, etanercept)

      b) Sirolimus

      c) IL-2 receptor antibodies (daclizumab, basiliximab)

      d) ATG

      e) Mesenchymal cells

      f) Alemtuzumab

      g) Pentostatin

      h) ECP

      i) Mycophenolate

    6. Antimicrobial prophylaxis should be considered: antibacterial, antiviral, antifungal, and prophylaxis for *Pneumocystis jiroveci* pneumonia (PCP).

    7. Some centers draw surveillance blood cultures weekly for patients on high-dose steroids and additional immunosuppression.

    8. Epstein-Barr virus (EBV), polymerase chain reactions (PCRs), and CMV should be monitored weekly.

    9. H_2 blockers should be administered with high-dose steroids.

V. Chronic GVHD (Alousi et al., 2007; Antin & Raley, 2013; Apperley & Masszi, 2012; Filipovich et al., 2005; Flowers & Martin, 2015; Jagasia et al., 2015; Lee & Flowers, 2008; Lee, Vogelsang, & Flowers, 2003; Martin et al., 2012; Maziarz & Abar, 2011; Mitchell, 2013; Peréz-Simón, Sánchez-Abarca, Díez-Campelo, Caballero, & San Miguel, 2006; Vogelsang, 2001)

A. Definition: Chronic GVHD is an immune-mediated disorder that occurs following allogeneic stem cell transplant. It has features that resemble autoimmune and immunodeficiency syndrome, such as scleroderma, Sjögren syndrome, primary biliary cirrhosis, wasting syndrome, bronchiolitis obliterans, immune cytopenias, and chronic immunodeficiency.

    1. It is a common late complication of allo-HSCT, significantly affecting overall survival and quality of life. It is the main cause of late, nonrelapse mortal-

ity and morbidity, primarily due to infections secondary to the disease itself or its treatment.

2. Clinical symptoms, not time of presentation following transplant, determine whether GVHD is acute or chronic.

3. It often requires long-term steroids, thereby putting patients at high risk for fatal infections.

4. It carries a reduced risk of recurrent disease by allowing benefit of graft-versus-disease (GVD) effect.

B. The major goal of treatment is to find a balance in controlling symptoms with the least amount of steroids or immunosuppressants.

C. Antimicrobial prophylaxis is recommended while on prolonged steroid/immuno-suppressive therapy.

1. Antifungal: Voriconazole, fluconazole, posaconazole

2. Viral: Herpes simplex virus (HSV) prophylaxis

   a) Acyclovir, valacyclovir

   b) Penicillin V potassium 250–500 mg BID

3. PCP prophylaxis: Trimethoprim-sulfamethoxazole, pentamidine, dapsone, atovaquone

4. Monitoring of CMV, EBV, PCR, and human herpesvirus 6 is recommended.

D. Pathophysiology (Apperley & Masszi, 2012; Ferrara et al., 2009; Jagasia et al., 2015; Min, 2011; Mitchell, 2013)

1. The pathophysiology of chronic GVHD is not clearly understood; however, T-lymphocyte imbalances, humoral immunity, activation of B cells, fibrosis, cytokine dysregulation, and high levels of IL-2, IL-6, interferon alpha, and TNF-α have been suggested.

2. Hypotheses from experimental studies (Flowers & Martin, 2015; Min, 2011)

   a) Thymic damage and defective negative selection of T cells: Normal functioning of thymus has been disrupted due to age and conditioning regimen.

   b) Autoantibody production by aberrant B cells: Secretion of inflammatory cytokines and fibrosing cytokines and B-cell pathways are activated, resulting in an immune response attack of tissues.

   c) Regulatory T-cell deficiencies: Inflammatory processes, as well as fibrosing processes, lead to tissue damage of the host. This essentially becomes a continued loop of inflammation and fibrosis.

E. Incidence and timing (Apperley & Masszi, 2012; Garnett et al., 2013; Jagasia et al., 2015; Lee & Flowers, 2008)

1. Chronic GVHD occurs in approximately 30%–70% of patients receiving an allogeneic transplant.

2. Most cases are diagnosed within the first year at a median of four to six months after HSCT, but 5%–10% of cases are initially diagnosed beyond the first year following transplant.

   a) Occurs in approximately 40% of patients receiving HLA-identical sibling transplants

   b) Occurs in more than 50% of mismatched related transplants

   c) Occurs in approximately 70% of matched unrelated transplants

3. Two categories of chronic GVHD: Classic chronic and overlap syndrome

   a) Classic chronic: Without any features of acute GVHD

   b) Overlap syndrome: Features of both acute and chronic manifestations occur

4. Approximately half of affected patients have three or more involved organs. Treatment typically requires immunosuppressive medications for a median of two to three years.

5. In a subset of patients, treatment is prolonged, with 15% still receiving immunosuppressive therapies at least seven or more years after the initial diagnosis of chronic GVHD.

6. Symptoms may involve one or multiple organs and be widespread.

7. Sequelae of chronic GVHD can be debilitating, including joint contractures, visual disturbances, and end-stage lung disease.

8. Early detection can prevent irreversible organ damage and improve survival and overall quality of life.

F. Risk factors (Apperley & Masszi, 2012; Atkinson et al., 1990; Flowers & Martin, 2015; Horwitz & Sullivan, 2006; Maziarz & Abar, 2011; Vogelsang, 2001)

1. Strongest risk factor is prior acute GVHD.

2. Risk of chronic GVHD increases progressively with increasing severity of acute GVHD.

3. More than 80% of patients who survive severe (grades 3–4) acute GVHD are expected to develop chronic GVHD.

4. Patients with mild grade 1 GVHD have a significantly increased risk of developing chronic GVHD compared with those with no acute GVHD.

5. Patients can, however, develop chronic GVHD without having had acute GVHD.

6. Other risk factors

   a) HLA-mismatched unrelated donors

   b) Increased age of both donor and recipient

   c) Type of pretransplant GVHD prophylaxis

   d) Use of non-T-cell-depleted graft and marrow

   e) Source of stem cells (mobilized PBSCs have a higher risk over bone marrow)

   f) Donor sex mismatched

   g) Parous female donors to male recipients are of the highest risk out of all possible donor–recipient combinations.

   h) Donor leukocyte infusions

   i) Bone marrow T-cell-depleted grafts have the lowest incidence.

   j) Splenectomy

G. Diagnosis and clinical manifestations (Filipovich et al., 2005; Horwitz & Sullivan, 2006; Jagasia et al., 2015)

1. Historically, chronic GVHD was diagnosed if symptoms were present following day 100 of stem cell transplant. This is no longer the case. Clinical manifestations and not time after transplant determine whether it is chronic or acute. No time limit is set for the diagnosis of chronic GVHD.

2. According to National Institutes of Health (NIH) criteria, the diagnosis of chronic GVHD requires the presence of at least one diagnostic manifestation of chronic GVHD or at least one distinctive sign confirmed by biopsy, radiographic, or other laboratory test (i.e., pulmonary function tests [PFTs]). It can involve one or more organs or sites.

3. Infection and other possible causes must be excluded.

4. Chronic GVHD can affect multiple organs; most common areas are skin and mouth, eyes, GI tract, and liver. Other organs include female genitalia, lungs, muscle, fascia, and joints.

H. Diagnostic manifestations of chronic GVHD by organ (Apperley & Masszi, 2012; Filipovich et al., 2005; Jagasia et al., 2015; Lee & Flowers, 2008; Maziarz & Abar, 2011)
  1. Skin
     a) Dyspigmentation
     b) Poikiloderma: Atrophy and changes in pigmentation
     c) Lichen planus: Erythematous/violaceous flat-topped papules or plaques with or without surface reticulations or with a silvery, shiny appearance in direct light
     d) Deep sclerotic features: Smooth, waxy, indurated skin, thickened or tight skin caused by diffuse sclerosis over a wide area, causing limitation of joint mobility
     e) Morphea-like superficial sclerotic lesions: Localized patchy areas of movable smooth or shiny skin with a leathery consistency, often with dyspigmentation
     f) Lichen sclerosus–like movable lesions: Ranges from discrete to coalescent gray to white moveable papules or plaques, often with follicular plugs and with a shiny appearance and leathery consistency
     g) Severe sclerotic features characterized by skin ulcers from minor trauma and thickened, tight, fragile skin that often is associated with poor wound healing
  2. Nails: Dystrophy characterized by longitudinal ridging, nail splitting or brittleness, onycholysis, and nail loss
  3. Scalp and body hair
     a) Alopecia (not due to chemotherapy or radiation therapy)
     b) Loss of body hair
     c) Premature graying, thinning, or brittleness
  4. Mouth
     a) Lichen planus–like changes (white hyperkeratotic and lacy-appearing lesions of the buccal mucosa, tongue, palate, or lips)
     b) Distinctive features of chronic GVHD (Infectious pathogens such as HSV and secondary malignancies must be excluded.)
        (1) Xerostomia (dry mouth)
        (2) Mucoceles
        (3) Mucosal atrophy
        (4) Ulcers
        (5) Pseudomembranes: Thin layer of cells that underlies organs, eyes, and other structures
     c) Both acute and chronic oral GVHD can present as gingivitis, mucositis, erythema, and pain.
  5. Eyes
     a) New-onset dry, gritty, or painful eyes
     b) Cicatricial conjunctivitis
     c) Keratoconjunctivitis sicca
     d) Confluent areas of punctate keratopathy
     e) Photophobia
     f) Periorbital hyperpigmentation
     g) Mucoid secretions (making it difficult to open eyes in the morning)
     h) Blepharitis (erythema of eyelids with edema)
     i) New ocular sicca (documented by low Schirmer test scores with a mean value of less than or equal to 5 mm at 5 minutes)

  j) New-onset keratoconjunctivitis sicca (documented by slit-lamp examination with a mean Schirmer test value of 6–10 mm)

6. Genitalia
    a) Lichen planus–like features
    b) Lichen sclerosus–like features
    c) Vaginal scarring or stenosis
    d) Clitoral or labial agglutination
    e) Phimosis and scarring or stenosis of male urethra or meatus
    f) Erosions, fissures, or ulcers
    g) Vulvar or vaginal dryness, burning, pruritus, or dyspareunia
    h) Patchy or generalized erythema or mucosal erosions

7. GI tract
    a) Esophageal web, stricture, or concentric rings documented by endoscopy or barium contrast
    b) Pancreatic exocrine insufficiency requiring enzyme supplements
    c) Nausea, vomiting, anorexia, diarrhea, weight loss, failure to thrive
    d) Wasting syndrome may be a symptom of chronic GVHD, but often is multifactorial (e.g., decreased caloric intake, poor intestinal absorption of macronutrients, increased resting energy expenditures, hypercatabolism).

8. Liver: No hepatic manifestations are either distinctive or diagnostic of chronic GVHD.
    a) Other causes such as drug, viral infections, and biliary obstruction must be considered.
    b) Chronic liver GVHD can be accompanied by manifestations of acute GVHD.
    c) Liver GVHD after day 100 can present, resembling acute hepatitis (rising alanine transaminase with or without jaundice) and occurring almost always after tapering immunosuppressants or receiving DLI. The second presentation is a slowly progressing cholestatic disorder with elevated serum alkaline phosphatase and gamma-glutamyl transpeptidase, followed by jaundice.

9. Lungs
    a) Bronchiolitis obliterans: Diagnosed with PFTs and radiologic testing
    b) New obstructive lung picture: Dyspnea on exertion, cough, wheezing
    c) Bronchiolitis obliterans may be used for diagnosis of chronic lung GVHD if the following criteria are met.
        (1) Ratio of forced expiratory volume in one second (FEV_1) to forced vital capacity (FVC) of less than 0.7 or the fifth percentile of predicted or FEV_1 less than 75% of predicted with greater than or equal to 10% decline over two years or less. FEV_1 should not correct to greater than 75% of predicted with albuterol.
        (2) Absence of respiratory tract infection documented by chest x-ray, CT scans, microbiologic cultures, bronchoalveolar lavage, respiratory tract viral screen, or sputum culture
        (3) Evidence of air trapping by PFTs: Residual volume greater than 120% of predicted or residual volume/total lung capacity

10. Musculoskeletal system
    a) Fascial involvement, often affecting forearms or legs and associated with sclerosis of overlying skin and subcutaneous tissue (resulting in joint stiffness or contractures)

      b) Fasciitis on examination with stiffness, restricted range of motion, wrist flex-
ion, or inability to assume a Buddha prayer position; edema of extremities
with or without erythema (early sign); peau d'orange (edematous skin with
prominent pores, resembling the surface of an orange)

      c) Clinical myositis with tender muscles and increased muscle enzymes:
A distinctive feature but not diagnostic of chronic GVHD. Evaluation
of myositis includes electromyography, creatine phosphokinase, and
aldolase.

      d) Myositis may present as proximal myopathy.

  11. Hematopoietic and immune system

      a) Hematopoietic abnormalities are associated with chronic GVHD but can-
not be used to establish a diagnosis.

      b) Lymphopenia (lymphocyte count less than 500/mm^3), eosinophilia (eosin-
ophil count 500/mm^3 or greater)

      c) Hypogammaglobulinemia or hypergammaglobulinemia

      d) Autoimmune hemolytic anemia

      e) Idiopathic thrombocytopenic purpura

      f) Thrombocytopenia (platelet count less than 100,000/mm^3) at the time of
diagnosis of chronic GVHD is a poor prognostic sign.

I. Classification (Filipovich et al., 2005; Lee & Flowers, 2008)

  1. Historically, chronic GVHD had been classified as limited or extensive.

  2. In 2005, NIH developed new categories of chronic GVHD.

      a) Classic chronic GVHD: No features or characteristics of acute GVHD

      b) Overlap syndrome: Diagnostic or distinctive features of chronic and acute
GVHD appearing together

  3. NIH developed a clinical scoring of organ systems, which is based on specific signs.

      a) The degree of organ involvement (mild, moderate, or severe)

      b) Laboratory data or histopathologic confirmation rather than time of onset
post-transplant

  4. Organ sites considered for scoring

      a) Skin (most commonly affected)

      b) Mouth (most commonly affected)

      c) Eyes

      d) GI tract

      e) Liver

      f) Lungs

      g) Joints and fascia

      h) Female genital tract

  5. Each individual organ or site is scored according to a 4-point scale (0–3), with 0
representing no involvement and 3 representing severe impairment.

  6. The effect of chronic GVHD on performance status also is considered on a 0–3
scale. Grading chronic GVHD is mild, moderate, or severe.

  7. The global scoring system assesses the following:

      a) Number of organs or sites involved

      b) Severity within each affected organ

      c) Global descriptions of mild, moderate, and severe reflect the degree of organ
impact and functional impairment caused by chronic GVHD.

(1) Mild chronic GVHD is the involvement of no more than two organs or sites (except for lung) with a maximum score of one.

(2) Moderate chronic GVHD involves at least one organ or site with a maximum score of 2; or three or more organs or sites with a maximum score of 1 in all affected sites (or a lung score of 1).

(3) Severe chronic GVHD occurs when a score of 3 is given to any organ (or a lung score of 2 or 3).

8. The global scoring system should be used after a diagnosis of chronic GVHD is confirmed and if a diagnostic feature is present. If a diagnostic feature is not present, at least one distinctive manifestation of chronic GVHD must be present, with the diagnosis supported by histologic, radiologic, or laboratory evidence of GVHD from any site.

J. Treatment (Couriel et al., 2006; Dignan, Amrolia, et al., 2012; Dignan, Scarisbrick, et al., 2012; Filipovich et al., 2005; Flowers & Martin, 2015; Garnett et al., 2013; Lee & Flowers, 2008; Maziarz & Abar, 2011; Mitchell, 2013)

1. Systemic therapy is the mainstay of treatment for moderate to severe chronic GVHD.

2. Treatment requires a multidisciplinary team of clinicians who are experts with knowledge of the management of chronic GVHD.

3. Mild GVHD may require and respond to topical treatment and not require additional systemic immunosuppression.

4. NIH guidelines recommend consideration of systemic treatment if three or more organs are involved or if any single organ has a severity score greater than 2.

5. For moderate to severe chronic GVHD, organ-specific topical therapies may be useful as adjuvant therapy.

6. Evaluation of response to therapy should occur at each clinic visit, and formal NIH staging should occur every three months.

7. Quality-of-life assessment also should be performed at each clinic visit or at least every three months.

K. Supportive care (Couriel et al., 2006; Dignan, Amrolia, et al., 2012; Dignan, Scarisbrick, et al., 2012; Maziarz & Abar, 2011; Treister, Duncan, Cutler, & Lehman, 2012)

1. Cutaneous chronic GVHD: Must rule out other etiology.
   a) Infection
   b) Vasculitis
   c) Drug reaction
   d) Dermatitis
   e) Skin cancer

2. Skin integrity in chronic GVHD is damaged, thus affecting temperature regulation and barriers.

3. Official dermatology consult should be requested.

4. Patients with chronic skin GVHD and on prolonged immunosuppression are at increased risk for developing a cutaneous malignancy.

5. Ultraviolet exposure should be minimized.

6. Routine skin examinations should be performed.

7. Nonintact skin
   a) Obtain cultures to rule out bacterial, viral, fungal, or mycobacterial infection.
   b) In denuded skin, wound dressings maintain a moist environment that enhances repair of the epithelium, lysis of necrotic tissue, and phagocytosis of necrotic debris.

    c) Protective films may be applied to prevent breakdown of fragile or compromised but not ulcerated skin.

    d) If indicated, topical antimicrobials, such as mupirocin ointment or silver-containing products, may be useful.

    e) Consider plastic surgery consult.

L. Treatment of chronic GVHD by organ/site

  1. Skin chronic GVHD (Wolff et al., 2010)

    a) Topical agents

      (1) Ointments and creams are better emollients than lotions and are less likely to sting when applied to erythematous areas.

      (2) For intact skin: Topical emollients, corticosteroids, antipruritic agents, and CNI creams

      (3) For erosions and ulcerations: Topical antimicrobials, protective film or dressings, wound care specialist consult

      (4) Nonsclerotic skin lesions without erosions or ulcerations (lichen planus–like) may respond well to topical steroids and emollients.

      (5) Topical steroid agents

        (a) From the neck down, treatment should begin with midstrength topical steroids (i.e., triamcinolone [0.1%] cream or ointment).

        (b) In cases that do not respond to midstrength topical steroids, short-term use of midstrength steroids with wet wraps can increase skin hydration and steroid penetration.

        (c) When wet wraps are not possible, higher-potency steroids (i.e., fluocinonide [0.05%] cream or ointment) may be used.

        (d) More potent steroids (i.e., clobetasol dipropionate [0.05%], halobetasol propionate [0.05%]) should not be used under occlusive dressing.

        (e) The use of wet wraps and high-potency steroids should be limited to 14 consecutive days, if possible.

        (f) Lower-potency steroids (hydrocortisone [1%–2.5%], desonide [0.05%]) should be used on the face, axillae, and groin and can be used for longer periods of time.

      (6) Topical therapy, including steroids or topical CNIs, is recommended as first-line ancillary and supportive care therapy.

      (7) Regular lubrication of dry but intact skin with emollients may decrease pruritus and maintain skin integrity.

      (8) Long-term use of topical steroids may cause atrophy and striae.

    b) Emollients may be used after the application of steroids. Emollients are occlusive and may increase the potency of steroids.

    c) Menthol-based creams and lotions may provide some relief as well as antipruritic topical immunosuppressants.

    d) Systemic antihistamines (diphenhydramine, hydroxyzine, and ranitidine)

    e) ECP is recommended as second-line systemic therapy for steroid-refractory GVHD.

    f) Physiotherapy is recommended with sclerodermoid disease.

    g) Phototherapy may be beneficial, but risk of cutaneous malignancy increases not only from phototherapy but also prolonged topical immunosuppression and history of previous chemotherapy.

    h) Support for atrophy or range of motion
      (1) Home physical therapy and occupational therapy
      (2) Support devices such as splints

2. Ocular chronic GVHD
    a) More common in chronic than acute
    b) Rule out other etiologies, including medications (e.g., anticholinergics, anti-depressants, psychotropic medications, antihistamines) and previous treatment (e.g., TBI, chemotherapy). Rule out infectious processes such as CMV retinitis, HSV, or varicella-zoster virus.
    c) Obtain an ophthalmology consult by an ophthalmologist familiar with GVHD.
    d) Diagnosis can be made early by clinical symptoms.
    e) Cataracts can develop from prolonged systemic steroid use and TBI.
    f) Complications, such as retinal hemorrhage and optic disc swelling, can occur.
    g) Supportive care focuses on increasing ocular surface moisture by lubrication and decreasing tear evaporation and tear drainage from the surface of the eye.
      (1) Lubrication: Preservative-free artificial tears to coat the ocular surface to minimize superficial dry spots on the cornea. Hydroxypropyl cellulose ophthalmic insert (prescription) can be inserted once or twice daily into the inferior cul-de-sac of the eye but may produce a constant foreign body sensation.
      (2) Decrease evaporation: Warm compresses and eyelid care may help to maximize the output of the meibomian glands, which produce the outer oil layer of the tear film and protect against evaporation.
        (a) Avoidance of low humidity
        (b) Use of eye protection (i.e., moisture chamber goggles)
        (c) Temporary or permanent occlusion of the tear duct puncta may provide relief for patients with severe sicca syndrome.
        (d) Permanent occlusion may be necessary, as the temporary plugs do fall out frequently.
      (3) Decrease inflammation: The benefit of topical cyclosporine on tear function in patients with GVHD has not been fully elucidated, but this type of treatment increases scores on the Schirmer test and decreases surface apoptosis in patients with other dry eye conditions. Ocular surface inflammation also may be decreased with autologous serum, but this treatment is available in only a limited number of centers.

3. Mouth and oral cavity chronic GVHD
    a) Second most common site after skin
    b) Three components of oral chronic GVHD
      (1) Mucosal involvement
      (2) Salivary gland involvement
      (3) Sclerotic involvement of mouth and surrounding tissues
    c) Oral chronic GVHD can cause pain, odynophagia, taste impairment, dryness, and decreased range of motion.
    d) Infectious etiology should be ruled out (e.g., HSV, human papillomavirus [HPV], *Candida*, other fungal organisms).
    e) Refer to an oral mucosal physician or dentist familiar with oral GVHD.

f) Topical steroids are given as the ancillary first-line therapy. Application of high-potency corticosteroid gel (fluocinonide, clobetasol, or betamethasone propionate) is the main treatment.

g) Application of tacrolimus ointment is an alternative to locally applied steroids.

h) Ancillary therapy may provide greater local benefit than systemic therapy alone.

i) Systemic therapy should be added early in treatment for severe oral cavity GVHD (sclerosis) and whenever isolated oral cavity GVHD fails to respond to supportive care.

j) ECP has been reported to be beneficial in managing oral GVHD.

k) Artificial saliva may be beneficial for hyposalivation.

l) Petroleum jelly–based ointments, such as topical tacrolimus, are generally less effective in the mouth than alcohol-based corticosteroid gels but are preferable for the treatment of chapped lips caused by GVHD.

m) Dexamethasone and other corticosteroid rinse formulations, such as prednisolone or triamcinolone, are held and swished in the mouth for four to six minutes and then expelled without swallowing. Treatment is four to six times per day. It is important to instruct patients to keep solution in the mouth for five minutes before expectorating and to avoid eating or drinking for 10–15 minutes after using the solution.

n) Use of children's toothpaste may be less sensitive, as it has less flavoring agents and no sodium lauryl sulfate. Avoid heavily flavored mouthwashes (especially those containing alcohol).

o) High-potency fluocinonide and very potent clobetasol gels can be applied directly to mucosa by applying gel to a gauze pad and leaving in place for several minutes four to six times per day.

p) Solutions and gels are hydrophilic and easily applied intraorally.

4. Salivary gland chronic GVHD
   a) Patients present with dry mouth and variable oral sensitivities to hot, cold, spicy, and acidic food, mint (e.g., mint toothpaste), and carbonated beverages.
   b) Patients also may develop mucoceles, which are recognized as painless blisters on the palate and inside lower lip.
   c) Treatment interventions include frequent water-sipping, salivary stimulants (sugar-free gum or candy), oral moisturizing agents, saliva substitutes, and avoidance of medications such as tricyclic antidepressants, selective serotonin reuptake inhibitors, antihistamines, and narcotics.
   d) For patients with mild salivary gland dysfunction, risk of tooth decay is increased; home fluoride treatments may be beneficial.

5. Sclerotic manifestations of chronic GVHD
   a) Topical therapy alone is insufficient.
   b) Systemic treatment is required.

6. Vulva and vaginal mucosa chronic GVHD
   a) Rule out other etiology, including HPV, yeast or bacterial infection, or estrogen deficiency.
   b) Instruct patients to practice good hygiene.
       (1) Clean genital area with warm water rather than with soap or feminine wash products.
       (2) Avoid mechanical and chemical irritants.

    (3) Apply a small amount of emollients or lanolin cream to the external genitalia; this may provide relief from itching and irritation.

    (4) Use vaginal moisturizers or other bacteriostatic gels in the vagina for comfort.

    (5) Consult with a gynecologist to evaluate for topical estrogen replacement.

  c) Topical therapy with high- or very high–dose steroids (clobetasol, beclomethasone) or immunosuppressive agents (tacrolimus ointment) has a high rate of success and is recommended as first-line therapy.

    (1) More rapid healing has been reported with addition of hormone replacement therapy.

    (2) Dilators and estrogen rings may be necessary for strictures.

    (3) Surgery may be required for severe cases of complete vaginal closure.

    (4) Sclerotic features require aggressive topical steroids and dilators.

7. GI chronic GVHD

  a) Upper GI

    (1) Odynophagia and dysphagia: Lubrication can ease discomfort caused by xerostomia.

    (2) Symptoms may present as dysphagia, nausea and vomiting, and anorexia.

    (3) Exclude other pathology by endoscopy or biopsy.

      (a) Strictures (esophageal web)

      (b) Radiation esophagitis

      (c) Fibrosis

      (d) Infections such as *Candida*

      (e) Acid reflux

      (f) Bile reflux

      (g) Small bowel bacterial overgrowth

    (4) May require esophageal dilatation

  b) Lower GI

    (1) Diarrhea is a common symptom of chronic GVHD.

    (2) Rule out other etiology for the diarrhea.

      (a) Infection

         i. The most important infections to rule out are CMV and *C. difficile* (e.g., CMV colitis may be present without the presence of an antigen [called *antigenemia*]).

        ii. Less common viruses include *Giardia*, *Rotavirus*, adenovirus, and fungi.

      (b) Colonoscopy should be performed for tissue biopsy.

    (3) For patients with an established diagnosis of GVHD, supportive care includes the following:

      (a) Antidiarrheal agents (loperamide [Imodium®] and diphenoxylate and atropine [Lomotil®])

      (b) Systemic immunosuppression

      (c) Nutrition consult

    (4) Malnutrition and an elevated body mass index are both risk factors for adverse outcomes following HSCT.

      (a) Malnutrition is associated with a decreased overall survival rate and increased risk of infection.

        (b) Nutritional requirements vary with age, gender, weight, and severity of chronic GVHD.

        (c) Electrolytes should be followed weekly.

        (d) Home TPN may be necessary.

    (5) Radiographic evaluation, including plain films and CT, may be necessary.

        (a) Colonoscopy and upper endoscopy

        (b) Trial of proton-pump inhibitor (e.g., omeprazole, pantoprazole)

        (c) Cytoprotective agent, such as sucralfate, if no response

8. Liver chronic GVHD

    a) Common; occurs in approximately 50% of HSCT recipients

    b) Hepatology referral may be necessary.

    c) Perform imaging studies to rule out gallbladder disease and exclude liver abscess.

    d) Obtain iron studies to rule out hemochromatosis.

    e) Primary management

        (1) Immunosuppression with high-dose steroids (2 mg/kg per day)

        (2) High-dose ursodeoxycholic acid (30–40 mg/kg per day)

9. Pulmonary chronic GVHD

    a) May be insidious, with slow progressive dyspnea and cough

    b) Differential diagnosis

        (1) Cryptogenic organizing pneumonia, which presents with fever, cough, and consolidated infiltrates on chest x-ray

        (2) Responds to steroid therapy

    c) Diagnostic recommendations

        (1) Pulmonary referral

        (2) Diagnostic measures of impairment

            (a) PFTs

            (b) Chest x-ray

            (c) High-resolution expiratory chest CT

            (d) Bronchoscopy

        (3) To exclude infection as etiology

            (a) PFTs: Demonstrate airflow obstruction with a reduced FEV_1 and FVC and FEV_1/FVC ratio. FEV_1 is the most sensitive marker for early obstructive changes, and a value of less than 45% is strongly predictive of poor outcome.

            (b) Chest x-ray: May be normal but can demonstrate ranges, including focal shadowing and more diffuse changes

            (c) High-resolution chest CT: Shows evidence of air trapping, small airway thickening, and bronchiectasis

            (d) Bronchoscopy to rule out infection

        (4) High-dose steroids: Oral prednisone 1 mg/kg

        (5) Severe symptoms may require a lung transplant.

    d) Prevention: Vaccinations

        (1) Pneumococcal (include 13- and 23-valent vaccines every five years)

        (2) Seasonal inactivated influenza

    e) Treatment

        (1) Imatinib: 100 mg initially, increased to 200 mg after one month in absence of toxicities

      (2) Inhaled steroids and leukotriene inhibitors (may be helpful as adjunct therapy; e.g., montelukast and azithromycin)

      (3) Bronchodilators

      (4) Supplemental oxygen

      (5) IV immunoglobulin

M. First-line systemic therapy for chronic GVHD: Corticosteroids (Apperley & Masszi, 2012; Dignan, Amrolia, et al., 2012; Dignan, Scarisbrick, et al., 2012; Flowers & Martin, 2015; Garnett et al., 2013; Lee & Flowers, 2008; Wolff et al., 2010)

  1. Corticosteroids are the standard initial systemic therapy.

  2. Dose is 1 mg/kg per day, followed by a taper to reach an alternate-day regimen with or without cyclosporine or tacrolimus. Institutional variance on dosing exists and can be up to 1 mg/kg BID; however, data are limited to support higher doses.

    a) Effect is likely caused by anti-inflammatory properties and lymphocytic effects.

    b) Alternate-day regimen also has an important role in facilitating adrenal recovery before the end of treatment.

  3. Tapering of steroids

    a) Strategies for tapering vary, with underlying general principle to use the least immunosuppressive dose that is sufficient to control GVHD symptoms. Recommendations include the following:

      (1) After two weeks, if the disease has not progressed, taper steroids by 25% per week to 1 mg/kg or prednisone on alternate days (Vogelsang, 2001).

      (2) Lee and Flowers (2008) recommend 1 mg/kg of steroids per day for approximately two weeks followed by a taper schedule to reach an alternate-day dose regimen as soon as possible following signs and symptoms.

      (3) Taper by 20%–30% every two weeks, with smaller decrements toward the end of the taper schedule (Flowers & Martin, 2015).

      (4) If chronic manifestations are severe, the patient has high-risk chronic GVHD features, or if the patient has less than a complete response, then the dose may be held at 1 mg/kg every other day for another two to three months and then tapered by 10%–20% per month for a total corticosteroid treatment course of nine months.

    b) Patients should be examined prior to each steroid dose reduction.

    c) If an exacerbation of recurrent chronic GVHD is evident at any step of the taper, the dose of prednisone is increased by two levels, with daily administration for two to four weeks followed by resumption of alternate-day schedule.

    d) Treatment should then be continued for at least three months before attempting to resume taper.

    e) The goal is to wean the steroids to the lowest dose or off to maintain control of symptoms of chronic GVHD.

    f) A combination of steroids with other immunosuppressive agents, such as CNIs, often is considered to minimize the toxicity of prolonged steroid use.

    g) Whenever possible, clinical trials should be offered to patients with chronic GVHD.

N. Secondary treatment (Cutler et al., 2008; Flowers & Martin, 2015; Flowers et al., 2008; Giaccone et al., 2005; Wolff et al., 2010)

1. Approximately 50%–60% of patients with chronic GVHD require a secondary treatment within two years after initial systemic therapy.
2. Indications for secondary treatment
   a) Worsening manifestations of chronic GVHD in a previously affected organ
   b) Development of chronic GVHD signs and symptoms in a previously unaffected organ
   c) Absence of improvement after one month of standard primary treatment
   d) Inability to decrease prednisone below 1 mg/kg per day within two months
   e) Significant treatment-related toxicity
3. No consensus exists on optimal secondary treatment for patients who have failed high-dose steroids; more clinical trials are needed.
4. Chronic GVHD is generally defined as either failure to improve after at least two months or progression after one month of standard corticosteroid-based immunosuppressive therapy.
5. Choice of second-line therapy often is physician preference.
6. Any of the medications used to treat acute GVHD also can be used to treat chronic GVHD. Steroids remain the mainstay. ATG, however, is not given for chronic GVHD.
7. Options for secondary treatment
   a) Tacrolimus or cyclosporine often is used in combination with steroids.
   b) ECP
   c) Sirolimus
   d) Low-dose MTX (anti-inflammatory and antiproliferative agent): 10 mg (range 7.5–15 mg) for a median of 25 weeks (range of 3–50 weeks) (Giaccone et al., 2005)
   e) Rituximab (mAb that targets and binds to B cells): 375 mg/m² every week for four weeks (Cutler et al., 2006)
      (1) Once bound to B cells, the host's immune system is triggered to attack those cells and to disable the cell to which it is bound.
      (2) Up to two additional four-week courses can be given as necessary.
      (3) In clinical studies, patients with cutaneous and musculoskeletal manifestations were the best responders.
      (4) Nursing considerations for administration
         (a) Infusion reactions manifested by rigors, hypotension, and SOB.
         (b) Patients should be premedicated with antihistamine and acetaminophen.
         (c) Some patients may require steroids.
      (5) Additional side effects
         (a) Progressive multifocal leukoencephalopathy
         (b) Reactivation of hepatitis B. Not recommended in patients who are hepatitis B core antibody positive.
   f) Mycophenolate mofetil
   g) Alefacept (Shapira et al., 2008)
      (1) Targeted to T lymphocytes and has been shown to have a selective effect on effector memory T cells
      (2) Dose: 30 mg intramuscular weekly
      (3) Best response in patients with GVHD of the skin, mucosa, vagina, and lung

        h) Alemtuzumab: 10 mg subcutaneous for six days
        i) Tyrosine kinase inhibitors (imatinib): Imatinib has antifibrotic and anti-inflammatory properties and carries potent immunomodulatory effects in both T-cell and B-cell response (Olivieri et al., 2009).
        j) Basiliximab (Dignan, Amrolia, et al., 2012; Dignan, Scarisbrick, et al., 2012; Wang et al., 2011)
           (1) Chimeric mAb that is an IL-2 receptor antagonist
           (2) Dose: 20 mg IV on days 1, 3, or 4 and weekly
        k) Pentostatin

VI. Chronic GVHD review of systems (Flowers & Martin, 2015)
    A. Skin: Feels tight or hard, increased dryness, pruritus or new rash, papules, discoloration, scar-like, scaly
    B. Sweat glands: Inability to sweat or keep body warm
    C. Skin appendages: Loss of hair on scalp or body, including brows or lashes, nail changes (ridges or brittleness), or nail loss
    D. Fascia and joints: Stiffness or pain in wrists, fingers, or other joints
    E. Eyes: Eye dryness or pain, sensitivity to wind or dry environments
    F. Mouth: Oral dryness, taste alterations, sensitivities (e.g., spicy food, carbonated drinks, toothpaste), ulcers, and sore pain
    G. Esophagus: Foods or pills get stuck when swallowing.
    H. Lungs: Cough, dyspnea (on exertion or rest), or wheezes
    I. Genital tract: Vaginal dryness, dyspareunia, pain, or dysuria caused by stenosis of urethra
    J. Weight loss: Unexplained weight loss or inability to gain weight (pancreatic insufficiency or hypermetabolism)

VII. Systematic comprehensive review of systems
    A. Comprehensive evaluations should take place at the time of initial diagnosis, at three- to six-month intervals thereafter, and with any major change in therapy.
    B. Close monitoring of all organs and potential sites of chronic GVHD will ensure early recognition and intervention. Routine PFTs, physiotherapy evaluation of range of motion, and dental, ophthalmology, gynecology, and dermatology examinations are recommended.

VIII. Transplant-related endocrine problems following allogeneic stem cell transplant are most often related to either the conditioning regimen or treatment for GVHD (Carpenter & Sanders, 2009; Kagoya, Seo, Nannya, & Kurokawa, 2012; Marini, Choi, Byersdorfer, Cronin, & Frame, 2015; Mohty & Apperley, 2010). These may develop any time following transplant but usually within the first few years.
    A. Growth failure with growth hormone deficiency
    B. Overt hypothyroidism (primarily from conditioning regimens)
    C. Primary gonadal failure
    D. Diabetes type 1 or 2
    E. Osteoporosis, osteopenia
    F. Hyperlipidemia
    G. Exocrine pancreatic insufficiency
        1. Osteoporosis and osteopenia can be major post-transplant complications.

a) Risk factors
   (1) Inactivity
   (2) TBI
   (3) Corticosteroid therapy (Bone loss is most rapid during the initial six months of glucocorticoid therapy and may occur with daily prednisone doses as low as 5 mg.)
   (4) GVHD
   (5) Hypogonadism
   (6) CNIs
b) Pathophysiology
   (1) Impaired bone mineralization through disturbances of calcium and vitamin D homeostasis
   (2) Imbalanced osteoblast and osteoclast formation
   (3) Deficiency in growth or gonadal hormone secretion
c) Diagnosis: Dual-photon densitometry at one year for adult women, all allogeneic HCT recipients, and patients who are at high risk for bone loss
   (1) Subsequent testing is needed to determine abnormalities, as well as response to therapy.
   (2) T-score for adults: Standard deviations (SDs) that are less than or equal to −2.5 below mean bone mineral density
   (3) Children: Osteopenia is a Z-score between −1 and −2 SD, and osteoporosis is a Z-score that is more than 2 SD below the mean.
d) Treatment
   (1) Calcium supplementation for patients on steroid therapy whenever daily calcium losses are increased or if low dietary intake of calcium
   (2) Recommended daily intake of elemental calcium
      (a) 800 mg for children aged 1–5 years
      (b) 1,200 mg for children aged 6–8 years
      (c) 1,500 mg for children aged 9 years and older
   (3) Recommended daily intake of oral vitamin D supplements
      (a) 400 IU for children aged 1–8 years
      (b) 400–800 IU for children aged 9 years and older
   (4) Check serum calcium, magnesium, and 1,25-dihydroxyvitamin D levels.
   (5) Recommend physical therapy for weight-bearing exercises.
   (6) Nutrition consult for dietary intervention
   (7) Gonadal failure may predate or exacerbate steroid-induced osteoporosis.
      (a) Hormone replacement therapy can increase bone mineral density in both women and men.
      (b) Women aged 50 years and older should consult with a gynecologist prior to starting hormone replacement therapy because of the potential for adverse risks.
      (c) Children: Growth hormone replacement or estrogen or testosterone replacement therapy can improve bone mineral density but should be coordinated with an endocrinologist.
   (8) Bisphosphonate therapy is indicated when hormone replacement therapy is inappropriate because of patient age, is otherwise contraindicated, or does not ameliorate reduced bone mineral density.

        (a) Enzymatic pathway in osteoclasts to inhibit bone resorption

        (b) Also may stimulate osteoblasts to promote bone formation

        (c) Forms of replacement

            i. Oral: Alendronate, risedronate. Must be taken with water while sitting or standing and in a fasting state to prevent esophagitis.

            ii. IV: Pamidronate, zoledronic acid. Requires dental clearance because of risk for osteonecrosis of the jaw.

            iii. Denosumab: Indicated for patients with osteoporosis

        (d) Duration of bisphosphonate therapy: Until normal bone mineral density is achieved and glucocorticoid therapy is discontinued

2. AVN

    a) AVN occurs a median of 12 months after transplantation.

    b) The hip is most frequently affected, although multiple joints may be involved.

    c) Joint involvement often is bilateral and more severe in glucocorticoid-associated AVN compared to idiopathic AVN.

    d) Diagnosis is determined by magnetic resonance imaging scan of the affected joint.

    e) Pathophysiology: Bone ischemia due to any combination of factors

        (1) Obliterative arteritis

        (2) Thrombophilia

        (3) Hyperlipidemia

        (4) Fat embolism

        (5) Repeated microfractures of weight-bearing bone

        (6) Increased intramedullary pressure that is possibly secondary in increased intramedullary fat

    f) Risk factors

        (1) Aged 16 years or older

        (2) Initial diagnosis of aplastic anemia or leukemia

        (3) Chronic GVHD

        (4) Glucocorticoid therapy (identified as most associated risk factor for developing AVN)

    g) Treatment

        (1) Pain relief

        (2) Early referral to orthopedic surgeon

        (3) Based on assumption that AVN results from bone ischemia secondary to an intramedullary compartment syndrome, core decompression may be used to promote revascularization of the femoral head. This procedure decompresses the medullary space by opening the area of dead bone from the outside, thereby restoring blood circulation to the necrotic bone and relieving pain.

        (4) Total joint replacement may be indicated. For children and young adults, avoid early replacement with artificial joints that have a finite life span.

3. Iatrogenic Cushing syndrome and adrenal insufficiency

    a) Etiology and characteristics

        (1) Prolonged steroid therapy to treat chronic GVHD

        (2) Poses cosmetic problems with young patients

        (3) More manageable with alternate-day steroid dosing

(4) Reversible given time off steroids, especially in younger patients

(5) Occurs with abrupt withdrawal of steroids (secondary adrenal insufficiency)

(6) Symptoms of fatigue and hypotension can be mild in some.

(7) Symptoms of adrenal insufficiency will likely occur in patients treated for longer than three weeks with daily steroid doses exceeding 7.5 mg prednisone or equivalent.

(8) Chronic suppression of hypothalamic-pituitary-adrenal axis causes adrenocortical atrophy and inability to generate sufficient cortisol, thus causing blunted cortisol response.

b) Diagnosis: Serum cortisol blood test at 7–9 am is less than 3.6 mcg/dl or serum cortisol at 30 or 60 minutes does not increase above 19 mcg/dl in response to a standard cosyntropin test.

c) Prevention and treatment

(1) A slow taper of steroids will decrease the risk of adrenal insufficiency.

(2) Hydrocortisone: 5–10 mg is preferred therapy to replace deficient production of adrenal cortisol.

(3) The total dose is divided into two to three daily doses, with one-half to two-thirds of the daily dose administered in the morning to physiologically mimic the cortisol secretion pattern (i.e., 10 mg in the morning and 5 mg at 5–7 pm).

(4) Hydrocortisone is the drug of choice for replacement therapy.

(5) Stress steroids need to be considered for illnesses that include fever, sepsis, vomiting, diarrhea, trauma, or major surgery.

(6) Recovery varies from days to several months.

(7) Secondary adrenal insufficiency should always be considered.

4. Hyperlipidemia (Kagoya et al., 2012; Marini et al., 2015)

a) Etiology

(1) A result of either intrahepatic cholestasis caused by chronic GVHD or secondary to medications

(2) Immunosuppressants such as CNIs, sirolimus, or steroids

b) Treatment

(1) No standard guidelines exist for the treatment of hyperlipidemia. Statins are used to decrease cholesterol and protect against premature cardiovascular disease. The lowest dose possible should be used to minimize potential drug–drug interactions (e.g., antifungal azoles, cyclosporine).

(2) Incidence of drug–drug interactions is higher in cyclosporine than other immunosuppressants and can cause elevation in LFTs, myopathy, and, in rare cases, rhabdomyolysis.

(3) Lifestyle modifications

(a) Low-fat diet

(b) Exercise

IX. Psychological aspects of transplant

A. A bone marrow transplant has a profound effect on the patient, caregivers, family, and friends.

B. Once this treatment modality is determined by all to be the best management strategy, life changes for the patient and those who are close to the patient occur and relationships are altered.

C. Many psychological and emotional issues surface, and both the patient and caregiver can experience significant physical and emotional challenges. A diagnosis of either acute or chronic GVHD adds to both the challenge as well as emotional burden. Some of these emotional and psychological challenges include the following:
   1. Adjusting to the fact that the patient has had a life-changing HSCT procedure and realizing that life for the patient, family, and caregiver has changed, most likely forever
   2. Coping with changes in self-image, especially if the patient has been diagnosed with chronic skin GVHD
   3. Dealing with medication-induced mood changes (e.g., labile emotions caused by steroids), which may cause anxiety, depression, and inability to sleep
      a) Anxiety and fear about the future (e.g., underlying disease returning, developing persistent acute or chronic GVHD, side effects of drugs used to treat GVHD, potential infectious complications with immunosuppression)
      b) Anxiety about becoming a "burden" to caregiver or family
      c) Anxiety over sexual intimacy with partner, ability and desire to perform, and fear over partner's response and desire
      d) Anxiety regarding financial strains, cost of medical care, and inability to work to meet those needs
      e) Anxiety and fear related to specific physical effects of either chronic or acute GVHD according to the organ(s) involved
         (1) GI: Volume and frequency of diarrhea
         (2) Acute or chronic skin GVHD: Degree of rash
         (3) Ocular GVHD: Visual problems
         (4) Pain or discomfort from local effects
         (5) Inability to gain weight
      f) Depression regarding lifestyle changes or an inability to engage in activities previously enjoyed
      g) Depression from worrying that the intended outcome of the transplant was not received or that the graft may be lost
D. Treatment and nursing interventions
   1. Screen for anxiety, depression, and suicidal tendencies among the patient and caregiver.
   2. Conduct a quality-of-life assessment at each visit or at least every three months.
   3. Establish psychiatric or psychology consult for psychotherapy.
   4. Establish social work consult for assistance with patient issues, such as transportation to and from clinic, hospital bills, and financial support.
   5. Provide a list of support groups for the patient.
E. Caregiver strain is common. Assessment of the mental, physical, and emotional health of the caregiver is critical. Antidepressants, anxiolytics, and medications that assist with normal sleeping patterns at night may help. Relaxation techniques (e.g., meditation, yoga, deep-breathing exercises) for the patient and caregiver to decrease stress and enhance emotional health also may be helpful.

Key Points

- Patient and family education on early identification of symptoms of graft-versus-host disease (GVHD) and prompt treatment is essential.
- Infection is one of the leading causes of death among patients with GVHD.
- Prevention of GVHD with immunosuppression before the allograft is critical.
- Antimicrobial prophylaxis should be considered, such as antibacterial, antiviral, antifungal, and prophylaxis for *Pneumocystis jiroveci* pneumonia.
- Some centers draw surveillance blood cultures weekly for patients on high-dose steroids and additional immunosuppression.
- Cytomegalovirus, Epstein-Barr virus, and polymerase chain reactions should be monitored weekly.
- An H_2 blocker should be administered with high-dose steroids.
- Patients should begin physical therapy or an exercise program to avoid deconditioning.
- Psychological and endocrine effects after transplant can be life threatening.
- Caregivers, as well as patients, should be supported.

References

Alousi, A.M., Bullinger, A., Couriel, D.R., Massaro, A., & Neumann, J.L. (2007). Graft-versus-host disease: Prevention and treatment. In R. Champlin & C. Ippoliti (Eds.), *Supportive care manual for blood and marrow transplantation* (pp. 97–138). Armonk, NY: Summit Communications.

Antin, J.H., & Raley, D.Y. (Eds.). (2013). *Manual of stem cell and bone marrow transplantation* (2nd ed.). New York, NY: Cambridge University Press.

Apperley, J., & Masszi, T. (2012). Graft-versus-host disease. In J. Apperley, E. Carreras, T. Gluckman, & T. Masszi (Eds.), *The EBMT-ESH handbook on hematopoietic stem cell transplantation* (6th ed., pp. 217–233). Retrieved from https://ebmtonline.forumservice.net/media/13/tex/content_alt/EBMT_Handbook2012_CHAP13.pdf

Atkinson, K., Horowitz, M.M., Gale, R.P., van Bekkum, D.W., Gluckman, E., Good, R.A., ... Ringdén, O. (1990). Risk factors for chronic graft-versus-host disease after HLA-identical sibling bone marrow transplantation. *Blood, 75*, 2459–2464.

Bechstein, W.O. (2000). Neurotoxicity of calcineurin inhibitors: Impact and clinical management. *Transplant International, 13*, 313–326. doi:10.1111/j.1432-2277.2000.tb01004.x

Carpenter, P.A., & Sanders, J.E. (2009). Endocrine and metabolic effects of chronic graft versus host disease. In G.B. Vogelsang & S.Z. Pavletic (Eds.), *Chronic graft versus host disease: Interdisciplinary management* (pp. 289–301). New York, NY: Cambridge University Press. doi:10.1017/CBO9780511576751.027

Chao, N.J. (2015). Clinical manifestations, diagnosis, and grading of acute graft-versus-host disease. UpToDate. Retrieved from http://www.uptodate.com/contents/clinical-manifestations-diagnosis-and-grading-of-acute-graft-versus-host-disease

Chapin, J., Shore, T., Forsberg, P., Desman, G., Van Besien, K., & Laurence, J. (2014). Hematopoietic transplant-associated thrombotic microangiopathy: Case report and review of diagnosis and treatments. *Clinical Advances in Hematology and Oncology, 12*, 565–573.

Charuhas, P.M. (2006). Medical nutrition therapy in hematopoietic cell transplantation. In L. Elliott, L.L. Molseed, P.D. McCallum, & Oncology Nutrition Dietetic Practice Group (Eds.), *The clinical guide to oncology nutrition* (2nd ed., pp. 126–137). Chicago, IL: American Dietetic Association.

Corella, E. (2011). Graft-versus-host disease prophylaxis. In R.T. Maziarz & S. Slater (Eds.), *Blood and marrow transplant handbook: Comprehensive guide for patient care* (pp. 83–100). New York, NY: Springer.

Couriel, D.R., Hosing, C., Saliba, R., Shpall, E.J., Anderlini, P., Rhodes, B., ... Donato, M. (2006). Extracorporeal photochemotherapy for the treatment of steroid-resistant chronic GVHD. *Blood, 107*, 3074–3080. doi:10.1182/blood-2005-09-3907

Cutler, C., Henry, N.L., Magee, C., Li, S., Kim, H.T., Alyea, E., ... Antin, J.H. (2005). Sirolimus and thrombotic microangiopathy after allogeneic hematopoietic stem cell transplantation. *Biology of Blood and Marrow Transplantation, 11,* 551–557. doi:10.1016/j.bbmt.2005.04.007

Cutler, C., Miklos, D., Kim, H.T., Treister, N., Woo, S.-B., Bienfang, D., ... Alyea, E. (2006). Rituximab for steroid-refractory chronic graft-versus-host disease. *Blood, 108,* 756–762. doi:10.1182/blood-2006-01-0233

Cutler, C., Stevenson, K., Kim, H.T., Richardson, P., Ho, V.T., Linden, E., ... Soiffer, R. (2008). Sirolimus is associated with veno-occlusive disease of the liver after myeloablative allogeneic stem cell transplantation. *Blood, 112,* 4425–4431. doi:10.1182/blood-2008-07-169342

Deeg, H.J. (2007). How I treat refractory acute GVHD. *Blood, 109,* 4119–4126. doi:10.1182/blood-2006-12-041889

Deeg, H.J., & Antin, J.H. (2006). The clinical spectrum of acute graft-versus-host disease. *Seminars in Hematology, 43,* 24–31. doi:10.1053/j.seminhematol.2005.09.003

Dignan, F.L., Amrolia, P., Clark, A., Cornish, J., Jackson, G., Mahendra, P., ... British Society for Blood and Marrow Transplantation. (2012). Diagnosis and management of chronic graft-versus-host disease. *British Journal of Haematology, 158,* 46–61. doi:10.1111/j.1365-2141.2012.09128.x

Dignan, F.L., Scarisbrick, J.J., Cornish, J., Clark, A., Amrolia, P., Jackson, G., ... British Society for Blood and Marrow Transplantation. (2012). Organ-specific management and supportive care in chronic graft-versus-host disease. *British Journal of Haematology, 158,* 62–78. doi:10.1111/j.1365-2141.2012.09131.x

Evans, S.O. (2009). The transplant pharmacopeia. In J. Treleaven & A.J. Barrett (Eds.), *Hematopoietic stem cell transplantation in clinical practice* (pp. 331–342). Edinburgh, Scotland: Elsevier Limited.

Ferrara, J.L.M., Levine, J.E., Reddy, P., & Holler, E. (2009). Graft-versus-host disease. *Lancet, 373,* 1550–1561. doi:10.1016/S0140-6736(09)60237-3

Ferrara, J.L.M., & Reddy, P. (2006). Pathophysiology of graft-versus-host disease. *Seminars in Hematology, 43,* 3–10. doi:10.1053/j.seminhematol.2005.09.001

Filipovich, A.H., Weisdorf, D., Pavletic, S., Socie, G., Wingard, J.R., Lee, S.J., ... Flowers, M.E.D. (2005). National Institutes of Health consensus development project on criteria for clinical trials in chronic graft-versus-host disease: I. Diagnosis and staging working group report. *Biology of Blood and Marrow Transplantation, 11,* 945–956. doi:10.1016/j.bbmt.2005.09.004

Flowers, M.E.D., & Martin, P.J. (2015). How we treat chronic graft-versus-host disease. *Blood, 125,* 606–615. doi:10.1182/blood-2014-08-551994

Flowers, M.E.D., Storer, B., Carpenter, P., Rezvani, A.R., Vigorito, A.C., Campregher, P.V., ... Martin, P.J. (2008). Treatment change as a predictor of outcome among patients with classic chronic graft-versus-host disease. *Biology of Blood and Marrow Transplantation, 14,* 1380–1384. doi:10.1016/j.bbmt.2008.09.017

Garnett, C., Apperley, J., & Pavlů, J. (2013). Treatment and management of graft-versus-host disease: Improving response and survival. *Therapeutic Advances in Hematology, 4,* 366–378. doi:10.1177/2040620713489842

Gauvreau, J.M., Lenssen, P., Cheney, C.L., Aker, S.N., Hutchinson, M.L., & Barale, K.V. (1981). Nutritional management of patients with intestinal graft-versus-host disease. *Journal of the American Dietetic Association, 79,* 673–677.

Giaccone, L., Martin, P., Carpenter, P., Moravec, C., Hooper, H., Funke, V.A.M., ... Flowers, M.E.D. (2005). Safety and potential efficacy of low-dose methotrexate for treatment of chronic graft-versus-host disease. *Bone Marrow Transplantation, 36,* 337–341. doi:10.1038/sj.bmt.1705022

Glucksberg, H., Storb, R., Fefer, A., Buckner, C.D., Neiman, P.E., Clift, R.A., ... Thomas, E.D. (1974). Clinical manifestations of graft-versus-host disease in human recipients of marrow from HLA-matched sibling donors. *Transplantation, 18,* 295–304.

Goker, H., Haznedaroglu, I.C., & Chao, N.J. (2001). Acute graft-vs-host disease: Pathobiology and management. *Experimental Hematology, 29,* 259–277.

Henry, L., & Loader, G. (2009). Nutrition support. In J. Treleaven & A.J. Barrett (Eds.), *Hematopoietic stem cell transplantation* (pp. 344–354). Edinburgh, Scotland: Elsevier Limited.

Horwitz, M.E., & Sullivan, K.M. (2006). Chronic graft-versus-host disease. *Blood Reviews, 20,* 15–27. doi:10.1016/j.blre.2005.01.007

Hsu, B., May, R., Carrum, G., Krance, R., & Przepiorka, D. (2001). Use of antithymocyte globulin for treatment of steroid-refractory acute graft-versus-host disease: An international practice survey. *Bone Marrow Transplantation, 28,* 945–950. doi:10.1038/sj.bmt.1703269

Ippoliti, C., & Massaro, A. (2007). Drugs and drug interactions. In R. Champlin & C. Ippoliti (Eds.), *Supportive care manual for blood and marrow transplantation* (pp. 9–39). Armonk, NY: Summit Communications.

Jacobsohn, D.A., & Vogelsang, G.B. (2007). Acute graft versus host disease. *Orphanet Journal of Rare Diseases, 2,* 35. doi:10.1186/1750-1172-2-35

Jagasia, M.H., Greinix, H.T., Arora, M., Williams, K.M., Wolff, D., Cowen, E.W., ... Flowers, M.E.D. (2015). National Institutes of Health consensus development project on criteria for clinical trials in chronic graft-versus-host disease: I. The 2014 Diagnosis and Staging Working Group Report. *Biology of Blood and Marrow Transplantation, 21,* 389–401. doi:10.1016/j.bbmt.2014.12.001

Kagoya, Y., Seo, S., Nannya, Y., & Kurokawa, M. (2012). Hyperlipidemia after allogeneic stem cell transplantation: Prevalence, risk factors, and impact on prognosis. *Clinical Transplantation, 26,* E168–E175. doi:10.1111/j.1399 -0012.2012.01628.x

Kalantari, B.N., Mortelé, K.J., Cantisani, V., Ondategui, S., Glickman, J.N., Gogate, A., … Silverman, S.G. (2003). CT features with pathologic correlation of acute gastrointestinal graft-versus-host disease after bone marrow transplantation in adults. *American Journal of Roentgenology, 181,* 1621–1625. doi:10.2214/ ajr.181.6.1811621

Kim, D.H., Sohn, S.K., Kim J.G., Suh, J.S., Lee, K.S., & Lee, K.B. (2004). Clinical impact of hyperacute graft-versus-host disease on results of allogeneic stem cell transplantation. *Bone Marrow Transplantation, 33,* 1025–1030. doi:10.1038/sj.bmt.1704479

Le Blanc, K., & Ringdén, O. (2006). Mesenchymal stem cells: Properties and role in clinical bone marrow transplantation. *Current Opinion in Immunology, 18,* 586–591. doi:10.1016/j.coi.2006.07.004

Lee, S.E., Cho, B.S., Kim, J.H., Yoon, J.H., Shin, S.H., Yahng, S.A., … Park, C.W. (2013). Risk and prognostic factors for acute GVHD based on NIH consensus criteria. *Bone Marrow Transplantation, 48,* 587–592. doi:10.1038/ bmt.2012.187

Lee, S.J., & Flowers, M.E.D. (2008). Recognizing and managing chronic graft-versus-host disease. *ASH Education Book, 2008,* 134–141. doi:10.1182/asheducation-2008.1.134

Lee, S.J., Vogelsang, G., & Flowers, M.E.D. (2003). Chronic graft-versus-host disease. *Biology of Blood and Marrow Transplantation, 9,* 215–233. doi:10.1053/bbmt.2003.50026

Levine, J.E., Paczesny, S., & Sarantopoulos, S. (2012). Clinical applications for biomarkers of acute and chronic graft-versus-host disease. *Biology of Blood and Marrow Transplantation, 18*(Suppl. 1), S116–S124. doi:10.1016/ j.bbmt.2011.10.019

Luznik, L., Bolaños-Meade, J., Zahurak, M., Chen, A.R., Smith, B.D., Brodsky, R., … Fuchs, E.J. (2010). High-dose cyclophosphamide as single-agent, short-course prophylaxis of graft-versus-host disease. *Blood, 115,* 3224–3230. doi:10.1182/blood-2009-11-251595

Luznik, L., O'Donnell, P.V., Symons, H.J., Chen, A.R., Leffell, M.S., Zahurak, M., … Fuchs, E.J. (2008). HLA-haploidentical bone marrow transplantation for hematologic malignancies using nonmyeloablative conditioning and high-dose, post-transplantation cyclophosphamide. *Biology of Blood and Marrow Transplantation, 14,* 641–650. doi:10.1016/j.bbmt.2008.03.005

Marini, B.L., Choi, S.W., Byersdorfer, C.A., Cronin, S., & Frame, D.G. (2015). Treatment of dyslipidemia in allogeneic hematopoietic stem cell transplant patients. *Biology of Blood and Marrow Transplantation, 21,* 809–820. doi:10.1016/j.bbmt.2014.10.027

Martin, P.J., Rizzo, J.D., Wingard, J.R., Ballen, K., Curtin, P.T., Cutler, C., … Carpenter, P.A. (2012). First- and second-line systemic treatment of acute graft-versus-host disease: Recommendations of the American Society of Blood and Marrow Transplantation. *Biology of Blood and Marrow Transplantation, 18,* 1150–1163. doi:10.1016/ j.bbmt.2012.04.005

Massenkeil, G., Rackwitz, S., Genvresse, I., Rosen, O., Dörken, B., & Arnold, R. (2002). Basiliximab is well tolerated and effective in the treatment of steroid-refractory acute graft-versus-host disease after allogeneic stem cell transplantation. *Bone Marrow Transplantation, 30,* 899–903. doi:10.1038/sj.bmt.1703737

Maziarz, R.T., & Abar, F. (2011). Chronic graft-versus-host disease. In R.T. Maziarz & S. Slater (Eds.), *Blood and marrow transplant handbook: Comprehensive guide for patient care* (pp. 189–212). New York, NY: Springer.

McCrudden, R., Williams, D.B., O'Connor, T., & Vickers, C.R. (2004). Gastrointestinal, hepatic, gallbladder, pancreatic, and perianal complications. In K. Atkinson, R. Champlin, J. Ritz, W.E. Fibbe, P. Ljungman, & M.K. Brenner (Eds.), *Clinical bone marrow and blood stem cell transplantation* (3rd ed., pp. 1417–1453). Cambridge, United Kingdom: Cambridge University Press.

Min, C.K. (2011). The pathophysiology of chronic graft-versus-host disease: The unveiling of an enigma. *Korean Journal of Hematology, 46,* 80–87. doi:10.5045/kjh.2011.46.2.80

Mitchell, S.A. (2013). Acute and chronic graft-versus-host disease. In S.A. Ezzone (Ed.), *Hematopoietic stem cell transplantation: A manual for nursing practice* (2nd ed., pp. 103–153). Pittsburgh, PA: Oncology Nursing Society.

Mohty, M., & Apperley, J.F. (2010). Long-term physiological side effects after allogeneic bone marrow transplantation. *ASH Education Book, 2010,* 229–236.

Olivieri, A., Locatelli, F., Zecca, M., Sanna, A., Cimminiello, M.R., Raimondi, R., … Bacigalupo, A. (2009). Imatinib for refractory chronic graft-versus-host disease with fibrotic features. *Blood, 114,* 709–718. doi:10.1182/blood -2009-02-204156

Parfitt, J.R., Jayakumar, S., & Driman, D.K. (2008). Mycophenolate mofetil-related gastrointestinal mucosal injury: Variable injury patterns, including graft-versus-host disease-like changes. *American Journal of Surgical Pathology, 32,* 1367–1372. doi:10.1097/PAS.0b013e31816bf3fe

Pasquini, M.C., & Zhu, X. (2015). Current uses and outcomes of hematopoietic stem cell transplantation. CIBMTR summary slides 2015. Retrieved from https://www.cibmtr.org/referencecenter/slidesreports/summaryslides/Pages/index.aspx

Peréz-Simón, J., Sánchez-Abarca, I., Díez-Campelo, M., Caballero, D., & San Miguel, J. (2006). Chronic graft-versus-host disease: Pathogenesis and clinical management. *Drugs, 66,* 1041–1057. doi:10.2165/00003495-200666080-00002

Peritt, D. (2006). Potential mechanisms of photopheresis in hematopoietic stem cell transplantation. *Biology of Blood and Marrow Transplantation, 12*(Suppl. 2), 7–12. doi:10.1016/j.bbmt.2005.11.005

Przepiorka, D., Kernan, N.A., Ippoliti, C., Papadopoulos, E., Giralt, S., Khouri, I., ... Light, S. (2000). Daclizumab, a humanized anti-interleukin-2 receptor alpha chain antibody, for treatment of acute graft-versus-host disease. *Blood, 95,* 83–89.

Przepiorka, D., Weisdorf, D., Martin, P., Klingemann, H.G., Beatty, P., Hows, J., & Thomas, E.D. (1995). 1994 consensus conference on acute GVHD grading. *Bone Marrow Transplantation, 15,* 825–828.

Selbst, M.K., Ahrens, W.A., Robert, M.E., Friedman, A., Proctor, D.D., & Jain, D. (2009). Spectrum of histologic changes in colonic biopsies in patients treated with mycophenolate mofetil. *Modern Pathology, 22,* 737–743. doi:10.1038/modpathol.2009.44

Shapira, M.Y., Abdul-Hai, A., Resnick, I.B., Bitan, M., Tsirigotis, P., Aker, M., ... Or, R. (2008). Alefacept treatment for refractory chronic extensive GVHD. *Bone Marrow Transplantation, 43,* 339–343. doi:10.1038/bmt.2008.324

Slater, S. (2011). Acute graft-versus-host disease. In R.T. Maziarz & S. Slater (Eds.), *Blood and marrow transplant handbook: Comprehensive patient care* (pp. 167–188). New York, NY: Springer.

Treister, N., Duncan, C., Cutler, C., & Lehmann, L. (2012). How we treat oral chronic graft-versus-host disease. *Blood, 120,* 3407–3418. doi:10.1182/blood-2012-05-393389

Vargas-Díez, E., Garcia-Díez, A., Marin, A., & Fernández-Herrera, J. (2005). Life-threatening graft-versus-host disease. *Clinics in Dermatology, 23,* 285–300. doi:10.1016/j.clindermatol.2004.06.005

Vogelsang, G.B. (2001). How I treat chronic graft-versus-host-disease. *Blood, 97,* 1196–1201. doi:10.1182/blood.V97.5.1196

Wang, J.Z., Liu, K.Y., Xu, L.P., Liu, D.H., Han, W., Chen, H., ... Huang, X.J. (2011). Basiliximab for the treatment of steroid-refractory acute graft-versus-host disease after unmanipulated HLA-mismatched/haploidentical hematopoietic stem cell transplantation. *Transplantation Proceedings, 43,* 1928–1933. doi:10.1016/j.transproceed.2011.03.044

Wolff, D., Gerbitz, A., Ayuk, F., Kiani, A., Hildebrandt, G.C., Vogelsang, G.B., ... Greinix, H. (2010). Consensus conference on clinical practice in chronic graft-versus-host disease (GVHD): First-line and topical treatment of chronic GVHD. *Biology of Blood and Marrow Transplantation, 16,* 1611–1628. doi:10.1016/j.bbmt.2010.06.015

Study Questions

1. T.R. is a 28-year-old woman with acute myeloid leukemia in her second complete remission who is admitted for a matched unrelated allogeneic stem cell transplantation. Her conditioning regimen is as follows:

   Myeloablation (busulfan/cyclophosphamide) and immunosuppression with tacrolimus and methotrexate (5 mg/m^2 on days +1, +3, +6, and +11).

   She did not receive methotrexate on day +11 because of severe mucositis. Her transplant course was complicated by mucositis, neutropenic fever, and *Clostridium difficile* diarrhea. T.R. had no symptoms of graft-versus-host disease (GVHD) during the hospital course. Her blood counts recovered, and she was discharged to home. Day +30 bone marrow showed 100% donor. A clinic visit on day +50 revealed a new maculopapular rash covering 40% of T.R.'s body. She is staged as grade 2. The skin biopsy is consistent with GVHD. What is the initial management?
   A. Check tacrolimus level.
   B. Start systemic steroids.
   C. Start topical steroids.
   D. A and C

2. T.R.'s tacrolimus level is therapeutic at 11. One week later, at the scheduled clinic visit, her rash has decreased to grade 1. T.R. reports "watery diarrhea" five times per day. She is admitted to the hospital for further evaluation and treatment. How should the patient be managed?

   (1) Continue PO medications. (2) Add antidiarrheal agents. (3) Rule out infectious etiology of diarrhea. (4) Change medications from PO to IV. (5) Request gastrointestinal (GI) consult. (6) Obtain accurate measurement of stool volume.
   A. 1, 2, 5
   B. 1, 3, 6
   C. 2, 3, 4, 5, 6
   D. 2, 3, 4, 5

3. T.R.'s tacrolimus level remains therapeutic at 11. The volume of diarrhea in 24 hours is 1,000 ml. Infectious etiology workup is negative. Colonoscopy was obtained, and the report describes erythema and ulcerations. Cytomegalovirus (CMV) and other viral strains are negative. The formal interpretation of biopsy shows consistency with GVHD. T.R. is therefore diagnosed with stage 2 acute GVHD. How should the patient be managed?
   A. Add systemic steroids (methylprednisolone 1–2 mg/kg per day).
   B. Add mycophenolate.
   C. Treat with infliximab.
   D. Treat with antithymocyte globulin (ATG).
   E. Add cyclosporine.

4. One week later, T.R.'s volume of diarrhea has increased to 3,000 ml per day. How should the patient be treated?
   A. Increase steroids.
   B. Add infliximab or ATG and attempt to taper steroids.
   C. Continue same treatment and wait.
   D. Start clear liquids PO to replace GI fluid loss.

5. What is the standard regimen of immunosuppression for myeloablative transplant?
   A. Steroids
   B. Tacrolimus and cyclosporine
   C. Steroids and tacrolimus
   D. Tacrolimus and methotrexate

6. C.W. presents to clinic on day 30 after allogeneic transplant (matched unrelated donor) with a rash on her arms and chest. Using the Rule of Nines, what stage is the patient?
   A. Stage 0
   B. Stage 1
   C. Stage 2
   D. Stage 1–2

7. C.W. returns with progression of rash on her face, chest, back, and arms. Diarrhea of approximately 1–2 L per day and a new elevation in serum bilirubin of 2 mg/dl are noted. The patient reports feeling weak and is having difficulty eating. She is able to get out of bed daily to sit in a chair, but her appetite is poor. She bathes without assistance. What overall grade is the patient?
   A. Grade 1
   B. Grade 2
   C. Grade 3
   D. Grade 4

8. L.K. is approximately two months status-post allogenic bone marrow transplantation using an unrelated donor. She comes to the clinic complaining of an itchy rash on her chest and arms. Her immunosuppression regimen is cyclosporine and mycophenolic acid. What would be the initial treatment?
   A. Admit for IV steroids.
   B. Check cyclosporine level.
   C. Use topical hydrocortisone and have her return in three days.
   D. B and C

9. Y.R. is a 25-year-old woman who has never been pregnant and will be receiving an unrelated transplant from a 40-year-old man. The graft is 9/10 human leukocyte antigen (HLA)-matched. Both donor and recipient are CMV positive. Y.R. has been transfused prior to transplant. What is the biggest risk factor for Y.R. developing GVHD?
   A. Age of donor
   B. Sex mismatch
   C. CMV positivity in both donor and recipient
   D. HLA mismatch

10. Cyclosporine and tacrolimus have many drug–drug interactions. A major interaction is with voriconazole, which is frequently used in the HSCT setting. When calculating the dose of calcineurin inhibitors (CNIs) for immunosuppression, what should be done?
    A. Calculate dose based on lean body weight and follow levels.
    B. Ask doctor to change voriconazole to an alternative.
    C. Give drugs at least four hours apart to avoid interaction, dose-reduce CNI by one-third to one-quarter, and follow levels closely.
    D. None of the above

11. Which graft source has a higher risk of developing acute GVHD?
    A. Peripheral blood stem cells
    B. Bone marrow
    C. Umbilical cord blood
    D. None of the above

12. What is the first organ usually involved with acute GVHD?
    A. Lungs
    B. Eyes
    C. GI tract
    D. Skin

13. What is the phenomenon that occurs approximately 7–14 days post-HSCT and has the following symptoms: fever, erythroderma, and noncardiogenic pulmonary edema?
    A. Acute GVHD
    B. Engraftment syndrome
    C. Hyperacute GVHD
    D. Early acute GVHD

14. GVHD can occur at the time of immunosuppression taper. What is this type of acute GVHD referred to as?
    A. Persistent recurring late GVHD
    B. Hyperacute GVHD
    C. Classic acute GVHD
    D. Overlap syndrome

15. What immunosuppressant can cause serum sickness?
    A. Mycophenolate
    B. Cyclosporine
    C. Steroids
    D. ATG

16. Long-term use of CNIs affects what part of the body?
    A. Bones
    B. Heart
    C. Kidneys
    D. Liver

17. Sirolimus can cause which of the following?
    A. Pulmonary toxicity
    B. Cardiomyopathy
    C. Renal insufficiency
    D. Liver toxicity

18. With which of the following does transplant-associated microangiopathy occur?
    A. Sirolimus alone
    B. Sirolimus and steroids
    C. Sirolimus and mycophenolate mofetil
    D. CNIs (tacrolimus and cyclosporine)

19. Which immunosuppressant can cause hirsutism?
    A. Tacrolimus
    B. Steroids
    C. Sirolimus
    D. Cyclosporine

20. Which drug is used to both prevent graft rejection and GVHD?
    A. ATG
    B. Cyclosporine
    C. Tacrolimus
    D. Sirolimus

21. Overlap syndrome is a classification of GVHD that consists of which of the following?
    A. Classic acute and persistent recurring late GVHD
    B. Hyperacute GVHD
    C. Features of both acute and chronic GVHD
    D. Chronic GVHD

22. Chronic GVHD carries a reduced risk of recurrent disease by allowing the benefit of graft-versus-leukemia effect.
    A. True
    B. False

23. Although the pathophysiology of chronic GVHD is unclear, some hypotheses include which of the following?
    A. B cells
    B. Cytokines including interleukin (IL)-2, IL-6, and tumor necrosis factor-alpha (TNF-α)
    C. T cells only
    D. A and B

24. Patients with chronic GVHD are at an increased risk for which of the following?
    A. Relapsed disease
    B. Infections
    C. Electrolyte abnormalities due to long-term CNIs
    D. Renal dysfunction

25. Chronic GVHD occurs most frequently when?
    A. Within 30 days of transplant
    B. Four to six months after transplant
    C. After day 100 post-HSCT
    D. Within the first year

26. What is the strongest risk factor for chronic GVHD?
    A. Prior acute GVHD
    B. HLA disparity
    C. Older donor
    D. Older recipient

27. An important poor prognostic feature of chronic GVHD is which of the following?
    A. White blood cell count less than 5,000/mm^3
    B. Platelet count less than 100,000/mm^3
    C. Hemoglobin level less than 7 g/dl
    D. Lymphocyte count less than 500/mm^3

28. What are the most commonly involved organs of chronic GVHD?
    A. Skin, mouth, and muscles
    B. Mouth, liver, and eyes
    C. Lung, GI tract, and joints
    D. Skin, liver, and mouth

29. What is one characteristic feature of chronic GVHD of the mouth?
    A. Open ulcers
    B. White lines and lacy-appearing lesions on the buccal mucosa and tongue palate
    C. Dry mucous membranes
    D. B and C

30. Chronic GVHD of eyes significantly affects quality of life after allogeneic HSCT. What usually is the first treatment modality?
    A. Preservative-free artificial tears
    B. Ophthalmic antibiotic ointment
    C. Lubrication
    D. Cyclosporine eye drops

31. Chronic GVHD can be manifested in the hematopoietic system and cytopenias including:
    A. Lymphocyte count less than 500/mm^3 and eosinophilia
    B. Anemia
    C. Thrombocytopenia
    D. All of the above

32. It is unlikely that someone will develop chronic GVHD without a history of acute GVHD.
    A. True
    B. False

33. Scoring of chronic GVHD involves which of the following?
    A. Specific organs and the number of organs involved
    B. Severity within each affected organ
    C. Functional impairment
    D. All of the above

34. What is the primary first-line therapy for moderate to severe chronic GVHD?
    A. Adding a CNI if patient is not on one
    B. Adding extracorporeal photopheresis
    C. Adding sirolimus
    D. Adding systemic steroids

35. National Institutes of Health guidelines recommend consideration of systemic treatment for chronic GVHD if
    A. Three or more organs are involved.
    B. One organ has a severity score that is greater than 2.
    C. Any organ has involvement of chronic GVHD.
    D. Major organ such as the eyes, lungs, or liver is involved.
    E. A and B

36. What is one of the major tasks in diagnosing either acute or chronic GVHD?
    A. Rule out other etiologies such as infection or drug reaction.
    B. Obtain a biopsy.
    C. Assess timing of symptoms.
    D. All of the above

37. For chronic GVHD of the skin, the use of topical agents may improve symptoms and clinical features. To treat GVHD that involves the face, topical agents include:
    A. High-potency steroids BID for no more than seven days.
    B. Emollients.
    C. Antipruritic creams.
    D. CNI creams such as tacrolimus.
    E. Low-potency steroids such as hydrocortisone (1%).
    F. B, C, D, E

38. What is the one organ that is involved more in chronic GVHD than acute GVHD?
    A. GI tract
    B. Skin
    C. Liver
    D. Eyes

39. When should a quality-of-life assessment in a patient with chronic GVHD occur?
    A. Annually
    B. At least every three months and whenever steroids are tapered
    C. Only if the patient reports a change
    D. None of the above

40. Why should rituximab be used for chronic GVHD therapy?
    A. Monoclonal antibodies are effective for both acute and chronic GVHD.
    B. Cells play a role in autoimmunity.
    C. Rituximab targets B cells.
    D. The degree of immunosuppression with rituximab is not high, and patients do not become neutropenic with it.
    E. B and C
    F. B and D

Post-Transplant Issues

Rebecca Norton, MSN, RN, CCRN,
Ima N. Garcia, RN, MSN, ACNP-BC, AOCNP®, and
Kimberly Noonan, RN, ANP, AOCN®

I. Post-transplant cardiac issues and immunologic issues
   A. Advances in hematopoietic stem cell transplantation (HSCT) have significantly improved over the last several decades. Although this has led to an improvement in survival rates, post-transplant complications have increased. It is essential that healthcare teams are aware of long-term cardiac and immunologic complications for patients following HSCT. This section will include the assessment, diagnosis, and management of cardiac and immunologic complications following HSCT.
      1. Cardiac complications are not as prevalent as other long-term HSCT complications; cardiovascular problems, however, may be underreported. Late cardiac effects may be detected years or decades after HSCT. Cardiac dysfunctions or complications may present as a questionable correlate because cardiovascular abnormalities are prevalent in the general population. Cardiovascular disease encompasses the entire arterial vascular network and includes post-HSCT cerebrovascular disease, ischemic heart disease, and peripheral arterial disease.
      2. Incidence of post-transplant cardiovascular disease (Chow et al., 2011; Martin et al., 2010; Tichelli et al., 2007)
         a) In a 2007 study, Tichelli et al. reported that the cumulative incidence of first arterial event after allogeneic HSCT (allo-HSCT) was 22.1% at 25 years.
         b) A study by Chow et al. (2011) that compared HSCT recipients to the general population reported an increase in cardiovascular death in HSCT recipients: HSCT recipients had an increased incidence of ischemic heart disease, cardiomyopathy, heart failure, stroke, vascular diseases, rhythm disorders, and related conditions that predispose people to more cardiovascular diseases, such as hypertension, renal disease, dyslipidemia, and diabetes.
         c) Mortality rates remained four to nine times higher than the expected population rate for at least 30 years post-transplant (Martin et al., 2010). In one study, it was estimated that HSCT recipients had a 30% lower life expectancy when compared to the general population, regardless of current age. The leading causes of excess deaths were second malignancies or recurrent disease. This was followed by infections, chronic graft-versus-host disease (GVHD), respiratory diseases, and cardiovascular diseases.

B. Types of cardiac disease commonly diagnosed in HSCT patients (Agarwal & Burkart, 2013; Aleman et al., 2007; Majhail et al., 2012; Marini, Choi, Byersdorfer, Cronin, & Frame, 2015; Novartis Pharmaceuticals, 2013; Pulsipher et al., 2012; Wyeth Pharmaceuticals, Inc., 2011)

   1. Cardiomyopathy, congestive heart failure, and arrhythmias
      a) These diseases often are related to previous anthracycline and radiation and are particularly noted in patients with lymphoma.
      b) High-dose cyclophosphamide therapy has been associated with congestive heart failure, pericarditis, and arrhythmias.
   2. Hypertension and dyslipidemia
      a) These diseases may be multifactorial and related to treatment, metabolic syndrome, and immunosuppression.
      b) Sedentary lifestyle or endocrine abnormalities, such as hypothyroidism or hypogonadism, also may be a factor.
      c) Many immunosuppressive medications can alter lipid homeostasis or cause other cardiac symptoms.
   3. Hypertension and hyperkalemia: Cyclosporine side effects
   4. Hyperlipidemia, hypertension, and peripheral edema: Sirolimus side effects
   5. Other cardiovascular diseases
      a) Myocardial infarction or ischemic heart disease
      b) Coronary heart disease
      c) Stroke
      d) Transient ischemic attack
C. Assessment of cardiac disease: Annual clinical assessment and physical examination should be obtained by the primary oncology team, bone marrow transplant provider, cardiologist, or primary care provider.
   1. History and physical examination: Report cardiac symptoms or abnormalities such as chest pain or chest pressure, increase in shortness of breath, dyspnea on exertion, paroxysmal nocturnal dyspnea, palpitations, rapid heart rate, syncope, fatigue, or peripheral edema.
   2. Document an increase in central venous pressure or presence of peripheral edema, digital clubbing, or abnormal heart sounds.
   3. Assess cardiovascular risk factors.
      a) Obesity
      b) Smoking
      c) Hyperlipidemia
      d) Diabetes
      e) Sedentary lifestyle
      f) Family history
   4. Include an intensive cardiac workup, if clinically indicated, with tests such as electrocardiogram (ECG), echocardiogram, chest x-ray, or stress test.
   5. Monitor vital signs: Laboratory values are based on clinical findings.
      a) Lipid profile
      b) Glucose/hemoglobin A1c
      c) Brain natriuretic peptide
      d) Thyroid function test
   6. Refer patients to cardiology as clinically indicated.
   7. Prevention and education

       a) Exercise
       b) Weight loss or healthy weight maintenance
       c) Dietary counseling
       d) Smoking cessation
       e) Medication adherence

D. Management of cardiac disease
   1. Medications
       a) Antihypertensives and antiarrhythmics
       b) Monitoring for statin interactions and statin therapy (should be held or dose-reduced)
       c) Hypoglycemic medications
       d) Thyroid medication
       e) Smoking cessation medication (e.g., varenicline, bupropion, nicotine products)
       f) Antianxiety medications
   2. Weight loss
       a) Exercise
       b) Nutrition counseling
       c) Smoking cessation
         (1) Medication
         (2) Smoking cessation programs
       d) Stress reduction (Pillay, Lee, Katona, Burney, & Avery, 2014)
         (1) In a recent study, approximately 11%–14% of patients reported clinical levels of depression or anxiety (Pillay et al., 2014).
         (2) Common strategies used in the management of depression and anxiety
           (a) Mindfulness exercises
           (b) Exercise
           (c) Counseling
           (d) Psychiatry
           (e) Social services
           (f) Support groups
           (g) Medications (if indicated)
              i. Anxiolytics
              ii. Antidepressants

E. Immunologic issues
   1. High-dose chemotherapy associated with the stem cell treatment process results in bone marrow failure caused by myeloablative effects. Infection-related complications remain a major cause of transplant-related mortality and morbidity.
       a) However, supportive care measures have significantly improved survival outcomes in HSCT recipients.
       b) International consensus guidelines for the prevention of infectious complications in HSCT recipients were published in 2009 (Tomblyn et al., 2009).
       c) Guidelines for vaccinations of the HSCT recipient also were developed to aid in preventing long-term infectious complications (Ljungman et al., 2009).
   2. Factors that influence risk of infection include personal history of infections, chemotherapy regimen intensity, and type of transplant (Kumar et al., 2015).

    a) Personal history
      (1) Infection history
      (2) Infectious disease markers
      (3) Current risk factors (central line–associated bloodstream infection)
      (4) Myeloablative or reduced-intensity chemotherapy (RIC) regimen
    b) Type of transplant (autologous or allogeneic): Donor factors
      (1) Infection history (e.g., cytomegalovirus [CMV] status)
      (2) Type of donor (matched related or matched unrelated)
      (3) Type of infection
        (a) Bacterial
        (b) Viral
        (c) Fungal
    c) Prevention and management
      (1) Environmental management
        (a) Limit public exposure when there is a known infectious illness.
        (b) Maintain good hand hygiene practices.
        (c) Avoid caring for pets.
      (2) Medications
        (a) Prophylactic antibiotics and antivirals
        (b) Treatment: Antibiotics, antivirals, and IV immunoglobulin
      (3) Ongoing surveillance, as the frequency of sepsis in HSCT was five times higher when compared to non-HSCT transplant patients
      (4) Vaccinations
3. Autologous HSCT (AHSCT)
    a) Although AHSCT infections are serious, the majority of infections are regimen-related, and few are caused by GVHD.
    b) Kumar et al. (2015) reported mortality-related sepsis in AHSCT at greater than 30%.
4. Allo-HSCT (Martin-Peña, Aguilar-Guisado, Espigado, Parody, & Cisneros, 2011)
    a) Time to recovery of other hematopoietic lineages typically occurs over the course of weeks following allo-HSCT.
    b) As a result, lymphocyte recovery is a prolonged process. The patient undergoing HSCT often is immunocompromised for several months. Some patients continue to demonstrate immune deficits for several years following HSCT.
    c) The development of GVHD is associated with an increase in the risk of infection.
    d) Martin-Peña et al. (2011) reported 1.36 infection-related episodes per patient in the first year after transplantation and 1.48 infection-related episodes per patient at two years after transplantation.
5. RIC or nonmyeloablative
    a) Although infection is common in nonmyeloablative HSCT, it also may be associated with fewer early infections. Early infections may not necessarily affect later infections (Bachanova et al., 2009).
    b) Although the magnitude of myelosuppression in patients undergoing nonmyeloablative HSCT is milder, the depth and extent of lymphodepletion tends to be similar to the prolonged periods of immune incompetence observed in recipients of myeloablative regimens (Tomblyn et al., 2009).

6. Myeloablative (Bachanova et al., 2009)
    a) Myeloablative HSCT is associated with a higher rate of infection-related mortality during the first year.
    b) Infections vary widely based on the conditioning regimen, donor type, immunosuppressive therapy, and host-related factors (e.g., age, comorbidities, malignancy).
7. Type of transplant conditioning regimen (Tomblyn et al., 2009)
    a) A higher risk of infection is present early post-transplant with highly myelosuppressive chemotherapy.
    b) An increase in infection risk exists with certain immunosuppressive drugs (e.g., corticosteroids, antithymocyte globulin [ATG], alemtuzumab).
8. Donor (Ljungman, 2014; Parody et al., 2015; Wagner et al., 2014)
    a) The use of an unrelated donor may increase the recipient's risk of infection.
    b) In a study by Parody et al. (2015), patients who received a single cord blood transplantation increased their risk of Epstein-Barr virus (EBV) and CMV infections when compared to unrelated bone marrow or peripheral blood stem cell (PBSC) recipients. This was caused by the patients' naïve immune systems.
    c) Neutrophil recovery and immune reconstitution may be prolonged with cord blood.
    d) CMV can be transmitted from a seropositive donor to a seronegative patient. This finding also increases transplant-related mortality rates and negatively affects the overall survival rate of recipients, as well as increases their transplant-related mortality rate (Ljungman, 2014).
    e) A higher risk of infection is present in donors who are human leukocyte antigen (HLA) mismatched, particularly with haploidentical donors.
    f) An increase in recipient comorbidity may negatively affect transplant outcome. Examples of comorbidity include the following:
        (1) Infection (increases with older individuals)
        (2) Previous splenectomy
        (3) Chronic GVHD
        (4) Cardiac disease
        (5) Diabetes
        (6) Chronic obstructive pulmonary disease
9. Common sites of infection
    a) Central line or bloodstream isolates
    b) Gastrointestinal (GI) tract
    c) Skin
    d) Respiratory
    e) Soft tissue
    f) Genitourinary tract
10. Types of infections (Hakki et al., 2007; Mikulska, Del Bono, & Viscoli, 2014; Willems et al., 2012)
    a) Bacterial
        (1) Patients are at risk for encapsulated bacterial infections. *Streptococcus pneumoniae* is the most common post-transplant infection and can cause pneumonia, meningitis, or sepsis.

(2) Although *Clostridium difficile* (*C. difficile*) infections are common in recipients during their first year following transplant, most *C. difficile* infection occurs during the acute phase of transplant.

(3) *Pseudomonas aeruginosa* is a common post-HSCT infection. In one study, the median time to diagnosis was 63 days (Hakki et al., 2007).

(4) Multidrug-resistant organisms are commonly experienced during the engraftment phase of transplant but should be considered in the post-transplant setting.

(5) Vancomycin-resistant *Enterococci*

(6) Methicillin-resistant *Staphylococcus aureus*

(7) Multidrug-resistant *Pseudomonas aeruginosa* or carbapenem-resistant *Pseudomonas aeruginosa*

(8) Extended-spectrum beta-lactamase–producing *Enterobacteriaceae*

(9) *Mycobacterium tuberculosis* (TB) and atypical mycobacteria are a concern, especially in patients with poor T-cell immunity. TB is increased in certain endemic areas and can occur in both AHSCT and allo-HSCT (Gea-Banacloche et al., 2009; Marr, 2012).

b) Viral (Blennow et al., 2014; Chemaly, Shah, & Boeckh, 2014; Dahi et al., 2015; Erard, Wald, Corey, Leisenring, & Boeckh, 2007; Marchesi et al., 2014; Martin-Peña et al., 2011; Vermont et al., 2014)

(1) CMV is the most common infection syndrome in HSCT.

    (*a*) CMV-seropositive patients had lower overall survival, lower leukemia-free survival, and higher nonrelapse mortality than CMV-seronegative patients receiving stem cells from CMV-seronegative donors (i.e., double negatives) (Ljungman, 2014).

    (*b*) In a 2014 study, Marchesi et al. found that patients with multiple myeloma who were treated with bortezomibbased regimens were at a higher risk of developing symptomatic CMV reactivation after AHSCT when compared to patients who received treatment with vincristine, doxorubicin, and dexamethasone.

    (*c*) Common treatments for CMV include ganciclovir, foscarnet, and valacyclovir.

(2) The development of varicella-zoster virus (VZV) is a long-term complication of HSCT. The incidence of VZV reactivation is estimated at 20%–25% within two years of an allo-HSCT. Common treatments for VZV include acyclovir, famciclovir, and valacyclovir.

(3) Herpes simplex virus (HSV) type 1 and 2 reactivation can occur both early and late after HSCT. It is estimated that when prophylaxis is not used, the incidence of HSV-1 or HSV-2 is approximately 30%.

(4) Influenza infection can be a late complication of HSCT and can lead to poor outcomes in recipients, specifically among those receiving augmented immunosuppression for GVHD. The influenza vaccine will aid in the prevention of influenza; it is not, however, fully protective. Other treatments include the following:

    (*a*) Respiratory syncytial virus often is treated with ribavirin.

    (*b*) Viral influenza can be treated with neuraminidase inhibitors, such as oseltamivir or zanamivir.

c) Fungal (Kontoyiannis et al., 2010; Muto, 2011; Tomblyn et al., 2009)

        (1) Aspergillosis is the most common late invasive fungal infection. Galactomannan antigen and beta-D-glucan serum testing often is obtained to diagnose invasive fungal infections, especially in patients with neutropenia. *Candida* fungal pathogens are commonly described in HSCT recipients.

        (2) Mucormycosis also is considered a serious post-transplant fungal infection.

        (3) *Pneumocystis jiroveci* pneumonia can occur in 4%–16% of HSCT recipients who are not on prophylaxis.

        (4) Guidelines for the use of antifungal prophylaxis for patients at risk of developing serious invasive fungal infections (engraftment and postengraftment phase) were revised in 2014 (Girmenia et al., 2014).

     d) Common treatments for fungal infections include voriconazole, micafungin, posaconazole, and liposomal amphotericin.

F. Prevention and management of infections (Miceli et al., 2013): Immunization

   1. Vaccine antibodies decline months to years after an allo-HSCT or AHSCT.

   2. International consensus guidelines for preventing infectious complications for HSCT recipients were published in 2009 (Tomblyn et al., 2009).

   3. Vaccinations are left to the discretion of the provider. For example, vaccinations for measles, mumps, and rubella may not be given if the patient is immunocompromised.

   4. The following vaccines may be given during the post-transplant setting (see Table 6-1).

     a) Pneumococcus

     b) Pertussis, tetanus, diphtheria

     c) *Haemophilus influenzae* type B

     d) Hepatitis B

     e) Meningococcus

     f) Influenza

     g) Measles, mumps, and rubella (24 months post-transplant)

     h) VZV (currently investigational)

G. Surveillance (Majhail et al., 2012)

   1. Helper T lymphocytes (CD4) counts and CD4/CD8 ratios can be obtained as one marker to assess immune reconstitution.

   2. Multidrug-resistant colonization status and the history of past infections should be documented and monitored in the outpatient setting.

   3. Appropriate contact isolation should be implemented in the post-transplant setting and precautions should be followed.

   4. Clearance of infection precautions should be considered per institutional policies and procedures.

   5. CMV reactivation screening should be based on risk factors. Immunosuppression and baseline CMV status of the recipient and donor is a strong consideration when implementing CMV screening.

H. Antibiotics

   1. Trimethoprim-sulfamethoxazole (TMP-SMX) is preferred primary care provider prophylaxis for six months or longer per transplant center policy.

   2. Consider prophylactic antibiotics targeting encapsulated organisms for patients with chronic GVHD while on aggressive immunosuppressive therapy (Mijhail et al., 2012).

   3. Consider prophylactic antibiotics following HSCT if treated with immunosuppressive therapy.

Table 6-1. Sample Post-Transplant Immunization Schedule

Organism	Vaccine	Suggested Schedule*	Dose and Route	Comments
Inactivated Vaccines				
Pneumococcal	PCV7/ PPSV23	9, 12, and 18 months	0.5 ml IM or SC	Can be given 6 months post-transplant
Diphtheria, tetanus, and pertussis	DTaP	9, 12, and 18 months	0.5 ml IM	Can be given 6 months post-transplant
Haemophilus influenzae type B	HIB	9, 12, and 18 months	0.5 ml IM	Can be given 6 months post-transplant
Hepatitis B (HBV)	–	12, 14, and 18 months	1 ml IM	Administer to patients who are HBV-negative.
Meningococcus	–	One dose after 6 months	0.5 ml SC	Recommended in areas with an increase in meningococcus
Influenza	–	One dose after 4–6 months	0.5 ml IM	Give annually as available in the fall months. May administer 4 months post-transplant; however, 2 doses of vaccine is suggested.
Live Virus Vaccines				
Measles, mumps, and rubella (MMR)	MMR	24 months	0.5 ml SC	Limit exposure to immunocompromised individuals. MMR vaccine may be held if patient is immunosuppressed.
Zoster vaccine	Shingles vaccine	24 months	0.65 ml SC	Safety investigation is ongoing; vaccine is not routinely administered. Limit exposure to immunocompromised individuals. May be held if patient is immunosuppressed.

* Individualized schedule per transplant center

IM—intramuscular injection; SC—subcutaneous injection

Note. Based on information from Centers for Disease Control and Prevention, 2011; Ljungman et al., 2009; Miceli et al., 2013; Rubin et al., 2014.

I. Antiviral and antifungal agents
   1. The prophylaxis of VZV should be administered post-HSCT.
   2. Lifestyle restrictions are unique to each transplant center. Along with the following safety measures, patients and their families should be educated about early signs and symptoms of infection, as well as the importance of seeking early medical attention.
      a) Practicing safe sex

  b) Staying hydrated

  c) Adhering to food safety standards

  d) Following travel guidelines

II. Ocular, musculoskeletal, and psychological complications and graft rejection and failure

 A. The use of bone marrow transplantation to treat oncologic and non-oncologic diseases in adults and children continues to expand. As the indications, incidence, and overall survival outcomes increase, so will the prevalence of transplant-related complications. Transplant-related side effects may influence overall survival and can affect the physicality and mentality of the patient. Common post-transplant issues may include ocular damage, musculoskeletal changes, psychosocial difficulties, and the possibility for graft rejection or graft failure. It is crucial that clinicians caring for transplant patients are aware of potential hurdles and are familiar with risk factors, clinical signs and symptoms, diagnoses, and management of transplant-related complications.

 B. Ocular damage following HSCT can involve all parts of the eye and may be a consequence of immunosuppression, conditioning regimens (e.g., chemotherapy, irradiation, or both), or underlying disease. This damage applies to both adult and pediatric populations (Balasubramaniam, Raja, Nau, Shen, & Schornack, 2015; Hirst, Jabs, Tutschka, Green, & Santos, 1983). Patients at risk may develop ocular complications associated with GVHD, dry eye syndrome, optic disc and retinal microvasculopathy, and opportunistic infections (Nassar, Tabbara, & Aljurf, 2013; Nassiri et al., 2013; Ogawa et al., 1999).

  1. GVHD is a major cause of ocular morbidity following allo-HSCT.

  2. Symptoms are common and include photophobia, hyperemia, hemorrhagic conjunctivitis, pseudomembrane formation, lagophthalmos, and corneal ulceration.

  3. Pathophysiology (Hessen & Akpek, 2012; Khanal & Tomlinson, 2012; Wang et al., 2010)

   a) The eye is a target organ for GVHD.

   b) The ocular surface undergoes major changes following allogeneic transplant, even when dry eyes are not apparent.

   c) Involvement in chronic GVHD appears as inflammatory destruction of the conjunctiva, fibrotic lacrimal glands, decreased goblet cell density, and decreased tear production.

   d) Late complications include retinal lesions and cataracts.

  4. Prevalence and risk factors (Kim, 2005, 2006; Tabarra et al., 2009)

   a) Ocular GVHD develops in approximately 40%–60% of patients following allo-HSCT and 60%–90% of patients with acute or chronic GVHD. Ocular damage may lead to severe ocular surface disease, which can significantly affect quality of life (QOL) and restrict activities of daily living (ADL).

   b) Ocular damage may be the initial manifestation of systemic GVHD.

   c) Risks are increased in the presence of skin or mouth involvement.

   d) Higher risk is detected in allogeneic transplants from related donors compared with unrelated donors. This is theoretically attributed to conditioning with ATG in the unrelated donor population.

   e) No clear correlation has been identified with respect to stem cell source.

  5. Manifestations (Filipovich et al., 2005)

   a) Affected tissues include the eyelid, periorbital skin, conjunctiva, cornea, lens, lacrimal system, sclera, uvea, and retina.

    b) New-onset eye dryness, grittiness, or pain, difficulty opening eyes in the morning because of mucoid secretions, cicatricial conjunctivitis, keratoconjunctivitis sicca, and confluent areas of punctate keratopathy are common.

    c) Changes in eyelid skin include maculopapular, erythematous exanthema, dermatitis, lagophthalmos, ectropion, poliosis, madarosis, and vitiligo.

6. Dry eye syndrome (keratoconjunctivitis sicca) (Hessen & Akpek, 2012)

    a) Dry eye syndrome is the most frequent complication, occurring in 40%–76% of patients with chronic GVHD.

    b) It can be the initial presentation and sole complication of GVHD.

    c) It also can occur in the absence of other systemic complications.

    d) The main source is lymphocytic infiltration of the accessory and major lacrimal glands, which may trigger fibrosis of the acini and ductules.

    e) Other causes include radiation, chemotherapy, immunosuppression, and infection.

    f) Risk factors for severe dry eye include meibomian gland disease and female-to-male HSCT.

    g) Dry eye syndrome can occur at any time, from a few weeks to years after transplantation; the median time of development is around six months.

    h) Subjective symptoms are characteristic of the disease and include dry eyes, foreign body sensation, ocular fatigue, discharge, and dull sensation.

    i) Symptoms often progress to severe dry eye that resembles Sjögren syndrome.

    j) Other symptoms include burning, stinging, itching, soreness, heaviness of eyelids, and photophobia.

    k) Grading: Symptoms of dry eye syndrome can be assigned a score of 0–3 based on severity.

       (1) 0 = No dry eye symptoms

       (2) 1 = Dry eye symptoms affecting ADL (eye drops three or fewer times per day) or asymptomatic signs of keratoconjunctivitis sicca

       (3) 2 = Dry eye symptoms partially affecting ADL (eye drops more than three times per day or punctal plugs) without vision impairment

       (4) 3 = Dry eye symptoms significantly affecting ADL (special eyewear to relieve pain) or unable to work because of ocular symptoms or loss of vision caused by keratoconjunctivitis sicca

7. Conjunctival disease (Nassar et al., 2013; Nassiri et al., 2013)

    a) Rare: Occurs in approximately 10% of ocular damage cases

    b) Indicative of severe systemic involvement

    c) Ranges from mild erythema to pseudomembranous and cicatrizing conjunctivitis

    d) More ulcerative and hemorrhagic in the setting of acute GVHD (typically leads to conjunctival scarring and symblepharon)

    e) Grading: Symptoms of conjunctivitis can be assigned a score of 0–4 based on severity.

       (1) 0 = None

       (2) 1 = Conjunctival hyperemia

       (3) 2 = Conjunctival hyperemia with chemotic response and serosanguinous exudate

       (4) 3 = Pseudomembranous conjunctivitis

       (5) 4 = Pseudomembranous conjunctivitis with corneal epithelial sloughing and subsequent conjunctival scar and symblepharon formation

8. Cataract (Allan et al., 2011; Hessen & Akpek, 2012; Kim, 2006)
    a) Attributed to radiation and steroid therapy and is not a direct result of GVHD itself
    b) Most common cause of visual acuity loss
    c) Higher risk for patients who received total body irradiation (TBI) versus fractionated TBI
    d) Eventually requires cataract surgery
    e) Grading: Symptoms of cataract can be assigned a score of 1–3 based on severity
        (1) 1 = Occasional subcapsular opacities and vacuoles in the central region of the lens
        (2) 2 = Small clusters of subcapsular opacities remaining discrete
        (3) 3 = Multiple clusters of subcapsular opacities that have mostly coalesced
9. Diagnosis and grading (Nassiri et al., 2013)
    a) Close monitoring, symptom assessment, and comprehensive ophthalmic examinations, including the following:
        (1) Visual acuity testing
        (2) Slit-lamp examination
        (3) Dry eye workup
        (4) Tonometry
        (5) Funduscopy
    b) Diagnosis can be made by conjunctival biopsy.
    c) Thorough history and physical examination are necessary.
10. Prophylaxis and treatment (Nassiri et al., 2013)
    a) Acute GVHD prophylaxis primarily consists of immunosuppression as single or combination therapy.
    b) Cyclosporine eye drops have shown efficacy in ocular GVHD.
    c) Eye shielding during TBI can suspend cataract development and diminish severity.
11. Systemic therapy (Nassar et al., 2013)
    a) Systemic immune suppression is the foundation of GVHD management.
    b) Topical steroids, cyclosporine, or tacrolimus may reduce cicatricial and fibrovascular scarring and prevent progression to stage 4 disease.
    c) Calcineurin inhibitors have been found to be useful to ameliorate the sequential signs of chronic ocular GVHD.
12. Local therapy (Nassar et al., 2013)
    a) Supportive ocular care is intended to minimize the need for systemic immunosuppressive therapy.
    b) Patient education should include environmental management such as humidifiers and lower room temperatures.
    c) Treatment goals are to lubricate eyes and decrease surface tearing, thus improving ocular surface moisture.
    d) Tear function can be improved by controlling lubrication, evaporation, and drainage. Using artificial tears is the most common approach.
    e) The use of topical steroids or cyclosporine may decrease ocular inflammation.
    f) Autologous serum eye drops have shown benefit in patients with dry eye syndrome and are recommended earlier in the course of the disease.
    g) Wearing eye protection, such as moisture chamber goggles, can help decrease evaporation.

h) Special contact lenses, including soft and hard scleral lenses, have been shown to be safe and effective for recalcitrant cases. They also may reduce dependency on lubricants, minimize symptoms, and improve QOL.

13. Surgical treatment in refractory cases (Johnson et al., 1999; Nassar et al., 2013)
    a) Tarsorrhaphy decreases the exposed surface area, thus minimizing dryness and evaporation.
    b) Temporary or permanent occlusion of the tear-duct puncta decreases drainage and may provide additional benefit.

14. Retinal microvasculopathy complications: Commonly exhibited in allogeneic transplant recipients and include retinal hemorrhage, cotton wool spots, and optic disc edema
    a) Pathophysiology: Findings usually are attributed to pancytopenia in the early post-transplant phase (vitreous or intraretinal hemorrhage), GVHD, cyclosporine, or conditioning regimens that contain TBI.
    b) Treatment: Symptoms generally resolve spontaneously within two to three months and are correlated with platelet count recovery.

15. Opportunistic infections (Ayuso et al., 2013)
    a) Pathophysiology: Can be viral, bacterial, or fungal. Attributed to neutropenia or immunosuppressive therapy and immunocompromised state.
        (1) Common viral reactivations include CMV, human herpesvirus type 6 (HHV-6), VZV, and EBV.
        (2) Opportunistic infections typically occur in older patients but also can be seen in the pediatric population.
    b) The use of prophylactic antivirals, antibacterials, and antifungals is recommended for immunocompromised patients.

C. Musculoskeletal complications
    1. The prevalence of autologous and allogeneic transplants has increased over the past 40 years. Improvements in therapy and infection prophylaxis have led to an observed decrease in transplant-related mortality. Increasingly larger numbers of long-term survivors have developed early and late transplant-related musculoskeletal complications, which include avascular necrosis (AVN), osteoporosis, fracture, and osteomyelitis. These complications can negatively affect mobility and exercise tolerance and worsen overall QOL (Serio et al., 2013).
    2. Osteoporosis (Campbell et al., 2009; Serio et al., 2013; Tauchmanovà et al., 2003)
        a) Pathophysiology: Osteoporosis is ascribed to the effect of numerous influences, including myeloablative conditioning regimens; cytokine release at the time of transplant; altered kidney, liver, and bowel function, resulting in decreased intake and altered metabolism of calcium and vitamin D; gonadal failure; and long-lasting steroid use and immunosuppression.
        b) Incidence
            (1) Osteoporosis occurs more frequently than AVN.
            (2) Affected areas include the femoral neck (50%) and lumbar spine (20%).
            (3) Early bone loss may consist of both demineralization and architectural damage with associated organic matrix deficit.
        c) Diagnosis
            (1) Dual-energy x-ray absorptiometry (DEXA) measures bone density and mineralization but does not provide information on architectural damage and bone formation.

(2) High-resolution computed tomography (CT) and magnetic resonance imaging (MRI) scans allow for three-dimensional assessment of trabecular structure; however, these techniques can be costly and time consuming.

(3) Ultrasonic evaluation permits assessment of physical properties of bone tissue and can account for more structural changes than DEXA. Ultrasonic evaluation by phalangeal ultrasound allows for the evaluation of bone density and elasticity, trabecular orientation, and cortical-to-trabecular ratio.

   d) Treatment: Prompt treatment consists of supportive measures, including lifestyle modification, calcium and vitamin D supplements, and bisphosphonates, as indicated.

3. AVN (Campbell et al., 2009; Tauchmanovà et al., 2003; Wiesmann et al., 1998)

   a) AVN of the bone is a painful and debilitating condition that develops when blood supply to the bone is disrupted. This usually arises in areas with terminal circulation, occurring most commonly in the femoral head.

   b) Pathophysiology: The condition is believed to be the result of vascular compromise, bone and cell tissue death, or disruption of bone repair mechanisms.

   c) Incidence

      (1) Multiple studies report an incidence of approximately 5%–20% in long-term allogeneic transplant survivors.

      (2) The mean time from transplant to diagnosis is approximately 12–13 months. It appears to occur earlier in transplant recipients than in patients treated with steroids for other chronic illnesses.

      (3) AVN is a progressive process that often results in joint destruction within three to five years if left untreated.

   d) Risk factors

      (1) GVHD

      (2) Older age

      (3) Primary diagnosis of acute leukemia

      (4) TBI

      (5) Steroid therapy

   e) Diagnosis: MRI preferred to conventional radiology

   f) Staging (see Table 6-2)

   g) Treatment

      (1) Conservative management includes rest, analgesics, and pulsing electromagnetic fields.

      (2) Surgical treatment includes core decompression or hip replacement.

Table 6-2. Staging of Avascular Necrosis by Magnetic Resonance Imaging (MRI) Scan

Stage	MRI Feature
I	Nonhomogeneous loss in T1 signal intensity
II	Wedge-shaped crescent sign
III	Crescent sign, sequestra, cortical collapse
IV	Degenerative changes with narrowed joint space

Note. Based on information from Wiesmann et al., 1998.

4. Pediatrics
   a) Skeletal complications in pediatric HSCT survivors can affect their ability to attend and perform well in school, interact with peers, lead healthy lifestyles, and ultimately, function normally in society.
   b) Multiple skeletal complications can occur following pediatric HSCT. The three primary obstacles are osteochondroma, AVN, and diminished bone marrow density (Ruble, 2008).
   (1) Osteochondroma (Ruble, 2008): Bony growths that consist of both bone and cartilage resulting from epiphyseal damage
      (a) Incidence: 20%–24%
      (b) Risks are greater in patients who receive TBI at a younger age.
      (c) Latency period for developing osteochondromas is 4.6–6 years following therapy.
      (d) Signs and symptoms
         i. Painless, bony lesions that can be located on the central or peripheral skeleton; multiple sites can be involved.
         ii. Diagnosis is typically made with plain radiographs or skeletal survey.
      (e) Treatment
         i. Surgical resection for pain control or impaired motor function may be warranted.
         ii. Malignant transformation can occur with higher doses of radiation (median of 4,500 cGy).
         iii. No established guidelines currently exist for screening or follow-up. History and physical examinations should include evaluation for skeletal abnormality. Lesions may be followed with serial examinations. Lesions that increase in size or become symptomatic require further evaluation.
   (2) AVN and osteonecrosis (Ruble, 2008)
      (a) Pathophysiology: Results from ischemia caused by microvascular alterations, affecting blood supply to the bone
      (b) Incidence: May be as high as 50%
      (c) Risk factors
         i. History of GVHD
         ii. Glucocorticoid use
         iii. Immunosuppression
         iv. Older age at time of HSCT
      (d) AVN occurs most frequently in the hip but also can occur in the knees and at multiple sites.
      (e) Patients often present with pain or functional limitations.
      (f) Diagnosis can be made with an MRI. Plain radiographs also have been used to identify and quantify necrotic changes (Wiesmann et al., 1998).
      (g) Treatment
         i. The early stage consists of non-weight-bearing, analgesics, and physical therapy. Surgical interventions include core decompression, arthroplasty, and joint replacement.

           ii. Recommendations for follow-up include yearly history and physical with focus on joint pain, swelling, range of motion, and immobility (Ruble, 2008; Wiesmann et al., 1998).

      (3) Diminished bone mineral density (Ruble, 2008)

         (a) Pathophysiology: Disruption of bone mineralization has been attributed to cytokine production in response to malignant processes and altered vitamin D metabolism. Cancer therapy affects the fragile balance between osteoblast (bone forming) and osteoclast (bone resorbing) activity responsible for normal bone mineral density. This disruption leads to bone turnover suppression and an imbalance between collagen synthesis and degradation.

         (b) Diminished bone mineral density poses a significant threat in children and adolescents who have not yet achieved their peak bone mass.

         (c) Glucocorticoids are known to disrupt osteoblast and osteoclast balance and can lead to Cushing syndrome. Skeletal effects of Cushing syndrome include muscle wasting, weakness, and diminished bone mineral density.

         (d) Calcium and vitamin D deficiencies related to poor dietary consumption, altered absorption and metabolism, lack of sun exposure, and renal dysfunction also may have a negative effect on bone mineral density.

         (e) Diminished physical activity and weight bearing have been associated with decreased bone mineral density.

         (f) Patients usually are asymptomatic, but studies have shown that the lumbar spine, femur, and femoral neck are at risk for osteopenia and fractures.

         (g) Baseline screening with DEXA scans or quantitative CT is recommended for long-term follow-up.

         (h) Treatment

           i. Nutritional supplementation with calcium and vitamin D

           ii. Correction of possible endocrinopathy or renal dysfunction

          iii. Bisphosphonates

   5. Osteomyelitis (Pandey, Maximin, & Bhargava, 2014)

     a) Osteomyelitis can be bacterial or fungal and may be lethal.

     b) Treatment consists of aggressive management with various drug combinations.

D. Psychosocial complications

   1. HSCT is a rigorous procedure that can have profound effects on patients and families. The psychological effect alone, both before and after HSCT, can be immense. Transplant demands may cause lingering psychological distress, unlike other experiences with patients with cancer (Andrykowski, 1994).

   2. Because of the distinct nature of the transplant experience, psychosocial assessment and interventions should be a high priority. Post-transplant recovery can come with protracted physical and psychological setbacks and place tremendous social and financial strain on the patient's caregivers, friends, and family members.

   3. Additionally, the transplant trajectory can include multiple hospital readmissions for acute complications, slow recovery, and long-term problems. In many cases,

psychological issues can present a greater challenge for the healthcare team than the medical concerns (Eldredge et al., 2006).

  a) Undergoing HSCT can be psychologically overwhelming. Healthcare professionals may frequently overlook or fail to grasp the enormity of trauma possible for patients (Cooke, Gemmill, Kravits, & Grant, 2009). Although the majority of patients maintain good global QOL following HSCT, recognizing those patients who are more psychologically vulnerable is imperative (Saleh & Brockopp, 2001). Risk factors can predict a poorer overall psychological outcome and include the following (Jacobsen et al., 2002; Saleh & Brockopp, 2001):

   (1) Prior psychiatric morbidity or history
   (2) Pretransplant nonadherence
   (3) Lack of stable social support
   (4) Younger age
   (5) Female gender
   (6) Avoidant coping strategies
   (7) Poor functional status upon admission
   (8) Pain
   (9) Recent smoking cessation prior to hospitalization
   (10) History of considerable regimen-related toxicity

  b) Physical domain (Cooke et al., 2009)
   (1) Post-transplant physical complications that patients encounter influence psychological functioning.
      (a) Increased depression rates are associated with slower physical recovery, as well as chronic GVHD.
      (b) Other causative factors
         i. Frequent, ongoing medical appointments
         ii. Medication side effects
      (c) Outstanding issues lasting more than one year after HSCT
         i. Thoughts of being disconnected from "normal" people and obstacles with reintegration
         ii. Sensation of being ill-equipped for post-transplant life
         iii. Difficulties with fatigue restraints
         iv. Taxing cognitive changes
   (2) Post-transplant sexual complications
      (a) Vaginal dryness
      (b) Erectile dysfunction
   (3) Cognitive dysfunction (Phillips et al., 2013)
      (a) Subjective reports of cognitive impairment are common in transplant recipients.
      (b) HSCT patients frequently recount trouble with concentration, memory, and word finding. However, studies of objective neuropsychological functioning in HSCT patients demonstrate varied results.
      (c) Numerous studies corroborate that several patients experience impaired functioning on neuropsychological testing before HSCT; nonetheless, inconsistencies exist in the literature regarding whether cognitive functioning improves, declines, or remains constant after transplant.

       (d) Patients who describe cognitive difficulties that impede daily functioning should be referred to a neuropsychologist for evaluation and management of cognitive deficits.

c) Psychological domain (Cooke et al., 2009)

    (1) Depression

       (a) The incidence of depression among the general cancer population ranges from 10% to 25%. In some studies, however, rates of depression in the transplant population are greater, ranging from 25% to 50%.

       (b) Longitudinal studies convey that depression intensifies soon after transplantation and then appears to even out over time. Even so, some studies continue to report rates as high as 25% one year post-transplant. Higher depression levels post-transplant may lead to prolonged psychological distress.

       (c) Post-transplant physical health symptoms

          i. Possible increase in symptom-related distress

          ii. May contribute to a higher suicide rate

          iii. May decrease survival

    (2) Distress (Cooke et al., 2009)

       (a) As a whole, transplant patients experience high levels of distress, which is frequently attributed to intensified therapy.

       (b) Pretransplant distress levels of 50% have been documented. These numbers are much higher than the general cancer population distress levels of 30%.

       (c) Psychological distress can encompass the following areas:

          i. Existential concerns

          ii. Obsessive-compulsiveness

          iii. Loneliness

          iv. Long-lasting health concerns (e.g., memory loss)

    (3) Post-traumatic stress disorder (PTSD) (Cooke et al., 2009; Widows, Jacobsen, Booth-Jones, & Fields, 2005)

       (a) Innovative research has been emerging in the psychosocial literature that examines the rates and characteristics of PTSD among transplant patients.

       (b) The transplant experience itself can be categorized as a "traumatic experience" that can generate long-lasting psychological effects. Widows et al. (2005) reported a rate of PTSD at 5% among transplant survivors. Patients who exhibited higher incidences of PTSD symptoms experienced the following:

          i. Negative assessments of the transplant experience

          ii. Avoidance-based coping strategies

          iii. Decreased social support

          iv. Increased social constraint

       (c) Examination of the association between social support and coping strategy used after transplantation corroborated that the existence of a supportive environment encouraged patients to exercise healthier methods of coping to process and manage the traumatic experience.

d) Social domain (Cooke et al., 2009; Frick et al., 2006; Rodrigue, Pearman, & Moreb, 1999; Sherman, Cooke, & Grant, 2005)

   (1) Social support is a principal component for post-transplant psychological recovery.

   (2) Sufficient social support predicts increased survival, improved QOL, lower incidences of depression, fewer symptoms of PTSD, and reduced psychosocial morbidity.

   (3) An additional issue in the social domain is the ability to return to school or work.

      (a) Syrjala, Langer, Abrams, Storer, and Martin (2005) reported that physical limitations peaked at 90 days post-transplant, followed by improvement at one year. No considerable change in improvement was noted at three and five years.

      (b) Of patients who worked outside the home, 20% returned to work full time by one year and 31% by two years. Risk factors for delay in returning to work included being female and having extensive chronic GVHD.

      (c) Descriptive data in the support group setting show that all patients modified their school or work experience after transplantation. Examples of adjustment include the following:

         i. Changing majors in school

         ii. Obtaining jobs that were less stressful

         iii. Decreasing hours

         iv. Facing fear of discrimination and not divulging the transplant history

         v. Finding meaningful work that was unlike the previous work setting

e) Spiritual domain

   (1) Post-traumatic growth (PTG) (Jacobsen et al., 2002; Widows et al., 2005), the notion that patients seek out meaning or benefit after transplantation, has been evolving in the literature.

   (2) By definition, the possibility for PTG entails that patients go through a stressful event and then undergo positive psychological results or advantages. Potential affirmative sequelae after transplantation include the following:

      (a) Development of a new philosophy of life

      (b) Greater appreciation of life

      (c) Making positive changes in personal characteristics

      (d) Improving relationships with family and friends

   (3) Potential predictors of PTG

      (a) Adequate social support

      (b) Capacity to approach social situations, daily challenges, and long-term obstacles, rather than avoid them

      (c) Young age

      (d) Less education

      (e) Superior use of positive reinterpretation or cognitive appraisal

      (f) Impression of mastery and self-efficacy

      (g) Ability to problem solve and seek alternative rewards

f) Survivorship (Cooke et al., 2009)

  (1) Although most long-term HSCT survivors report contentment with their QOL and consider themselves to be productive, stable, and well adjusted, most do not return to their preillness state of health.

  (2) Studies report that survivors continue to suffer psychological distress related to concerns about relapse or development of secondary malignancies, altered body image, sexual dysfunction, anxiety about their families, and ambiguity regarding the future and professional reintegration.

g) Suggested interventions (Cooke et al., 2009; Sherman et al., 2005)

  (1) Antidepressants are valuable for treatment of depression, presuming that the healthcare professional possesses the ability to assess the situation, make the diagnosis, and treat appropriately.

  (2) The National Comprehensive Cancer Network® Distress Thermometer (Vachon, 2006) is a simple tool developed for assessment of patient distress. It has been shown to compare favorably with longer measures for anxiety and depression and can be used to screen and identify distress successfully throughout transplant recovery across various domains of QOL.

  (3) Psychoeducational interventions are nurse-led sessions that can include problem-solving techniques, education regarding depression and available therapies, and counseling on improving communication with healthcare professionals concerning symptom control and management.

  (4) Support groups

    (a) A support group environment may benefit patients who would gain from a shared unique experience, particularly in situations in which family and friends may not be able to identify.

    (b) Group therapy can be effective to reduce depression and psychiatric symptoms and improve QOL.

  (5) Complementary and alternative medicine (Cooke et al., 2009)

    (a) The use of relaxation techniques has been found to be useful in reducing anxiety and depression.

    (b) There also has been a movement in the field of psychosocial oncology to examine the "Eastern approach" to health and healing. In this setting, trauma can be viewed as an opportunity for growth, thus encouraging a positive attitude toward cancer, life, and the reestablishment of energy and balance. Possible interventions include diet modifications, meditation, massage, exercise, self-care, cognitive restructuring, promotion of emotional expression, visualization of positive outcomes, counting blessings, giving back, and disclosing experiences through verbal, artistic, or written expression.

E. Graft rejection and graft failure

  1. Graft rejection and graft failure are noteworthy complications following allo-HSCT. The incidence ranges from 1% to 20%, and prognosis is poor (Jabbour et al., 2007). It may present as primary graft failure, which is characterized as a lack of initial engraftment of donor cells, or secondary graft failure, which is

the loss of donor cells after initial engraftment. In the setting of secondary graft failure, autologous stem cell recovery may appear or marrow aplasia and pancytopenia may develop. This leaves the patient at risk for life-threatening complications, including infection and hemorrhage, which can subsequently increase the duration and cost of hospitalization (Jabbour et al., 2007; Mattsson, Ringdén, & Storb, 2008; Weisdorf et al., 1995). Factors influencing graft failure or graft rejection include the following (Mattsson et al., 2008; Wolff, 2002; Woodard et al., 2003):

   a) Rejection is attributed to the recipient's immune response against donor immunohematopoietic cells.
   b) Rejection is supported by the presence of recipient lymphocytes, preferentially T cells, and the absence of donor cells in the blood or bone marrow.
2. Other causes of graft failure
   a) Primary disease
   b) HLA disparity
   c) Inadequate number of stem cells
   d) Immunosuppression
   e) Use of T-cell depletion
   f) Immune-mediated processes
   g) Septicemia
   h) ABO incompatibility
   i) Viral infections (specifically CMV, HHV-6, and parvovirus)
   j) Drug toxicity
   k) Source of stem cells (Incidence is higher in cord blood and is as high as 20%. This is due to smaller stem cell volume in cord blood unit and less stringent guidelines for HLA matching.)
3. Molecular diagnosis of engraftment (Jabbour et al., 2007; Mattsson et al., 2008)
   a) Polymerase chain reaction amplification of variable number tandem repeat loci is a precise technique used to identify donor and recipient cells following allo-HSCT.
   b) A rise in recipient T cells precedes graft rejection. In the setting of RIC regimens, it may be particularly beneficial to follow T-cell chimerism, where high numbers of recipient T cells on day +28 may be an indicator of graft rejection.
4. Prevention of graft failure (Mattsson et al., 2008; Patel & Zimring, 2013)
   a) In patients with increased possibility of graft failure, using a more intensified conditioning regimen, such as those incorporating total lymphoid irradiation, thoracoabdominal irradiation, or TBI, has been suggested.
   b) Other areas of study include augmenting cell dose by giving donors buffy coat cell transfusions, administering granulocyte–colony-stimulating factor–mobilized PBSCs as an alternative to bone marrow, employing ATG in combination with cyclophosphamide for aplastic anemia, and reducing the frequency of pretransplant blood transfusions.
5. Management of graft dysfunction (Tang et al., 2014; Wolff, 2002; Yoshihara et al., 2012)
   a) Regardless of etiology, graft failure should be detected early by assessing blood counts and monitoring therapeutic blood levels of antirejection medications.
   b) Graft failure is identified as a serious and life-threatening process requiring intervention.

  c) Cytokine support has demonstrated various outcomes. Numerous patients respond to cytokines with an increase in absolute neutrophil count (ANC), with some responders sustaining counts even after cessation of growth factor. Optimal results are noted in patients who possess at least partial donor hematopoietic chimerism or receive a second stem cell infusion.

  d) Because inadequate stem cell dose is related to the occurrence of graft dysfunction, increasing the dose has been presumed to reduce this possibility. However, the ideal stem cell dose recommended to prevent graft dysfunction has not been established, and increasing doses may be ineffective.

  e) For patients who will not undergo autologous recovery, salvage transplantation should be performed early to achieve engraftment and full hematopoiesis.

  f) In the majority of recent studies examining salvage transplantation for graft failure, fludarabine and either ATG or alemtuzumab were incorporated in the preparative regimen. These agents are extremely immunosuppressive and anticipated to suppress host immunocompetent cells, including T and natural killer cells, which are involved in the mechanism of immune-mediated graft rejection. Furthermore, the use of ATG or alemtuzumab lessens the risk for GVHD following salvage transplantation.

  g) Questions remain regarding the need for additional conditioning and immunosuppression, hematopoietic stem cell source, and the role of using a different donor.

  h) The benefit of autologous backup also is being looked at as a practical approach to achieve neutrophil recovery and allow for ample time to prepare the patient for a second stem cell transplant if needed.

6. Cellular therapy to overcome graft failure (Mattsson et al., 2008)

  a) Donor lymphocyte infusion (DLI) may be used to overcome rejection in cases with decreasing donor T-cell chimerism. Side effects of DLI include GVHD and marrow aplasia. DLI has a potent immunologic effect and, when combined with anti-CD3 monoclonal antibody receptor (OKT3), may reverse imminent rejection even in patients with a 5/6 HLA-mismatched unrelated graft.

  b) In patients with persistent poor graft function and in the absence of graft rejection, a boost of donor stem cells without additional preparative chemotherapy may be indicated. Because this procedure may induce GVHD, T-cell depletion of the stem cells should be considered to reduce the incidence of GVHD and improve survival.

III. Hydration and electrolyte complications

 A. Maintaining adequate hydration and fluid balance is an essential part of supportive care for HSCT recipients. Fluid and electrolyte imbalances can occur throughout the entire transplantation process, especially in the pre- and post-transplant phases. Metabolic disturbances may be life threatening and can be a direct result of medications, high-dose chemotherapy regimens, cancer-related disease processes, and complications. Additionally, HSCT recipients are at risk due to poor oral intake, increased fluid loss from emesis or diarrhea (regimen related), or febrile episodes. Although common electrolyte abnormalities are expected—which include decreased potassium, phosphorus, magnesium, and calcium levels—the most challenging electrolyte abnormality is hyponatremia during cyclophosphamide administration. Bone marrow transplant nurses must closely monitor HSCT recipients for changes in hydration status as well as electrolyte imbalances to ensure interventions are provided in a timely manner for optimal patient outcomes and safety.

B. Hydration
1. Definition
    a) Hydration is the normal balance at which the body survives and maintains all functions (e.g., regulates body temperature, regulates waste, lubricates joints).
    b) It is an important factor in HSCT supportive care management (Doig & Huether, 2014).
2. Physiology and pathophysiology (De Pas et al., 2001; Doig & Huether, 2014; Flores et al., 2008; Khan, 2015; Mackenzie, 2002; Mitchell, 2013; Park & Roe, 2000; Ritchie, Ledue, & Craig, 2007)
    a) Normal: Total body water (TBW) is the percentage of total body weight that is water; the TBW of a normal adult is approximately 60%. The TBW increases during infancy and starts to decrease in older adults.
        (1) TBW estimates adequate hydration when the recipient's morning body weight is near admission weight (baseline), fluid intake and urine volume are normal, and urine color is pale yellow.
        (2) Water balance is regulated by the secretion of antidiuretic hormone (ADH) and the perception of thirst.
    b) Abnormal
        (1) Dehydration occurs when patients decrease their fluid intake, experience excessive water loss greater than sodium loss, or a combination of both factors.
        (2) Fluid and electrolyte imbalances occur in the majority of transplant recipients and are caused by medications, including the preparative regimen, medical interventions, and complications following HSCT.
        (3) Changes in body weight provide a simplistic assessment of hydration status in real time.
        (4) Fluid shifts between extracellular and intracellular compartments can affect laboratory results and lead to misinterpretation, causing errors in medical decision making.
    c) Fluid balance in HSCT recipients
        (1) The fluid balance of HSCT recipients needs to be closely monitored in the pre- and early post-transplant period because continuous fluctuations related to poor oral intake, medication regimens, nausea and vomiting, diarrhea, infectious complications (e.g., *C. difficile*, CMV), and renal insufficiency can occur.
        (2) Assessment methods include obtaining weight on admission and monitoring daily intake (food and IV fluids), output (stool, urine, and emesis), and daily weights.
        (3) The goal during the preparative regimen and early post-transplant period is to maintain the patient's admission weight achieved by diuresis to prevent fluid volume overload or adequate hydration with administration of IV fluids or fluid intake.
        (4) Fluid overload during IV fluid administration may expose recipients to increased risk for respiratory failure.
            (a) Capillary leak syndrome may occur in HSCT recipients receiving conditioning regimens and also can occur during engraftment syndrome.

Engraftment syndrome is a rare disorder characterized by episodes of transient vascular collapse caused by endothelial cell injury in which plasma leaks from the intravascular space to the interstitial space.

    (b) Symptoms include rapidly developing edema, pulmonary edema, weight gain, renal shutdown, anasarca, and hypovolemic shock.

  (5) HSCT recipients may experience acute renal failure caused by one of the following:

    (a) Acute tubular necrosis

    (b) Sinusoidal obstruction syndrome (SOS, formerly known as veno-occlusive disease)

    (c) Septic shock (i.e., nephrotoxic agents)

    (d) TBI: More likely to cause dysfunction when combined with nephrotoxic drugs versus TBI alone

3. Clinical features (Armstrong, 2007; De Pas et al., 2001; Flores et al., 2008; Khan, 2015; Mackenzie, 2002; Mitchell, 2013; Park & Roe, 2000; Porth, 2014; Thompson, 2002)

  a) Etiology

    (1) HSCT

    (2) Conditioning regimens

    (3) Medication regimens

    (4) Nausea and vomiting, diarrhea

    (5) GVHD (grades 3–4)

    (6) SOS

  b) Signs and symptoms

    (1) Fluid overload

      (a) Acute weight gain (percentage of body weight): Assess for mild volume excess (2%), moderate volume excess (5%), and severe volume excess (greater than 8%).

      (b) Assess for increased respiratory rate, dyspnea, rales, and rhonchi.

      (c) Assess for edema.

      (d) Vascular volume excess: Assess for full, bounding pulse, jugular vein distension, pulmonary edema (severe excess), shortness of breath, dyspnea, crackles in lungs, and cough.

    (2) Dehydration

      (a) Acute weight loss, percentage of body weight: Assess for mild dehydration (2%), moderate dehydration (5%), and severe dehydration (greater than 8%).

      (b) Interstitial fluid volume deficit: Assess for decreased skin turgor, dry mucous membranes, and sunken eyeballs.

      (c) Vascular volume deficit: Assess for postural hypotension; weak, rapid pulse; decreased venous return; decreased urine output; weakness; increased hematocrit; hypotension and shock (severe dehydration).

4. Diagnostic tests (Armstrong, 2007; De Pas et al., 2001; Flores et al., 2008; Khan, 2015; Mackenzie, 2002; Mitchell, 2013; Park & Roe, 2000; Porth, 2014; Thompson, 2002): Basic metabolic panel (blood urea nitrogen, creatinine) and liver enzyme studies

5. Treatment (Khan, 2015; Mitchell, 2013)

  a) IV fluids

        b) Aggressive diuresis for fluid volume excess

        c) Adequate fluid intake and output for hydration

   6. Patient education

        a) Adequate intake and output

        b) Causes of dehydration and fluid volume overload

        c) Treatment options

        d) Signs to report to caregiver (increased shortness of breath, presence of edema)

C. Hyponatremia

   1. Definition (Berendt & D'Agostino, 2005)

        a) A sodium level less than 120 mEq/L

        b) Electrolyte complications, sodium deficiency

   2. Physiology and pathophysiology (Berendt & D'Agostino, 2005; Ezzone, 2013; Khan, 2015; Philibert, Desmeules, Filion, Poirier, & Agharazii, 2008)

        a) Normal

           (1) Normal sodium level is 136–146 mEq/L.

           (2) Sodium is the primary cation in the plasma and extracellular fluid.

        b) Abnormal

           (1) In recipients with acute myeloid leukemia (AML), Hodgkin lymphoma, and acute lymphoblastic leukemia, an elevated ADH is present that is associated with syndrome of inappropriate antidiuretic hormone secretion (SIADH), leading to severe hyponatremia.

           (2) Cyclophosphamide in high doses can induce hyponatremia, weight gain, and urine with low osmolality (known as hyponatremic syndrome). It can begin 4–12 hours following infusion and last up to 20 hours. It is proposed that the active metabolites produce the syndrome rather than the actual drug.

              (a) It is possible for SIADH to occur after high-dose cyclophosphamide on rare occasions.

              (b) The principal mechanism is not an increase in the secretion of ADH but may be the potential renal effects of ADH or a direct effect of the chemotherapy agent on the distal tubule, resulting in increased permeability to water in the kidneys.

                 i. ADH (vasopressin) is produced in the hypothalamus and stored in the posterior pituitary gland. It plays a key role in regulating water and sodium in the body.

                 ii. An up-and-down regulatory system exists in which the posterior pituitary gland will sense too little water and release ADH. This causes the collecting ducts in the kidneys to reabsorb water, thus creating a balance.

                 iii. When the body has too much water, it stops releasing ADH and the kidneys excrete more water. SIADH is an inappropriate release of ADH and causes water reabsorption and hyponatremia, also known as *water intoxication.*

           (3) Vincristine and vinblastine administration may have similar effects.

              (a) Vincristine-induced SIADH, in which plasma ADH levels are elevated, can occur within two to three days following administration and last up to one month.

(b) Because the drug disrupts microtubules in peripheral nerves, vincristine may have the same effects on the posterior lobe of the pituitary gland that stores vasopressin. These effects have been associated with permanent neurotoxicity.

(4) A complication related to SOS can cause hyponatremia in patients undergoing autologous or allogeneic HSCT.

(5) It is a common electrolyte alteration in patients with cancer.

3. Clinical features (Armstrong, 2007; De Pas et al., 2001; Ezzone, 2013; Flores et al., 2008; Hannon & Thompson, 2010; Khan, 2015; Mackenzie, 2002; Park & Roe, 2000; Porth, 2014; Thompson, 2002; Vaidya, Ho, & Freda, 2010)

   a) Etiology: Cyclophosphamide, vincristine, vinblastine, and diuretic therapy (see Table 6-3)

   b) Signs and symptoms

     (1) Hyponatremia: Headache, anorexia, myalgias, nausea and vomiting, and slight alterations in neurologic functioning. With sodium levels less than 115 mEq/L, the patient may experience mental status changes, obtundation, seizures, and possibly death.

     (2) SIADH: The hallmark symptom is weight gain in the absence of edema.

4. Diagnostic tests (Armstrong, 2007; De Pas et al., 2001; Ezzone, 2013; Flores et al., 2008; Hannon & Thompson, 2010; Khan, 2015; Mackenzie, 2002; Park & Roe, 2000; Porth, 2014; Thompson, 2002; Vaidya et al., 2010)

   a) Monitor serum sodium levels frequently.

   b) Assess urine and serum osmolality and urine sodium.

5. Treatment (Armstrong, 2007; De Pas et al., 2001; Doig & Huether, 2014; Ezzone, 2013; Flores et al., 2008; Hannon & Thompson, 2010; Khan, 2015; Mackenzie, 2002; Park & Roe, 2000; Porth, 2014; Thompson, 2002; Vaidya et al., 2010): The mainstay of treatment for correcting the underlying cause (i.e., SIADH) includes fluid restriction (usually less than 1,000 ml per day, depending on severity), loop diuretics, salt tablets, and, in severe cases, hypertonic saline (3%) with caution.

6. Patient education

   a) Causes of SIADH

   b) Signs and symptoms to report

   c) Seizure precautions

   d) Fluid restriction

   e) Potential cognitive changes and altered gait

D. Hypernatremia

1. Definition: Hypernatremia results from hyponatremic syndrome caused by water loss or excess sodium. It is a sodium level greater than 160 mEq/L.

2. Physiology and pathophysiology (Berendt & D'Agostino, 2005; Doig & Huether, 2014; Ezzone, 2013; Khan, 2015; Mount, 2012; Philibert et al., 2008)

   a) Normal

     (1) Sodium is the major cation, accounting for approximately 90% of the cations in the extracellular fluid.

     (2) Hormonal regulation of salt occurs because aldosterone is secreted in the adrenal cortex. Aldosterone is released when circulating sodium levels are low, potassium levels are high, and perfusion in the kidneys has decreased.

Table 6-3. Common Electrolyte Complications of Hematopoietic Stem Cell Transplantation

Electrolyte Complication	Possible Causes	Signs and Symptoms*	Treatment

Hyponatremia	• Acute renal injury
	• Drugs
	  – Carboplatin
	  – Cisplatin
	  – Cyclophosphamide
	  – Cytarabine
	  – Diuretics (thiazides, loops)
	  – Ifosfamide
	  – Melphalan
	  – Opioid analgesics
	  – TMP-SMX
	  – Vinca alkaloids
	• Low albumin
	• SIADH
	• Volume depletion
	  – Diarrhea
	  – Hemorrhage
	  – Nausea, vomiting
	• VOD
		Asymptomatic: Serum Na may be ≥ 125 mEq/L.
		Complications (less severe): May be < 125 mEq/L
		• CNS abnormalities
		  – Disorientation
		  – Headaches
		  – Lethargy
		• Muscle cramps
		• Nausea, vomiting
		• Volume depletion (hypovolemia)
		  – Dry mucous membranes
		  – Orthostatic hypotension
		  – Poor skin turgor
		  – Tachycardia
		Complications (more severe): May be < 115 mEq/L
		• CNS abnormalities
		  – Brain-stem herniation
		  – Coma
		  – Impaired mental status
		  – Seizures
		• Death
		• Respiratory arrest
			Normal range: 136–146 mEq/L
			• Assessment of volume status and tonicity essential
			  – Hypo-, eu-, hypervolemia
			  – Hypo-, iso-, hypertonic
			• **Hypotonic eu- or hypervolemia:**
			  – Treat underlying cause/discontinue offending agent.
			  – Water restriction for several days (for asymptomatic, less severe)
			  – 0.9% sodium chloride in water (for less severe)
			  – 3% sodium chloride in water plus loop diuretic (for more severe)
			  – Vasopressin receptor antagonist (for more severe)
			  * Selective V₂: tolvaptan at 15 mg PO daily (max 60 mg)
			  * Nonselective: conivaptan at 20 mg IV (load) over 30 minutes followed by 20 mg per day CIVI for 2–4 days (max 40 mg/day CIVI)
			• **Hypotonic hypovolemia:**
			  – Treat underlying cause/discontinue offending agent.
			  – 0.9% sodium chloride in water
			• **Nonhypotonic:**
			  – Treat underlying cause/discontinue offending agent.
			• **Maximum rate of correction:**
			  – Na 8–12 mEq/L/24 hours (0.33–0.5 mEq/L per hour) to avoid development of osmotic demyelination syndrome

(Continued on next page)

Table 6-3. Common Electrolyte Complications of Hematopoietic Stem Cell Transplantation *(Continued)*

Electrolyte Complication	Possible Causes	Signs and Symptoms*	Treatment

Hypokalemia	• Cellular reuptake
	• Decreased intake
	• Drugs
	  – Aminoglycosides
	  – Amphotericin B
	  – Carboplatin
	  – Cidofovir
	  – Cisplatin
	  – Foscarnet
	  – Ifosfamide
	  – Loop diuretics
	  – Penicillin
	• Gastrointestinal loss
	  – Diarrhea
	  – Nausea/vomiting
	• Renal dysfunction
		Asymptomatic
		Complications (less severe)
		• Constipation
		• Generalized weakness, lassitude
		• Muscle cramps
		Complications (more severe)
		• Ascending paralysis
		• Cardiac arrhythmias
		• Impairment of respiratory function
		• Muscle necrosis
			Normal range: 3.5–5 mEq/L
			• 3–3.4 mEq/L
			  – Potassium chloride 40–80 mEq PO in divided doses or IV at 20 mEq/hour
			• ≤2.9 mEq/L
			  – Potassium chloride 10–20 mEq IV per hour for at least 5 hours

Hyperkalemia	• Acute renal failure
	  – Drugs
	  – Leukemic infiltration of kidneys
	• Contrast-induced neuropathy
	• Drugs: TMP-SMX
	• Sepsis
	• TLS
		Asymptomatic
		Complications (less severe)
		• Abdominal distension
		• Fatigue, weakness
		Complications (more severe)
		• Cardiac arrhythmias
		• Nausea/vomiting
			Normal range: 3.5–5 mEq/L
			• 5.1–6 mEq/L
			  – Diuretics: furosemide 20–40 mg IV once
			• 6.1–6.9 mEq/L
			  – Glucose (1 amp) plus short-acting insulin (10 units)
			  – Inhaled beta-2 agonists (albuterol 10–20 mg nebulized over 10 minutes)
			  – Sodium bicarbonate (if due to acidosis) 50–100 mEq IV over 10–20 minutes
			  – Sodium polystyrene sulfonate 15–30 g PO or rectally

(Continued on next page)

Table 6-3. Common Electrolyte Complications of Hematopoietic Stem Cell Transplantation (Continued)

Electrolyte Complication	Possible Causes	Signs and Symptoms*	Treatment

Hyperkalemia *(cont.)*			• ≥ 7 mEq/L
			  – Calcium gluconate 10% (for cardiac protection)
			  – Glucose/insulin
			  – Inhaled beta-2 agonists
			  – Sodium bicarbonate
			  – Sodium polystyrene sulfonate 45–60 g PO or rectally
			  – Dialysis

Hypercalcemia	• HHM
	• Bone resorption (MM, lymphoma)
	• Drugs
	  – Cyclosporine
	  – Ganciclovir
	  – Lithium
	  – Thiazides
	  – Vitamin D
	• PTH secretion by tumors
	• Secretion of vitamin D (by HL, leukemia, lymphoma, myeloma, solid tumors [lung, breast])
		Asymptomatic: Serum Ca may be < 13 mg/dl.
		Complications (less severe)
		• Anorexia
		• Constipation
		• Nausea/vomiting
		• Polydipsia/polyuria
		• Severe dehydration
		Complications (more severe)
		• Acute renal failure
		• CNS abnormalities
		  – AMS
		  – Coma
		  – Confusion
		  – Lethargy
		  – Memory loss
		  – Seizures
		  – Stupor
		• Cardiac abnormalities
		  – AV block
		  – Bradycardia
		• Death
		• Pancreatitis
		• Tetany
			Normal range: 8.7–10.2 mg/dl
			• Mild to moderate (10.3–12 mg/dl)
			  – Rehydration (200–500 ml/hour 0.9% normal saline daily) plus furosemide (20–40 mg IV after hydration every 12–24 hours)
			  – Bisphosphonates
			  * Pamidronate (60–90 mg IV over 2–4 hours once)
			  * Zoledronate (4 mg IV over 15–30 minutes once)
			• Moderate to severe (> 12 mg/dl)
			  – Rehydration (200–500 ml/hour 0.9% normal saline daily) plus furosemide (20–40 mg IV after hydration every 12–24 hours)
			  – Calcitonin (4–8 IU/kg SC every 12–24 hours)
			  – Dialysis
			  – Bisphosphonates
			  * Pamidronate (60–90 mg IV over 2–4 hours once)
			  * Zoledronate (4 mg IV over 15–30 minutes once)

(Continued on next page)

Table 6-3. Common Electrolyte Complications of Hematopoietic Stem Cell Transplantation *(Continued)*

Electrolyte Complication	Possible Causes	Signs and Symptoms*	Treatment

Hypocalcemia	• Apheresis
	• Decreased intake
	• Drugs
	  – Aminoglycosides
	  – Bisphosphonates
	  – Foscarnet
	    * L-asparaginase
	    * Loop diuretics
	    * Pentamidine
	• Precipitation of calcium-phosphate complex
	• Renal dysfunction
		Asymptomatic
		Complications (less severe)
		• Chills
		• Headache
		• Muscle cramping
		• Numbness of the extremities or lips
		Complications (more severe)
		• Cardiac abnormalities
		  – Arrhythmia
		  – Bradycardia
		  – Chest pain
		• Laryngeal spasm
		• Muscle abnormalities
		  – Tetany
		  – Paresthesia
		  – Seizures
		• Nausea/vomiting
			Normal range: 8.7–10.2 mg/dl (corrected)
			• < 8.7 mg/dl (corrected)
			  – Asymptomatic
			    * Oral calcium carbonate 1–3 g/day PO
			  – Symptomatic
			    * 1–2 g calcium gluconate (10%) (10–20 ml IV over 10–15 minutes) followed by infusion of 6 g calcium gluconate in 500 ml 5% dextrose over 4–6 hours
			    * May use calcium chloride (10%)

Hypomagnesemia	• Decreased intake
	• Drugs
	  – Aminoglycosides
	  – Amphotericin B
	  – Carboplatin
	  – Cisplatin
	  – Cyclosporine
	  – Foscarnet
	  – Ifosfamide
	  – Loop diuretics
	  – Pentamidine
	  – Prednisone
	  – Tacrolimus
		Asymptomatic
		Complications (less severe)
		• CNS abnormalities
		  – Apathy
		  – Dizziness
		  – Lethargy
		• Muscle abnormalities
		  – Cramps
		  – Weakness
		  – Tremors
		Complications (more severe)
		• CNS abnormalities
		  – Coma
		  – Seizures
			Normal range: 0.69–1.07 mmol/L
			• Maintenance of normal range
			  – Elemental magnesium 250–500 mg PO 2–4 times daily
			  – Note: Diarrhea may be a side effect and should be monitored.
			• 0.51–0.68 mmol/L
			  – Magnesium sulfate 2–4 g IV over 1–4 hours (rate depends on severity of symptoms)
			• ≤ 0.5 mmol/L
			  – Magnesium sulfate 5 g IV over 1–5 hours (rate depends on severity of symptoms and if cardiac abnormalities present)

(Continued on next page)

Table 6-3. Common Electrolyte Complications of Hematopoietic Stem Cell Transplantation *(Continued)*

Electrolyte Complication	Possible Causes	Signs and Symptoms*	Treatment

Hypomagnesemia *(cont.)*	• Nausea/vomiting
	• Renal dysfunction
		• Dysrhythmias
		• Muscle abnormalities
		  – Hyperreflexia
		  – Tetany	

Hypophospha-temia	• Bence Jones proteins (MM) resulting in proximal renal tubular dysfunction
	• Cellular reuptake/shift
	• Decreased intake
	• Drugs
	  – Foscarnet
	  – Ifosfamide
	• Hypercalcemia
	• Nausea/vomiting
	• Renal dysfunction
		Asymptomatic
		Complications (more severe)
		• CNS abnormalities
		  – Coma
		  – Confusion
		  – Seizures
		• Impaired energy metabolism from decreased ATP production
		• Muscle abnormalities
		  – Impaired cardiac contractibility
		  – Respiratory depression
		  – Rhabdomyolysis
		  – Weakness
			Normal range: 2.5–4.3 mg/dl
			• Maintenance of normal range
			  – PO phosphate supplementation
			• 1.5–2.4 mg/dl
			  – Potassium phosphate 10 mmol/L once over 2–4 hours
			• ≤ 1.4 mg/dl
			  – Potassium phosphate 15–30 mmol/L once over 3–5 hours
			• If potassium > 4 mmol/L, use sodium phosphate as alternative.

* Dependent on the acuity and depth of electrolyte loss or gain

AMS—altered mental status; ATP—adenosine triphosphate; AV—atrioventricular; Ca—calcium; CIVI—continuous intravenous infusion; CNS—central nervous system; HHM—humoral hypercalcemia of malignancy; HL—Hodgkin lymphoma; IV—intravenous; MM—multiple myeloma; Na—sodium; PO—orally; PTH—parathyroid hormone; SC—subcutaneous; SIADH—syndrome of inappropriate antidiuretic hormone; TLS—tumor lysis syndrome; TMP-SMX—trimethoprim-sulfamethoxazole; VOD—veno-occlusive disease

(3) Osmotic gradient changes are a result of sodium gain or loss and known as changes in tonicity (changes in salt in relation to water).

(4) These alterations are classified as hypertonic (hyperosmolar), isotonic (iso-osmolar), or hypotonic (hypo-osmolar).

(5) Serum osmolality is maintained at 286–294 mOsm.

   b) Abnormal

(1) The most common cause of hypernatremia in HSCT recipients is decreased fluid intake.

(2) Essential hypernatremia (absence of thirst) occurs when the thirst center of the brain is disrupted (i.e., tumors), leading to severe dehydration without other symptoms. Secondary causes result in neurologic changes, such as irritability, lethargy, seizures, and coma.

(3) Although it is rare, diabetes insipidus can occur with systemic cancers, such as leukemia and lymphoma.

(4) Hypernatremia can be exhibited after transplantation as a result of corticosteroids (see Table 6-3).

3. Clinical features (Armstrong, 2007; De Pas et al., 2001; Ezzone, 2013; Flores et al., 2008; Khan, 2015; Mackenzie, 2002; Park & Roe, 2000; Porth, 2014; Thompson, 2002)

   a) Etiology

(1) Hypernatremia occurs in HSCT recipients when thirst is impaired or when they are severely ill or exhibiting signs of nausea and vomiting, diarrhea, dehydration, impaired renal function, or insensible water losses (e.g., fever, respiratory infections).

(2) Drugs are common causes of hypernatremia in the HSCT setting.

   b) Signs and symptoms

(1) Polyuria and polydipsia

(2) Low-grade temperatures

(3) Edema

(4) Neurologic symptoms (e.g., disorientation, convulsions, stupor, coma)

(5) Irritability, depression, and lethargy

(6) Muscle weakness

(7) Dry mucous membranes

(8) Flushing

4. Diagnostic tests (Armstrong, 2007; De Pas et al., 2001; Ezzone, 2013; Flores et al., 2008; Khan, 2015; Mackenzie, 2002; Park & Roe, 2000; Porth, 2014; Thompson, 2002)

   a) Monitor serum sodium levels frequently.

   b) Monitor urine and serum osmolality and urine sodium.

5. Treatment (Ezzone, 2013; Khan, 2015): The mainstay of treatment includes hypotonic IV fluids (i.e., 5% dextrose and 0.45% normal saline).

6. Patient education

   a) Causes of hypernatremia

   b) Signs and symptoms to report

   c) Importance of preventing dehydration

   d) Medications that may contribute to hypernatremia

E. Hypokalemia

1. Definition: A potassium level less than 3 mEq/L. A reciprocal relationship occurs with sodium (potassium decreases and sodium increases).

2. Physiology and pathophysiology (Berendt & D'Agostino, 2005; Doig & Huether, 2014; Ezzone, 2013; Khan, 2015; Philibert et al., 2008)

   a) Normal

      (1) Potassium is the major intracellular cation, which influences many cellular processes, including membrane polarization and enzymatic processes in the cell.

      (2) Intracellular potassium is greater than extracellular potassium, with several mechanisms in place to ensure adequate distribution in the different bodily fluids.

   b) Abnormal

      (1) The use of high-dose corticosteroids can produce a similar effect found in hyperaldosteronism or diuretic use, resulting in high aldosterone levels in the presence of low renin levels and showing a primary hyperaldosteronism state.

      (2) GI losses from vomiting and diarrhea contribute to hypokalemia. Diarrhea causing hypokalemia can result in metabolic acidosis, creating low urinary sodium.

      (3) Shifting of potassium from the extracellular space to the intracellular space is primarily a result of either insulin administration or metabolic alkalosis.

3. Clinical features (Armstrong, 2007; De Pas et al., 2001; Doig & Huether, 2014; Ezzone, 2013; Flores et al., 2008; Khan, 2015; Mackenzie, 2002; Park & Roe, 2000; Porth, 2014; Thompson, 2002)

   a) Etiology

      (1) One of the major causes of hypokalemia in HSCT recipients is diuresis after periods of excessive fluid overload. Other causes include GI losses, shifting of potassium from the extracellular to the intracellular space, decreased dietary intake, and renal tubular dysfunction in recipients with AML.

      (2) Drugs used in the transplant setting are common causes of hypokalemia (see Table 6-3).

   b) Signs and symptoms

      (1) Anorexia

      (2) Rapid, irregular pulse, ECG changes (i.e., flattened T wave, ST segment depression)

      (3) Muscle weakness

      (4) Hypotension

      (5) Paresthesia

4. Diagnostic tests (Armstrong, 2007; De Pas et al., 2001; Doig & Huether, 2014; Ezzone, 2013; Flores et al., 2008; Khan, 2015; Mackenzie, 2002; Park & Roe, 2000; Porth, 2014; Thompson, 2002)

   a) Monitor basic metabolic panel frequently.

   b) Monitor pH levels.

5. Treatment (Ezzone, 2013; Khan, 2015): The mainstay of treatment for potassium replacements (orally or intravenously) includes supplementation (medication and nutritious diet).

6. Patient education

   a) Risks for decreased potassium

   b) When to notify nurse (exhibiting signs of weakness, fatigue, decreased appetite, or heart palpitations)

F. Hyperkalemia
  1. Definition: A potassium level greater than 5 mEq/L. A reciprocal relationship occurs with sodium (potassium increases and sodium decreases).
  2. Pathophysiology (Berendt & D'Agostino, 2005; Doig & Huether, 2014; Ezzone, 2013; Khan, 2015; Philibert et al., 2008): Hyperkalemia is caused by an increased intake of potassium, decreased urinary excretion of potassium, or movement of potassium out of the cells.
    a) Dietary excesses of potassium are uncommon.
    b) If impaired renal function is chronic, there may be adaptation. However, in acute renal failure, oliguria (urine output of less than 30 ml/hour) can occur, accompanied by increased serum potassium.
    c) Movement of intracellular potassium to the extracellular environment occurs with cell trauma or a change in cell permeability (e.g., acidosis, cellular hypoxia).
  3. Clinical features (Armstrong, 2007; De Pas et al., 2001; Doig & Huether, 2014; Ezzone, 2013; Flores et al., 2008; Khan, 2015; Mackenzie, 2002; Park & Roe, 2000; Porth, 2014; Thompson, 2002)
    a) Etiology: In transplant recipients, the cause of hyperkalemia is related to dehydration, compromised renal function, acidosis (i.e., sepsis), and medications (i.e., amphotericin B) (see Table 6-3).
    b) Signs and symptoms
      (1) Anxiety
      (2) Abdominal cramping
      (3) Diarrhea
      (4) Weakness (especially in lower extremities)
      (5) Paresthesia
      (6) Irregular pulse
  4. Diagnostic tests (Armstrong, 2007; De Pas et al., 2001; Ezzone, 2013; Flores et al., 2008; Khan, 2015; Mackenzie, 2002; Park & Roe, 2000; Porth, 2014; Thompson, 2002)
    a) Laboratory: Monitor basic metabolic panel frequently.
    b) Diagnostics: Obtain 12-lead ECG.
  5. Treatment (Doig & Huether, 2014; Ezzone, 2001; Khan, 2015): The mainstay of treatment for hyperkalemia is hydration and diuresis simultaneously to increase urine output to approximately 3 L per day.
    a) Administer 50% glucose, as ordered, to increase plasma insulin levels, resulting in intracellular shift of potassium.
    b) Administer sodium polystyrene sulfonate, as ordered, to promote potassium loss in the feces.
  6. Patient education
    a) Causes of hyperkalemia
    b) Signs and symptoms to report (muscle weakness, numbness in hands or feet, or diarrhea)
G. Hypophosphatemia
  1. Definition (Berendt & D'Agostino, 2005): A phosphate level less than 2 mg/dl
  2. Physiology and pathophysiology (Berendt & D'Agostino, 2005; Doig & Huether, 2014; Ezzone, 2013; Khan, 2015; Philibert et al., 2008)
    a) Normal
      (1) Normal phosphate levels are 2.5–4.5 mg/dl.

(2) Phosphate is fundamental to metabolic processes and is primarily located in the cells.

(3) Calcium and phosphate have an inverse relationship; as one increases, the other decreases.

b) Abnormal

(1) The most common causes of hypophosphatemia are intestinal malabsorption, increased renal excretion, and inadequate absorption associated with vitamin D deficiency.

(2) Increased renal excretion is related to hyperparathyroidism.

(3) The consequences of hypophosphatemia are related to decreased capacity for oxygen transport of red blood cells (RBCs). When phosphate levels are low, 2,3-diphosphoglycerate and adenosine triphosphate levels become low and diminish release of oxygen to the tissues, causing an oxyhemoglobin curve shift to the left.

(4) Leukocyte and platelet dysfunctions may be associated with hypophosphatemia, with increased risk for blood clotting alterations and infection.

(5) Low levels of serum phosphate levels can increase serum calcium levels.

3. Clinical features (Armstrong, 2007; De Pas et al., 2001; Doig & Huether, 2014; Ezzone, 2013; Flores et al., 2008; Khan, 2015; Mackenzie, 2002; Park & Roe, 2000; Porth, 2014; Thompson, 2002)

a) Etiology: The most common causes in HSCT recipients are drug related (see Table 6-3).

b) Signs and symptoms: Irritability, confusion, numbness, and coma with severe losses

4. Diagnostic tests (Armstrong, 2007; De Pas et al., 2001; Ezzone, 2013; Flores et al., 2008; Khan, 2015; Mackenzie, 2002; Park & Roe, 2000; Porth, 2014; Thompson, 2002)

a) Monitor serum phosphate level daily.

b) Monitor serum calcium level daily.

5. Treatment (Ezzone, 2013; Khan, 2015): The mainstay of treatment is to identify the underlying cause and treat with phosphate replacement.

6. Patient education: Educate patients and families about causes of hypophosphatemia and signs and symptoms. However, the patient may be asymptomatic or symptoms may be nonspecific and depend on cause, duration, and severity.

H. Hyperphosphatemia

1. Definition (Berendt & D'Agostino, 2005): A phosphate level greater than 5 mg/dl

2. Physiology and pathophysiology (Berendt & D'Agostino, 2005; Doig & Huether, 2014; Ezzone, 2013; Khan, 2015; Philibert et al., 2008)

a) Normal: Phosphate levels are 2.5–4.5 mg/dl.

b) Abnormal

(1) Hyperphosphatemia develops when a significant loss of glomerular filtration in the kidneys has occurred.

(2) Due to cellular destruction as a result of the conditioning regimen, large amounts of phosphate are released into the blood.

(3) High serum phosphate levels can lower serum calcium levels.

3. Clinical features (Armstrong, 2007; De Pas et al., 2001; Doig & Huether, 2014; Ezzone, 2013; Flores et al., 2008; Khan, 2015; Mackenzie, 2002; Park & Roe, 2000; Porth, 2014; Thompson, 2002)

a) Etiology: Conditioning regimens cause a release of phosphate from cells into the blood (see Table 6-3).

b) Signs and symptoms: Symptoms are primarily associated with hypocalcemia, such as muscle cramps, tetany, and periorbital numbness or tingling.

4. Diagnostic tests (Armstrong, 2007; De Pas et al., 2001; Doig & Huether, 2014; Ezzone, 2013; Flores et al., 2008; Khan, 2015; Mackenzie, 2002; Park & Roe, 2000; Porth, 2014; Thompson, 2002)

   a) Monitor serum phosphate level daily.

   b) Monitor serum calcium level daily.

5. Treatment (Doig & Huether, 2014; Ezzone, 2013; Khan, 2015): The mainstay of treatment for hyperphosphatemia is aluminum hydroxide because it binds phosphate in the GI tract and is eliminated in the feces.

6. Patient education: Educate patients and families on causes of hyperphosphatemia and signs and symptoms to report.

I. Hypocalcemia (Doig & Huether, 2014; Philibert et al., 2008)

1. Definition

   a) A total corrected calcium level less than 8.5 mg/dl and ionized levels less than 4 mg/dl

   b) Calculation of calcium level: Corrected calcium = serum calcium + 0.8 × (4 − serum albumin)

2. Physiology and pathophysiology (Berendt & D'Agostino, 2005; Doig & Huether, 2014; Ezzone, 2013; Khan, 2015; Philibert et al., 2008)

   a) Normal

   (1) Normal calcium range is 4.5–5.5 mEq/L.

   (2) Calcium is the most plentiful inorganic electrolyte in the body and is responsible for many metabolic, physiologic, and structural processes.

   (3) It is primarily located in the bone and contributes to bone strength and rigidity.

   (4) Calcium regulates skeletal, cardiac, and smooth muscle and nerve transmissions.

   (5) Total body calcium is approximately 1,200 g.

   (6) Approximately 45% of the body's calcium is ionized and contributes to the most important physiologic body functions.

   b) Abnormal

   (1) Hypocalcemia may result from hypoparathyroidism, hypomagnesemia, malabsorption, nutritional (e.g., vitamin D) deficiencies, blood administration, nephrotic syndrome, renal failure, rhabdomyolysis, osteoblastic metastasis, hyperphosphatemia, and tumor lysis syndrome.

   (2) Hypocalcemia also may be caused by calcium deficiency from lack of green, leafy vegetables in the diet.

   (3) An excessive amount of dietary phosphorus binds with calcium; neither of the minerals is absorbed.

   (4) Blood transfusions contain citrate, which binds with calcium.

   (5) Drugs used in the HSCT setting may contribute to hypocalcemia (see Table 6-3).

3. Clinical features (Armstrong, 2007; De Pas et al., 2001; Doig & Huether, 2014; Ezzone, 2013; Flores et al., 2008; Khan, 2015; Mackenzie, 2002; Park & Roe, 2000; Porth, 2014; Thompson, 2002)

     a) Etiology: The primary causes in the HSCT setting are reduction of intake and medication related (see Table 6-3).

     b) Signs and symptoms

       (1) Tetany

       (2) Neuromuscular excitability

       (3) Seizures

       (4) Prolonged QT and ST intervals

       (5) Paresthesia

       (6) Chvostek sign and Trousseau sign (cardinal signs)

  4. Diagnostic tests (Armstrong, 2007; De Pas et al., 2001; Doig & Huether, 2014; Ezzone, 2013; Flores et al., 2008; Khan, 2015; Mackenzie, 2002; Park & Roe, 2000; Porth, 2014; Thompson, 2002)

     a) Monitor serum calcium, phosphorus, and magnesium levels daily.

     b) Ensure a baseline vitamin D level has been drawn to assess for low vitamin D.

  5. Treatment (Doig & Huether, 2014; Ezzone, 2013; Khan, 2015): The mainstay of treatment for hypocalcemia is IV calcium gluconate (for severe deficiency) or oral calcium replacements.

  6. Patient education

     a) Causes of hypocalcemia

     b) Medications that cause decreased calcium levels

     c) Signs and symptoms to report (e.g., numbness around the mouth)

J. Hypercalcemia

  1. Definition

     a) A calcium level greater than 12 mg/dl or corrected serum calcium greater than 13 mg/dl

     b) Classified as mild, moderate, or severe

  2. Physiology and pathophysiology (Berendt & D'Agostino, 2005; Doig & Huether, 2014; Ezzone, 2013; Khan, 2015; Philibert et al., 2008)

     a) Normal: Serum calcium levels are 8.5–10.2 mg/dl.

     b) Abnormal

       (1) Two of the most common causes of hypercalcemia are hyperparathyroidism and bone metastases with calcium reabsorption (i.e., multiple myeloma).

       (2) The primary cause of hypercalcemia in recipients with hematologic cancers is local osteolytic hypercalcemia, which is caused by increased bone resorption from direct bone destruction, as seen in multiple myeloma. Local osteolytic hypercalcemia releases calcium in the blood, usually seen in advanced disease.

  3. Clinical features (Armstrong, 2007; De Pas et al., 2001; Doig & Huether, 2014; Ezzone, 2013; Flores et al., 2008; Khan, 2015; Mackenzie, 2002; Park & Roe, 2000; Porth, 2014; Thompson, 2002; Wilkes, 2016)

     a) Etiology: Hypercalcemia is commonly seen in hematologic malignancies (i.e., multiple myeloma) and other electrolyte abnormalities. It also can be drug related (see Table 6-3).

     b) Signs and symptoms

       (1) Drowsiness

       (2) Lethargy

       (3) Anorexia

       (4) Nausea

          (5) Constipation

          (6) Muscle weakness

          (7) Delusions

          (8) Hallucinations

          (9) Impaired renal concentration

4. Diagnostic tests (Armstrong, 2007; De Pas et al., 2001; Doig & Huether, 2014; Ezzone, 2013; Flores et al., 2008; Khan, 2015; Mackenzie, 2002; Park & Roe, 2000; Porth, 2014; Thompson, 2002)

    a) Monitor serum calcium levels daily.

    b) Monitor serum magnesium and phosphorus levels daily.

    c) Monitor serum creatinine to assess kidney function; other electrolytes (such as potassium and magnesium) should be monitored daily as the kidneys can become overwhelmed by the calcium cations.

5. Treatment (Doig & Huether, 2014; Ezzone, 2013; Khan, 2015): The mainstay of treatment is hydration with normal saline at a rate of 200 ml/hour. Other treatments include calcitonin, glucocorticoids, and phosphates; treat underlying disease.

6. Patient education

    a) Causes of hypercalcemia

    b) Sign and symptoms to report (e.g., fatigue, lethargy, weakness, constipation, nausea and vomiting)

K. Hypomagnesemia

1. Definition (Berendt & D'Agostino, 2005; Doig & Huether, 2014; Khan, 2015)

    a) Magnesium is the fourth most abundant intracellular cation, with approximately 30% stored in cells, 1% stored in blood, and 40%–60% stored in muscles and bones.

    b) Normal magnesium levels are 1.8–2.4 mEq/L.

2. Physiology and pathophysiology (Berendt & D'Agostino, 2005; Doig & Huether, 2014; Ezzone, 2013; Khan, 2015; Philibert et al., 2008)

    a) Normal

        (1) One-third of magnesium is bound to plasma proteins, with the remaining in ionized form.

        (2) Magnesium plays a role in intracellular enzymatic reactions, nucleic acid stability, and neuromuscular excitability and reacts with calcium at the cellular level.

        (3) The kidneys conserve magnesium during low blood levels.

    b) Abnormal

        (1) Hypomagnesemia occurs when blood levels are less than 1.5 mEq/L, with additional decreases with tetany and neuromuscular excitability.

        (2) Hypomagnesemia levels are associated with low levels of phosphate.

3. Clinical features (Armstrong, 2007; Berendt & D'Agostino, 2005; De Pas et al., 2001; Doig & Huether, 2014; Ezzone, 2013; Flores et al., 2008; Khan, 2015; Mackenzie, 2002; Park & Roe, 2000; Porth, 2014; Thompson, 2002; Wilkes, 2016)

    a) Etiology

        (1) Hypomagnesemia is associated with diabetes mellitus, renal tubular dysfunction, malnutrition, malabsorption syndromes, and alcoholism.

        (2) Low levels of magnesium in the HSCT setting can be caused by cisplatin-induced renal wasting, diuretics, amphotericin B, some antibiotics, and conditions affecting the kidneys (see Table 6-3).

    b) Signs and symptoms

   (1) Confusion

   (2) Seizures

  4. Diagnostic tests (Armstrong, 2007; De Pas et al., 2001; Doig & Huether, 2014; Ezzone, 2013; Flores et al., 2008; Khan, 2015; Mackenzie, 2002; Park & Roe, 2000; Porth, 2014; Thompson, 2002): Monitor basic metabolic panel daily.

  5. Treatment (Doig & Huether, 2014; Ezzone, 2013; Khan, 2015): The mainstay of treatment is oral or IV magnesium sulfate replacement.

  6. Patient education

   a) Causes of decreased magnesium levels

   b) Symptoms to report (e.g., numbness around mouth, paresthesia of fingers and toes)

   c) Possible side effect of bowel changes (i.e., diarrhea) while taking oral magnesium supplements

L. Hypermagnesemia

 1. Pathophysiology (Berendt & D'Agostino, 2005; Doig & Huether, 2014; Ezzone, 2013; Khan, 2015; Philibert et al., 2008)

  a) A magnesium level greater than 2.5 mEq/L, primarily due to renal failure

  b) Excess magnesium taken orally can depress skeletal muscle contraction and nerve function.

 2. Clinical features (Armstrong, 2007; Berendt & D'Agostino, 2005; De Pas et al., 2001; Doig & Huether, 2014; Flores et al., 2008; Khan, 2015; Mackenzie, 2002; Park & Roe, 2000; Porth, 2014; Thompson, 2002; Wilkes, 2016)

  a) Etiology: Magnesium-containing antacids and renal failure are the causes of hypermagnesemia.

  b) Signs and symptoms

   (1) Nausea and vomiting

   (2) Hypotension

   (3) Muscle weakness

   (4) Bradycardia

   (5) Respiratory depression

 3. Diagnostic tests (Armstrong, 2007; Berendt & D'Agostino, 2005; De Pas et al., 2001; Doig & Huether, 2014; Ezzone, 2013; Flores et al., 2008; Khan, 2015; Mackenzie, 2002; Park & Roe, 2000; Porth, 2014; Thompson, 2002): Monitor magnesium levels daily or as needed.

 4. Treatment: The mainstay of treatment for hypermagnesemia is kidney dialysis or avoidance of magnesium-containing supplements.

 5. Patient education

  a) Symptoms, supplements, and the importance of hydration

   (1) Diaphoresis

   (2) Flushing

   (3) Lethargy

   (4) Hypotension

   (5) Bradycardia

   (6) Diminished deep tendon reflexes

  b) Importance of avoiding over-the-counter supplements that include magnesium (such as milk of magnesia [magnesium hydroxide])

  c) Importance of staying hydrated to protect kidneys if experiencing diarrhea from the magnesium

IV. Hematologic complications
- A. In HSCT recipients, neutropenia poses a significant risk for infectious complications. Both allogeneic and autologous HSCT recipients are at an increased risk for infectious complications; however, recipients of autologous HSCT have a lesser degree of risk than recipients who have undergone allogeneic HSCT, based on exposures and the level of immunosuppression. Infection increases substantially in the pre-engraftment period in the presence of neutropenia and mucosal barrier breakdown. During the postengraftment period, prolonged neutropenia in combination with other conditions, such as GVHD, graft rejection, invasive central lines, and nutritional deficits, can significantly increase morbidity and mortality because of lack of cell-mediated immunity. Gram-positive and gram-negative pathogens are the most common during the neutropenic period and associated with neutropenic fever. Other opportunistic infections that cause additional risk are fungal, viral, and respiratory complications. The prevention of infection from opportunistic sources is of paramount importance in the care of HSCT recipients.
- B. Neutropenia
  - 1. Definition (Camp-Sorrell, 2005, 2011; Gobel & O'Leary, 2007; Marrs, 2006; Rosselet, 2013): Neutropenia is a significant decrease in the number of circulating neutrophils. It can be caused by disease state or treatment. Varying degrees of neutropenia exist, but in all cases, the ANC is less than 1,000/mm³.
  - 2. Physiology and pathophysiology (Antunes, Pereira, & Cunha, 2013; Camp-Sorrell, 2005, 2011; Gobel & O'Leary, 2007; Goldman & Schafer, 2012; Hartung, Olson, & Bessler, 2013; Rosselet, 2013; Rothaermel & Baum, 2009; Seely, Pascual, & Christou, 2003; Tomblyn et al., 2009)
    - a) Normal
      - (1) The body's main lines of defense against infectious organisms include the skin, mucosal barriers, and white blood cells (WBCs).
      - (2) WBCs are made up of a five-part differential that includes several types of cells (such as neutrophils, basophils, eosinophils, and monocytes).
        - (a) Neutrophils are a type of granulocyte, or WBC, that aid in eliminating infections as part of the innate immune system. This type of granulocyte is produced from the myeloid lineage of granulocyte-monocyte progenitor cells and is identified by the presence of granules in its cytoplasm.
        - (b) The plasma membrane on the cells contains sensors and receptors to attack and destroy microorganisms.
          - i. Three types of granulocytes exist: neutrophils, basophils, and eosinophils.
          - ii. Neutrophils are the most abundant WBC, ranging from 50%–60%.
          - iii. Neutrophils engulf foreign particles in a process called *phagocytosis*.
          - iv. Neutrophils may be subdivided (e.g., segmented neutrophils, segmented bands).
          - v. Neutrophils are first to respond to infection or inflammation.
          - vi. Approximately 25% of neutrophils are found in the circulating blood. The remaining neutrophils are located in the

bone marrow, where they become a reserve in the event of an injury or infection.

(3) The formation of mature granulocytes in the bone marrow is achieved by a process called *granulopoiesis*. An important function in granulopoiesis is the granulocyte–colony-stimulating factor (G-CSF), which stimulates the longevity, proliferation, maturity, and functional activation of these cells. Therefore, the role of G-CSF in patients with neutropenia is significant. When no G-CSFs are present—which can occur in myeloid disorders such as myelodysplastic syndrome (MDS)—neutrophils in the circulating blood and bone marrow decrease. An increase in the proportion of neutrophil progenitors experiencing apoptosis, or cell death, is then present.

b) Abnormal

(1) Neutropenia following HSCT is the most common complication associated with high-risk morbidity and mortality and increased healthcare cost. Neutropenia may be congenital or acquired.

(a) Congenital: Severe congenital neutropenia results from abnormal chromosomal patterns of inheritance with a neutrophil count of less than 500/mm³ in the neonatal period. During this time, the infant will experience bacterial infections, such as perirectal abscess or omphalitis, infection in the umbilical stump. A bone marrow biopsy will reveal neutrophils that have maturation arrest and lack mature elements.

(b) Acquired: Chemotherapy- or radiation therapy–induced neutropenia is the most common cause of toxicity in the HSCT setting. It occurs within days of completing the chemotherapy drug or radiation conditioning regimen. Other forms of acquired neutropenia include disease state (myeloid disorders such as MDS and AML), infections (viral, bacterial, or fungal), and supportive treatment (antiviral therapies).

(2) Key factors related to the duration of neutropenia include previous chemotherapy agents and radiation (with or without chemotherapy), source of stem cells, number of stem cells infused, use of growth factors, corticosteroid medications, and the occurrence of post-transplant complications.

(3) The underlying disease state, such as myelofibrosis, can result in prolonged neutropenia, even with a satisfactory graft.

(4) The complications from prolonged neutropenia combined with other conditions, such as mucositis, GVHD, graft rejection, invasive central lines, and nutritional deficits, can significantly increase morbidity and mortality in the transplant recipient.

(5) Calculate the neutrophil count to measure the ANC (see Figure 6-1).

(a) To calculate the ANC, multiply the WBC count by the sum of the percentage of bands and percentage of neutrophils.

(b) The ANC determines the relative risk for developing an infection.

(c) An ANC of less than 100/mm³ is profound neutropenia, and the risk for infection is high, especially in HSCT patients receiving high-dose chemotherapy or radiation therapy as part of their conditioning regimen.

Figure 6-1. Formula for Calculating the Absolute Neutrophil Count

ANC calculation:
(% bands + % neutrophils) × total WBC = ANC

Recipient counts:
45% bands; 10% neutrophils; total WBC = 1,200
(0.45 + 0.10) × 1,200 = 660
ANC = 660/mm^3

ANC—absolute neutrophil count; WBC—white blood cell

Note. Based on information from Camp-Sorrell, 2011; Marrs, 2006.

     (d) ANC related to infection risk
        i. Minimal risk: ANC = 1,000–1,500/mm^3
        ii. Moderate risk: ANC = 500–1,000/mm^3
        iii. Severe risk: ANC ≤ 500/mm^3

3. Clinical features (Camp-Sorrell, 2011; Goldman & Schafer, 2012; Polovich, Olsen, & LeFebvre, 2014; Rosselet, 2013): The severity and duration associated with neutropenia directly correlate with the incidence of infections leading to life-threatening complications in the transplant recipient.
    a) Risk factors
       (1) Recipient
       (2) Conditioning regimen
       (3) Depressed T-cell and B-cell function
       (4) Interferences in anatomic barriers (e.g., central line catheters, mucosal barrier of the GI tract)
       (5) Immunosuppressive medications (e.g., cyclosporine, steroids, ATG, methotrexate)
       (6) Bone marrow transplant
    b) Recipient factors
       (1) Age greater than 65 years (increased distribution of fat cells versus stem cells in the marrow)
       (2) Tumor invasion in the cellular marrow
       (3) Previous treatments with chemotherapy or radiation therapy
       (4) Diseases affecting the marrow (aplastic anemia)
       (5) Previous or current infection status (e.g., CMV, bacterial or fungal infections)
    c) Conditioning regimens
       (1) Chemotherapy agents (reduced intensity or high dose) result in pancytopenia of the cellular environment.
       (2) Radiation therapy fields with doses of 20 Gy or greater interrupt bone marrow production sites in the long bones, ilia, ribs, and sternum.
       (3) Biotherapy agents can modify the immune system.
       (4) Steroidal medications may inhibit migration of neutrophils to infection sites and alter processes in phagocytic enzymes.
    d) Immunosuppressants: Steroids reduce the activity of the immune system, preventing phagocytosis and neutrophil activity.

4. Signs and symptoms related to neutropenic fever or prolonged neutropenia (Camp-Sorrell, 2011; Rosselet, 2013)
   a) Neutropenic fever (pre-engraftment)
      (1) Neutropenic fever occurs in the majority of patients during the pre-engraftment phase. It usually occurs in autologous HSCT recipients in 10–14 days. With myeloablative allogeneic HSCT recipients, it usually occurs in 14–21 days because of an infectious source.
      (2) Fever may be the only clinical symptom; therefore, it should promptly be evaluated and treated empirically with antibiotics. Generally, the organism is a gram-positive source and less virulent (i.e., alpha *Streptococcus*, *Staphylococcus epidermidis*); however, more virulent sources have been identified, such as multiresistant bacterial strains.
      (3) The most virulent are the gram-negative rods with bacteremia, leading to sepsis and septic shock in a few hours.
      (4) In most cases, fever subsides with neutrophil engraftment; however, it may continue as a result of an occult infection. The infection is evident because of recovery of the inflammatory responses related to pneumonia or abscess.
   b) Prolonged neutropenia (postengraftment)
      (1) Prolonged neutropenia may result in a systemic inflammatory response syndrome, as manifested by the following:
         (a) Temperature greater than 100.4°F (38°C)
         (b) Heart rate greater than 90 beats per minute
         (c) Respiratory rate greater than 20 breaths per minute
         (d) WBC count greater than 12,000/mm³ or less than 4,000/mm³ and/or more than 10% bands in the peripheral blood precipitated by bacteria, viruses, and fungi.
      (2) The symptoms of sepsis are related to the release of proinflammatory actions of cytokines.
      (3) Typhlitis, also known as neutropenic enterocolitis, is a rare, life-threatening syndrome of clinical manifestations that includes abdominal pain, nausea, and bloody diarrhea. Bacteremia is noted in approximately 10%–50% of HSCT recipients with prolonged neutropenia, with one of the following organisms: *Pseudomonas aeruginosa*, Enterobacteriaceae, *Bacteroides fragilis*, viridans streptococci, enterococci, and *Candida*.
      (4) Pneumonia can be infectious or noninfectious. Noninfectious pneumonia types are common prior to engraftment. The infectious types are more prominent during the neutropenic period.
      (5) Acute respiratory distress syndrome can manifest and is generally a result of conditioning regimen toxicity or may be associated with sepsis.
      (6) Increased morbidity and mortality in HSCT is a result of infectious complications.
   c) Physical examination and medical history
      (1) Previous type of induction or conditioning regimen
      (2) Current antibiotic, antifungal, or antiviral medications that may be related to WBC suppression (e.g., amphotericin B, TMP-SMX)
      (3) Current use of G-CSF
      (4) Exposure to any person who may be ill (e.g., visitor, family member, healthcare worker)

5. Diagnostic tests (Rosselet, 2013)
    a) Laboratory
        (1) Pan cultures (blood [two sets]; urinalysis; urine culture, if symptomatic; any suspicious wound site; sputum culture; complete blood count [CBC]; serum creatinine; hepatic transaminases) identify source of infection.
        (2) Mixed venous oxygen saturation from central venous access evaluates tissue oxygenation.
        (3) Lactic acid evaluates anaerobic metabolism of the tissues.
    b) Radiology
        (1) As indicated based on symptoms
        (2) Imaging usually includes a chest radiograph or ultrasound of the abdomen or extremity if thrombus is suspected.
    c) Diagnostic: Obtain CT or MRI scan based on findings.
    d) Differential diagnosis (Gobel, Peterson, & Hoffner, 2013; Rosselet, 2013): Systemic inflammatory response syndrome, sepsis, septic shock, and engraftment syndrome
6. Treatment (Antin & Raley, 2013; Jubelirer, 2011; Marrs, 2006; Rosselet, 2013)
    a) The mainstay of treatment for neutropenic fever is prompt initiation of antimicrobials, such as cefepime, imipenem, meropenem, piperacillin/tazobactam, or aminoglycoside (fluoroquinolone plus clindamycin or aztreonam plus vancomycin, if allergic to penicillin).
    b) Antibiotic therapy is maintained for a minimum of seven days and continued until blood cultures are negative for three consecutive days or the causative organism is eradicated.
    c) Antibiotic therapy is generally continued until ANC is greater than 500/mm^3.
    d) Antivirals are recommended for recipients with suspected viruses, such as herpes family, or if mucosal lesions are present.
    e) Antifungal agents are initiated for fevers lasting for more than three days without a known cause.
    f) A neutropenic diet is considered strict in the transplant recipient population in some centers because of the potential increase in food-related bacterial infections and is continued until ANC is greater than 1,000/mm^3. Food safety is of paramount importance.
        (1) Generally, autologous and allogeneic HSCT recipients also should avoid botanical and herbal supplements until day +45 or until immunosuppressants are discontinued for at least one month.
        (2) One recent small pilot study conducted in a single center suggested that a neutropenic diet may not be necessary, but further research in other institutions is warranted (Lassiter & Schneider, 2015).
7. Patient education (Camp-Sorrell, 2011; Rosselet, 2013)
    a) Education should focus on teaching the recipient and caregiver about hygiene measures, signs and symptoms of infection, inspecting the catheter site and mucosal lining of the mouth, ensuring a clean environment, minimizing microbes on high-touch surfaces, practicing good personal hygiene, and continuing medications to prevent infections.
    b) Frequent hand washing, diligent oral care, and screening for sick visitors also should be encouraged.

c) Guidelines for preventing infectious complications among HSCT recipients were cosponsored by many organizations (Tomblyn et al., 2009). The guidelines are a joint effort to summarize current recommendations for users worldwide as a reference in infection prevention in HSCT.

C. Transplant-associated infections (Angarone & Ison, 2008; Beyer et al., 1995; Camus & Costabel, 2005; Coomes, Hubbard, & Moore, 2011; Goldman & Schafer, 2012; Leather & Wingard, 2001; Mackall et al., 2009; Marr et al., 2009; Mitchell, 2009; O'Donnell, 2009; Reiner, 2008; Rimkus, 2009; Rosselet, 2013; Soubani & Pandya, 2010; Tomblyn et al., 2009): HSCT-related infections are caused by neutropenia related to the myeloablative conditioning regimens. Three phases pose a high risk for a variety of opportunistic infections (see Figure 6-2).

   1. Phase I (pre-engraftment): Less than 15–45 days following transplant and engraftment

     a) This phase can vary according to the type of transplant received.

     b) Autologous bone marrow transplant recipients achieve neutrophil engraftment first, followed by allogeneic PBSC transplantation and bone marrow harvest transplant recipients. Matched unrelated donor (MUD) PBSC,

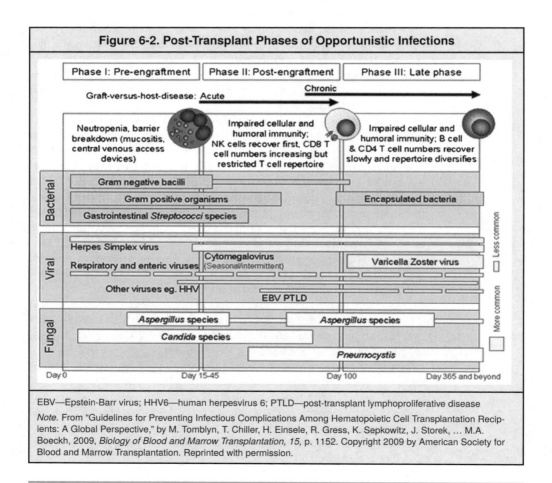

Figure 6-2. Post-Transplant Phases of Opportunistic Infections

EBV—Epstein-Barr virus; HHV6—human herpesvirus 6; PTLD—post-transplant lymphoproliferative disease

Note. From "Guidelines for Preventing Infectious Complications Among Hematopoietic Cell Transplantation Recipients: A Global Perspective," by M. Tomblyn, T. Chiller, H. Einsele, R. Gress, K. Sepkowitz, J. Storek, ... M.A. Boeckh, 2009, *Biology of Blood and Marrow Transplantation, 15,* p. 1152. Copyright 2009 by American Society for Blood and Marrow Transplantation. Reprinted with permission.

cord blood, and MUD bone marrow transplant recipients are typically last to achieve neutrophil engraftment.

c) During the pre-engraftment phase, there is loss of neutrophils to effectively fight infection. This is a result of the preparative regimen destroying normal cells, neutrophils, monocytes, and macrophages, as well as the diseased cells.

d) Recipients may develop a neutropenic fever, which is most likely caused by a bacterial pathogen, although negative cultures may be obtained.

e) Viral reactivation or fungal infections may occur during this phase.

f) With prolonged neutropenia in the first 45 days, the risk of *Aspergillus* infections can be problematic and should be monitored.

g) G-CSF and nonmyeloablative preparative regimens are instrumental in improving cellular recovery and fighting against early infections and complications.

h) Using mobilized PBSCs versus bone marrow greatly reduces the risk of infection in autologous recipients. Additionally, using mobilized PBSCs instead of bone marrow in allogeneic recipients results in earlier engraftment at a median time of 14 days, as opposed to 19 days.

i) The cell dose, which is the number of CD34+ progenitor cells given during transplant, is directly related to the rate of neutrophil recovery and is a marker for successful engraftment.

j) Colonized bacteria on the recipient's skin poses a significant risk for opportunist infections related to chemotherapy agents and central venous catheters.

k) Previous exposure to virogens, such as HSV, herpes zoster, and CMV, as well as other factors (e.g., type of transplant, specific disease, HLA match, medical history, and conditioning regimen) can significantly increase the risk of developing an infection during this phase.

l) Bacterial organisms (gram positive and gram negative) account for 90% of infections within the neutropenic period.

m) The most common locations for infection are the oral mucosa and the bloodstream because of catheter-associated bloodstream infections.

n) Bacterial opportunistic infections

    (1) Gram-positive organisms are associated with disruptions in the skin, oropharynx, and indwelling catheters.

    (2) Opportunistic gram-positive cocci are *Staphylococcus epidermidis*, *Staphylococcus aureus*, and viridans streptococci (*Streptococcus mitis* and *Enterococcus* species).

    (3) Gram-negative rod infections are a result of *Escherichia coli* (*E. coli*), *Klebsiella pneumoniae*, *Pseudomonas aeruginosa*, etc.

    (4) No indication currently exists for prophylactic treatment in the pediatric transplant population.

    (5) A fluoroquinolone antibiotic is administered for bacterial prophylaxis in adults with neutropenia for more than seven days.

    (6) Oral antibiotic prophylaxis should be discontinued when a transplant recipient develops a fever. Broad-spectrum (gram positive and gram negative) IV antibiotic coverage, such as third- and fourth-generation cephalosporins, quinolones, aminoglycosides, and vancomycin, should be initiated immediately.

    (7) Vancomycin-resistant *Enterococcus* (VRE) is a common cause of infection. VRE bacteremia (VREB) is the leading cause of bacteremia in the

pre-engraftment phase (median day 7) following HSCT and is associated with a high mortality rate.

(8) Pre-HSCT VRE screening and weekly surveillance have identified VREB in patients at risk.

(9) Four antibiotics have been approved by the U.S. Food and Drug Administration for treatment of VRE and VREB: quinupristin and dalfopristin, linezolid, daptomycin, and tigecycline.

(10) Vancomycin use should be discontinued after sensitivity is obtained and when not indicated for treatment in patients with VRE.

o) Fungal and candidal opportunistic infections

(1) Two main species exist: *Candida albicans*, affecting the oral mucosa, and *Aspergillus*, affecting the sinuses and lungs.

(2) Fluconazole, a fungal prophylaxis medication, is used for invasive candidiasis before engraftment. Micafungin and posaconazole are used for molds or fluconazole-resistant *Candida* species with an alternative of voriconazole.

(3) Invasive aspergillosis requires treatment with voriconazole, micafungin, posaconazole, and liposomal amphotericin.

(4) For invasive candidiasis, posaconazole or voriconazole is indicated for patients receiving immunosuppressant medications for chronic GVHD, such as steroids; those with prolonged neutropenia; and those at high risk for fungal infections.

(5) The Foundation for the Accreditation of Cellular Therapy standards recommend that hospitals use HEPA filtration, positive air pressure, and private rooms with appropriately sealed doors to recipients' rooms and the unit. This includes 12 air exchanges per hour with removal of particulate 0.3 mcm or greater in diameter in each private patient room, with a 99.7% efficiency.

(6) Recipients' bathrooms should be kept clean and free of mold at all times.

p) Viral opportunistic infections

(1) Recipients are at an increased risk for community-acquired respiratory viral (CRV) infections, HHV (i.e., CMV, HSV, VZV, EBV, HHV-6, HHV-7, and HHV-8), which are all associated with significant morbidity and mortality in transplant recipients, especially those who are seropositive.

(2) Prophylactic medications include acyclovir for HSV-seropositive allogeneic recipients.

(3) Ganciclovir also is given as preemptive therapy and treatment of CMV-seronegative recipients with seropositive donors. It is recommended that HSCT recipients and potential recipients with possible CRVs receiving conditioning treatment be placed on contact and droplet precautions until the organism is isolated. Following the institution's pathogen-specific guidelines is recommended. Each recipient and potential recipient with signs and symptoms should be tested for CRVs with viral cultures or rapid diagnostic tests.

(4) To prevent reactivation of HSV in the pre-engraftment phase, allogeneic transplant recipients who are HSV seropositive should receive antiviral prophylaxis along with the conditioning regimen and continue the regimen for approximately 30 days following HSCT.

(5) Allogeneic HSCT recipients have a greater risk for CMV than autologous recipients and should receive ganciclovir prophylaxis (i.e., front-line therapy) for the prevention of HSV-1 and HSV-2. This is especially necessary for those recipients with acute GVHD greater than grade 1. However, ganciclovir should be discontinued prior to transplant and restarted after the engraftment phase because it lowers the WBC count.

(6) HSV can manifest as mucositis in the phase I period. Prophylactic medication (acyclovir, valacyclovir) is administered for HSV and herpes zoster virus.

(7) CMV surveillance through laboratory testing should occur weekly for up to 60 days for early diagnosis and treatment. Currently, several laboratory tests for CMV are available, including testing of the CMV antigen pp65, CMV DNA, and CMV RNA.

(8) Allogeneic and autologous HSCT recipients at risk for *Pneumocystis jiroveci* pneumonia (PCP) are treated with TMP-SMX prior to transplant and until the discontinuation of immunosuppressants. However, this medication can cause pancytopenia during the pre-engraftment phase and should be stopped. Other medications substituted during this phase are dapsone, pentamidine, and atovaquone.

(9) Adenovirus is a common concern and may cause hemorrhagic cystitis, pneumonitis, or hepatitis in transplant recipients.

(10) The BK virus is a common virus found dormant in the kidneys and can manifest after transplant, causing hemorrhagic cystitis.

2. Phase II (postengraftment): 30–100 days following transplant

   a) During phase II, infection in allogeneic HSCT recipients is related to abnormal responses in cell-mediated and humoral immunity involving the release of cytokines, phagocytes, and cytotoxic and helper T lymphocytes.

   b) Infection is directly related to effects of immunosuppressive therapy and GVHD.

   c) Common pathogens include herpes viruses, CMV, EBV, PCP, adenovirus, BK virus, disseminated or hepatosplenic candidiasis, and *Aspergillus* species (sinuses and lungs).

      (1) HSV

         (a) HSV reacts most often in seropositive recipients after HSCT, especially in the presence of mucositis. Acyclovir is the agent of choice.

         (b) CMV is a major risk factor after HSCT and includes T-cell depletion, GVHD, and CMV viremia, with seropositive recipients being at greatest risk for reactivation (70%) followed by seronegative recipients with seronegative donors.

            i. However, seronegative recipients with seronegative donors are at a very low risk. These recipients should receive blood products that are CMV negative to reduce risk.

            ii. CMV GI disease and pneumonia are most common. For recipients with visual changes, CMV retinitis should be considered; however, this is uncommon.

            iii. Treatment is aimed at prevention in seropositive recipients, with antiviral chemoprophylaxis and preemptive therapy (virologic monitoring and antiviral treatment).

     (2) Post-transplant lymphoproliferative disorder (PTLD) is the most significant disease related to EBV.

         (a) Although rare, PTLD is more prevalent in allogeneic recipients who do not undergo T-cell depletion or receive an umbilical cord blood transplant.

         (b) Treatment includes monitoring for DNA load using a serum EBV, DNA, or polymerase chain reaction assay. If viral load increases, a CD20 monoclonal antibody (i.e., rituximab) should be administered.

     (3) Other common respiratory infections

         (a) Aspergillosis

         (b) PCP

         (c) Respiratory syncytial virus (i.e., parainfluenza viruses, influenza A virus)

         (d) Toxoplasmosis

  d) Differences between autologous and allogeneic transplants and the risks for infection are noted with a decrease in the autologous recipient and an increase in the allogeneic recipient secondary to GVHD and continued immunosuppression.

3. Phase III (late phase): More than 100 days following transplant. This phase will be discussed later in the section (see Figure 6-2).

  a) Definition (Rosselet, 2013; Zuckerman, 2009): Opportunistic infections occurring after day 100 following HSCT

  b) Physiology and pathophysiology (Rosselet, 2013)

     (1) Late post-transplant infections are generally due to the ongoing therapy for acute GVHD. These recipients are at risk for early engraftment complications because immunotherapies are tapered, resulting in the risk of reactivation of CMV, VZV, and HSV. Hepatitis B and C occur from GVHD. This is a common complication of T-cell impairment.

     (2) This concludes the last phase of the HSCT process. The majority of recipients have achieved engraftment of their WBCs and are not at risk for major infectious complications.

     (3) Recipients with ongoing complications (i.e., GVHD, graft failure, or disease relapse) are at a greater risk for major infectious complications.

     (4) The most common infections during the late phase include *Streptococcus pneumoniae, Haemophilus influenzae, Neisseria meningitidis*, sinusitis, and VZV.

  c) Nursing implications (Rosselet, 2013)

     (1) During the late phase, patient education is essential regarding infectious complications, assessment, medication dispensing, and care planning.

     (2) Referral to the physician who will resume care regarding transplant course and ongoing monitoring for complications is essential.

4. Engraftment

  a) Definition: Engraftment occurs when the stem cells of the donor have been taken up in the patient's bone marrow (autologous or allogeneic).

(1) The desired result is the engraftment of all cell lineages.

(2) There must be interaction of components between the host and the autograft or allograft following the pretransplant conditioning regimen (myeloablative or nonmyeloablative).

(3) It generally takes approximately 14–21 days for engraftment to occur. This is known as *homing*, as the hematopoietic stem cells find their home in the bone marrow from the peripheral blood.

(4) Neutrophil counts may fluctuate slightly until a steady state of 500/mm^3 for three consecutive days is achieved. This is known as *neutrophil engraftment*.

(5) Platelet engraftment occurs when the platelet count reaches 20,000/mm^3 or greater. Platelets are the last cell line to engraft following transplantation.

(6) Erythroid engraftment occurs when reticulocyte count reaches greater than 30,000/mm^3 or greater than 1% reticulocytes in a recipient who has not been transfused.

(7) T-cell engraftment occurs after mixed donor–recipient chimerism (i.e., presence of cells from two different individuals) is detected.

(8) Recovery of the recipient's hematologic and immune cells is influenced by factors such as the disease, preparative regimen, GVHD immunosuppressants, and viruses.

b) *Graft failure* is a term used to describe lack of neutrophil recovery at day 28 for myeloablative transplants. In cord blood transplants, the cutoff point for graft failure is day 42, which is based on the time that neutrophil engraftment occurs in most recipients.

c) Engraftment syndrome may develop during the pre-engraftment phase after myeloablative transplant in the absence of demonstrable infection.

(1) The syndrome is characterized by rash, fever, and endothelial injury (capillary leak) secondary to pulmonary edema.

(2) It primarily occurs in autologous transplant recipients but also may occur in allogeneic transplant recipients.

(3) Engraftment syndrome precedes neutrophil engraftment by several days and is associated with a rapid increase in the rate of neutrophils in the peripheral blood.

(4) Following the presence of neutrophils is the appearance of lymphocytes.

(5) Symptoms such as rash, fever, and hypoxia resolve after three to five days of high-dose corticosteroids followed by rapid taper (see Figure 6-3).

D. Thrombocytopenia

1. Definition (Camp-Sorrell, 2011; Gobel & O'Leary, 2007; Rosselet, 2013): Thrombocytopenia is a platelet count less than 100,000/mm^3 (see Table 6-4).

2. Physiology and pathophysiology (Burgunder, 2007; Douglas & Shelton, 2007; Gobel & O'Leary, 2007; Goldman & Schafer, 2012; Hillman, Ault, Leporrier, & Rinder, 2011; Hovinga & Lämmle, 2012; National Cancer Institute Cancer Therapy Evaluation Program [NCI CTEP], 2010; Rosselet, 2013; Shelton, 2016; Yldrm et al., 2015)

a) Normal

Figure 6-3. Major and Minor Manifestations for Diagnosis of Engraftment Syndrome*

Major Manifestations
- Fever ≥ 38.3°C (100.94°F) without identifiable infection source
- Rash involving > 25% of body surface without evidence of a medication reaction
- Pulmonary edema (noncardiogenic) as evidenced by pulmonary infiltrates (absence of cardiac dysfunction and infection) and hypoxia (oxygen saturation < 90%)

Minor Manifestations
- Total bilirubin ≥ 2 mg/dl or transaminase levels twice the normal level
- Serum creatinine twice the baseline level
- Weight gain
- Transient encephalopathy

* Engraftment syndrome is suspected by the manifestation of three major or two major and one or more minor.

Note. Based on information from O'Donnell, 2009.

Table 6-4. Common Terminology Criteria for Adverse Events Grading of Thrombocytopenia

Grade	Platelet Count
1	< LLN–75,000/mm³; < LLN–75.0 × 10⁹/L
2	< 75,000–50,000/mm³; < 75.0–50.0 × 10⁹/L
3	< 50,000–25,000/mm³; < 50.0–25.0 × 10⁹/L
4	< 25,000/mm³; < 25 × 10⁹/L
5	–

LLN—lower limit of normal

Note. From *Common Terminology Criteria for Adverse Events* [v.4.03], by National Cancer Institute Cancer Therapy Evaluation Program, 2010. Retrieved from http://evs.nci.nih.gov/ftp1/CTCAE/CTCAE_4.03_2010-06-14_QuickReference_8.5x11.pdf.

---

(1) Platelets, also known as thrombocytes, are small fragments developed in the bone marrow and regulated by a hormone-like substance called thrombopoietin produced by the kidneys.

(2) Platelets have a life span of approximately 8–10 days.

(3) A normal platelet count is considered to be between 150,000/mm³ and 400,000/mm³.

(4) Platelets function to maintain homeostasis and vascular integrity and prevent bleeding through clotting mechanisms.

(5) The spleen is a reservoir for approximately one-third of the total platelet volume.

(6) The spleen removes unused platelets from the circulation in approximately 10 days.

   b) Abnormal

      (1) Myelodysplasia is a common cause of impaired normal megakaryocyte proliferation, leading to thrombocytopenia.

    (2) Platelet count less than 10,000/mm^3 can be life threatening because of the potential for intracranial or GI bleeding.

    (3) Splenomegaly occurs when an abnormally large distribution of platelets is present; this results in thrombocytopenia in patients with lymphoma and in others with portal hypertension.

    (4) Other causes include fever, systemic infections (e.g., CMV, EBV, HHV-6, HIV, mycoplasma, mycobacteria), and common drugs (e.g., nonsteroidal medications, aspirin, TMP-SMX, heparin, furosemide, vancomycin, penicillin, cyclosporine A, ganciclovir), resulting in accelerated destruction or consumption of platelets in transplant recipients.

    (5) Acute blood loss or platelet production disorders also are causes of thrombocytopenia.

  c) Congenital: Congenital amegakaryocytic thrombocytopenia is a rare bone marrow failure syndrome caused by an autosomal recessive gene identified in the infantile period.

  d) Idiopathic

    (1) Idiopathic thrombocytopenic purpura (ITP) is caused by circulating antiplatelet autoantibodies that result from low-grade lymphoproliferative disorders such as chronic lymphocytic leukemia.

    (2) Thrombotic thrombocytopenic purpura (TTP) is considered to be an endothelial cell injury and is most likely associated with an acquired deficiency of ADAMTS13, an enzyme involved in blood clotting.

      (a) A hereditary autosomal recessive deficiency of ADAMTS13, called *congenital TTP*, can be present in children.

      (b) TTP associated with cancer is less pronounced, and recipients may not present with the full syndrome.

    (3) TTP/hemolytic uremic syndrome (HUS) can be associated with post-thrombocytopenia.

      (a) According to the Common Terminology Criteria for Adverse Events (NCI CTEP, 2010), TTP/HUS is a form of thrombotic microangiopathy accompanied by renal failure, hemolytic anemia, and severe thrombocytopenia occurring 3–12 months following transplantation (see Table 6-5).

      (b) This subacute chronic process occurs after endothelial vascular injury in which there is release of von Willebrand factor and microthrombi located in the vasculature.

    (4) Disseminated intravascular coagulation is a syndrome characterized by the systemic activation of coagulation. This leads to widespread thrombosis, compromising organ perfusion and resulting in organ death. The ongoing activation of coagulation will deplete platelets, contributing to a hypocoagulable state and bleeding.

    (5) Diffuse alveolar hemorrhage is a complication of severe thrombocytopenia secondary to *Aspergillus* species pneumonia, causing damage to the pulmonary small vessels and leading to blood collecting in the alveoli.

  e) Nonidiopathic

    (1) Drug-induced thrombocytopenia is caused by an immune-mediated destruction of platelets. This disorder is exhibited when all elements of the CBC are normal except for the platelet count. The etiology is

Grade	Description
1	Evidence of red blood cell destruction (schistocytosis) without clinical consequences
2	–
3	Laboratory findings with clinical consequences (i.e., renal insufficiency, petechiae)
4	Life-threatening consequences (e.g., central nervous system hemorrhage, thrombosis/embolism, renal failure)
5	Death

Table 6-5. Common Terminology Criteria for Adverse Events Grading of Hemolytic Uremic Syndrome

Note. From *Common Terminology Criteria for Adverse Events* [v.4.03], by National Cancer Institute Cancer Therapy Evaluation Program, 2010. Retrieved from http://evs.nci.nih.gov/ftp1/CTCAE/CTCAE_4.03_2010-06-14_QuickReference_8.5x11.pdf.

either an infection (viral or bacterial) or drug (antibiotic or antiviral) resulting from an immune reaction from the drug or its metabolites (see Figure 6-4).

(2) Cancers of the cell lineage, such as lymphoma, multiple myeloma, and leukemia, affect platelet production and can result in thrombocytopenia.

(3) Chemotherapy and radiation therapy can cause rapid destruction of platelets in the bone marrow from 7–14 days with combined regimens.

(4) Fever, endotoxins released from bacteria, and some medications (e.g., aspirin, heparin, phenytoin, tetracycline, digoxin) can lead to altered platelet development.

(5) The apheresis and mobilization processes in autologous transplant recipients may cause transient thrombocytopenia.

3. Clinical features (Camp-Sorrell, 2011; Rosselet, 2013)

a) History

(1) Recent cancer treatment such as radiation therapy, chemotherapy, or multimodal therapy

(2) Current medication use with drugs known to alter platelet production

(3) Septicemias that release endotoxins in the blood, altering or damaging platelets

Figure 6-4. Common Drugs Associated With Drug-Induced Thrombocytopenia

- Aspirin and aspirin-containing drugs
- Busulfan
- Carboplatin
- Cephalosporin
- Cyclophosphamide
- Cytarabine
- Etoposide
- Ganciclovir
- Linezolid
- Melphalan
- Nonsteroidal anti-inflammatory drugs
- Penicillin
- Sulfonamides/sulfonylureas
- Thiotepa
- Trimethoprim-sulfamethoxazole
- Valacyclovir
- Vancomycin

Note. Based on information from Camp-Sorrell, 2011; Ezzone, 2013.

(4) Recent apheresis or mobilization of stem cells in autologous transplant recipients

   b) Signs and symptoms

      (1) Bleeding from body orifices (nose, ears, mouth, rectum)

      (2) Platelet level less than 100,000/mm^3

   c) Physical examination

      (1) Assess for bleeding in urine, stool, and vomitus.

      (2) Assess for petechiae on upper and lower extremities and over pressure points (oral palate, elbows).

      (3) Assess skin for purpura, bruising, or bleeding at puncture sites.

      (4) Monitor platelet count. Platelet count less than 20,000/mm^3 is associated with major hemorrhage in the brain, lungs, and GI tract.

4. Diagnostic tests (Camp-Sorrell, 2011; Rosselet, 2013)

   a) Monitor platelet count.

   b) Monitor coagulation studies (i.e., prothrombin time, partial thromboplastin time, and fibrinogen).

   c) A bone marrow aspirate and biopsy may be warranted for prolonged thrombocytopenia to assess for decreased megakaryocyte production in the bone marrow or to rule out other causes (such as active cancer).

5. Treatment (Despotis, Zhang, & Lublin, 2007; Ezzone, 2009; Khan et al., 2007; Lemoine & Gobel, 2011; Rosselet, 2013; Sekhon & Roy, 2006)

   a) Nursing management includes supportive care for bleeding risk or bleeding.

   b) Interventions to minimize bleeding include avoidance of invasive procedures and use of tourniquet, blood pressure cuff, finger sticks, intramuscular injections, and rectal thermometers when platelet count is less than 20,000/mm^3.

   c) A trigger for transfusion may be set by the physician for recipients receiving a chemotherapy regimen in the HSCT setting. However, some recipients may need an increased trigger because of chronic anticoagulation therapy, active bleeding, or brain injury.

   d) Platelets are transfused when the platelet count reaches 10,000–20,000/mm^3 or patient is symptomatic or actively bleeding. A platelet transfusion is indicated for recipients with platelet counts less than 10,000/mm^3; the risk is high for spontaneous bleeding below this level.

   e) Recipients with thrombocytopenia generally will receive platelet transfusions during their course of disease.

      (1) Prophylactic platelet transfusion may be ordered and administered with multiple random donors (pooled platelets), single donor platelets, or an HLA-matched single donor.

      (2) Transfusion of platelets causes more adverse reactions than RBCs due to the possibility of WBCs being present in the product.

      (3) The most common adverse reactions during platelet transfusion are fever, allergic reactions, and, on rare occasions, related to a specific antigen.

      (4) Acetaminophen and diphenhydramine may be given as premedications if the recipient reports history of reaction prior to platelet administration.

      (5) Each unit of platelets transfused may increase the platelet count by 20%–50%.

(6) Platelet transfusions do not warrant the same ABO/Rh compatibility as RBC transfusions but should be leukopoor and irradiated. Exceptions include body weight lower than 40 kg (88.1 lbs) or platelet transfusion volume greater than 600 ml of unmatched platelets within a 24-hour period.

(7) Platelet refractoriness may have multiple causes such as sepsis, splenomegaly, disseminated intravascular coagulation, medication, fever, and bleeding. The response to platelets is measured by a corrected count increment. It is important to select the appropriate platelet components for transfusion, especially in some alloimmunized recipients.

6. Patient education
   a) Educate patients to notify their nurse or physician if exhibiting signs or symptoms of bleeding.
   b) Educate patients about bleeding precautions.
   c) Educate patients to avoid activities or injuries that may increase risk for bleeding.
   d) Educate patients to anticipate platelet transfusion as an expected part of the transplant process.

E. Anemia
   1. Definition (Baker, 2000; Camp-Sorrell, 2011; Gobel & O'Leary, 2007; Hillman et al., 2011; Lemoine & Gobel, 2011; Mehta & Hoffbrand, 2013; Munker, Hiller, & Paquette, 2007; Roy, 2010; Shelton, 2016): Anemia is a symptom of decreased circulating RBCs by one-third or greater than normal, identified on an initial screening examination in recipients with a hemoglobin level of less than 11 g/dl.
   2. Physiology and pathophysiology (Broadway-Duren & Klaassen, 2013; Chouinard & Finn, 2007; Helbig et al., 2007; Hillman et al., 2011; Marks & Glader, 2009; Munker et al., 2007; Rosselet, 2013; Worel et al., 2007)
      a) Normal
         (1) The main function of erythrocytes (commonly known as RBCs) is to transport oxygen to the tissues. Oxygen attaches to the hemoglobin, which contains a red compound (iron and porphyrin–containing substance) called *heme* of the cell. Normal adult hemoglobin is known as hemoglobin A (HbA). Between 200 and 300 million molecules of hemoglobin per erythrocyte are present and chemically combine with oxygen to form oxyhemoglobin and carbon dioxide. This chemical process enables the erythrocytes to transport oxygen to the tissues and carbon dioxide to the alveoli in the lungs to be exhaled into the air.
         (2) Approximately $5,000,000/mm^3$ erythrocytes within the blood plasma are present.
         (3) The average life span of an erythrocyte is 120 days.
         (4) To maintain an adequate number of erythrocytes, the bone marrow must produce and release approximately 2.5 billion erythrocytes per kilogram of body weight daily.
      b) Abnormal
         (1) Several causative factors affect HSCT recipients (e.g., bleeding, bone marrow suppression, hemolysis, type of malignancy, malnutrition, HUS, kidney failure, conditioning regimens, thrombotic microangiopathy) (see Figure 6-5).

Figure 6-5. Bleeding Complications and Etiologies That May Contribute to Anemia in Transplant Recipients

Pathophysiology	Etiology	Signs/Symptoms	Management
• Myelosuppression induced by preparative regimen • Delayed platelet engraftment • Marrow-suppressive medications • Coagulation abnormalities • Platelet autoantibodies • Graft rejection	• Graft-versus-host disease • Cyclosporine • Veno-occlusive disease • Altered mucosal barriers • Delayed or failed engraftment • Viral infection • ABO-incompatible bone marrow transplantation	• Skin/mucosa: petechiae, ecchymoses, bruising, scleral hemorrhage, epistaxis • Genitourinary: hematuria, menorrhagia • Gastrointestinal: guaiac-positive stool/emesis, abdominal distension or discomfort • Pulmonary: epistaxis, hemoptysis, change in breathing pattern • Intracranial: headache, restlessness, change in pupil response, seizure, change in mental status/level of consciousness	• Perform frequent assessment. • Monitor hemoglobin/hematocrit, platelets, and coagulation studies. • Minimize blood loss. • Administer blood products. • Avoid medications that inhibit platelet production or function. • Avoid invasive procedures. • Follow bleeding precautions.

Note. Based on information from Ezzone, 2009.

From "Hematologic Effects" (p. 166), by R.M. Rosselet in S.A. Ezzone (Ed.), *Hematopoietic Stem Cell Transplantation: A Manual for Nursing Practice* (2nd ed.), 2013, Pittsburgh, PA: Oncology Nursing Society. Copyright 2013 by Oncology Nursing Society. Reprinted with permission.

(2) With the decreased oxygen-carrying capacity and oxygen tension in the tissues, hypoxia occurs in the cells and tissues. Erythropoietin is stimulated by an up-and-down feedback mechanism. When hypoxia occurs, interstitial renal cells and central vein hepatocyte receptors signal an expression of the erythropoietin gene, which increases erythropoietin production. The increased production in the blood signals the erythrocyte precursor cells to produce RBCs.

(3) A hemoglobin level less than 10 g/dl in HSCT recipients should be evaluated, and a level of 7 g/dl should warrant transfusion of RBCs. A transfusion would be indicated with a hemoglobin level greater than 9 g/dl in patients with symptomatic anemia. Special considerations may be given to recipients with cardiovascular risk factors or older recipients. The expectation would be to increase HbA 1 g/dl for one RBC unit (10–15 ml/kg) (if recipient is not bleeding or hemolyzing).

(4) A kinetic approach uses the causative mechanism, including loss of RBCs (e.g., trauma, acute or chronic hemorrhage), decreased production of RBCs (i.e., lack of erythropoiesis, as in kidney disease), iron deficiency, folate deficiency, chemotherapy, radiation therapy, or malignancies of the bone marrow, and increased destruction of RBCs (i.e., hemolytic anemias, inherited or acquired).

(5) Anemia in bone marrow transplant recipients can be caused by hemolysis, bleeding, preparative regimens (i.e., chemotherapy or radiation

therapy to long bones suppressing bone marrow), type of malignancy, HUS, nutritional deficiency leading to poor dietary intake, acute renal failure (i.e., preparative regimens and other medications), and thrombotic microangiopathy.

  (a) Hemolytic anemias develop in one-third of all allogeneic transplant recipients and result from an acute hemolytic reaction.

  (b) It is considered a serious complication of HSCT. Donor–recipient ABO incompatibility can be major or minor.

  (c) Manifestations include chills, increased temperature, dyspnea, chest or back pain, abnormal blood loss, and shock.

  (d) The donor–recipient ABO incompatibilities may result in prolonged red cell destruction, continued hemolysis, and pure red cell aplasia.

(6) Prolonged red cell destruction is caused by alloantibodies in the recipient that react with the antigens in the donor's RBCs.

(7) ABO blood group antibodies can carry many risks and can mediate prolonged hemolysis following hematopoietic progenitor cell transplantation in which donor-derived antibodies are directed against antigens on the recipient's erythrocytes, causing active lysis of the cells.

(8) Pure red cell aplasia results in maturation arrest in the formation of red cells; erythroblasts are essentially absent in the bone marrow, which can last months to years.

(9) Taking preventive measures and anticipating risk factors in transplant recipients are essential for improving outcomes.

3. Clinical features (Camp-Sorrell, 2011; Rosselet, 2013)

  a) History of presenting signs and symptoms is contingent on the following:

  (1) Age of recipient

  (2) Acute or chronic blood loss

  (3) Compensatory mechanisms

  (4) Activity levels

  (5) Nutritional status

  (6) Dehydration level (may falsely elevate laboratory levels)

  b) Signs and symptoms

  (1) Fatigue (hallmark symptom)

  (2) Dyspnea on exertion

  (3) Pallor (nail beds, conjunctivae)

  (4) Weakness

  (5) Headache

  (6) Tachycardia

  (7) Tachypnea

  (8) Listlessness

  c) Physical examination

  (1) Anemia grade and documentation (per NCI CTEP's Common Terminology Criteria for Adverse Events) (see Table 6-6)

  (2) General appearance and orientation

  (3) Vital signs

  (4) Pale conjunctivae and nail beds

  (5) Cardiovascular (may auscultate systolic ejection murmur)

Table 6-6. Common Terminology Criteria for Adverse Events Grading of Anemia	
Grade	Description
1	Hemoglobin (Hgb) < LLN–10.0 g/dl; < LLN–6.2 mmol/L; < LLN–100 g/L
2	Hgb < 10.0–8.0 g/dl; < 6.2–4.9 mmol/L; < 100–80 g/L
3	Hgb < 8.0 g/dl; < 4.9 mmol/L; < 80 g/L; transfusion indicated
4	Life-threatening consequences; urgent intervention indicated
5	Death

LLN—lower limit of normal

Note. From *Common Terminology Criteria for Adverse Events* [v.4.03], by National Cancer Institute Cancer Therapy Evaluation Program, 2010. Retrieved from http://evs.nci.nih.gov/ftp1/CTCAE/CTCAE_4.03_2010-06-14_QuickReference_8.5x11.pdf.

     (6) Skin pallor, dryness, and brittle hair
  4. Diagnostic tests (Camp-Sorrell, 2011; Lemoine & Gobel, 2011; Rosselet, 2013)
    a) Daily hemoglobin and hematocrit levels should be monitored throughout the anemia period. Laboratory tests should be completed more frequently if the recipient is actively bleeding or if bleeding is suspected.
    b) Hemolytic anemia workup, such as CBC, urinalysis, lactate dehydrogenase, direct and indirect Coombs test, and fractionated bilirubin, should be ordered, if applicable, for transfusion reactions.
    c) Anemia studies, such as iron, ferritin, folate, erythropoietin, and reticulocyte count (if not assessed), should be considered.
  5. Treatment (Hillman et al., 2011; Lemoine & Gobel, 2011; Rosselet, 2013)
    a) The mainstay of treatment for anemia is RBC transfusion if symptomatic and management of symptoms.
    b) Nursing management related to blood transfusions in the HSCT setting
      (1) HSCT recipients will require multiple RBC transfusions until recovery of the RBC lineage.
      (2) Although blood transfusions are safe, risks are associated (e.g., transmission of infectious disease, alloimmunization, febrile nonhemolytic reactions).
        (a) Infectious diseases include viruses (i.e., hepatitis A, B, and C; EBV; CMV), bacteria, and protozoa.
        (b) Alloimmunization may occur in the event that antibodies are developed, which leads to destruction of the transfused blood products (i.e., platelets). This is secondary to multiple transfusions and may result in refractory thrombocytopenia.
        (c) Febrile nonhemolytic reactions occur most often with platelet transfusion at any point during the transfusion and several hours following the transfusion. This is thought to occur either because antibodies create a reaction with the WBCs or as a result of the cytokine action in the product. Or, they are developed by the recipient after transfusion. Risk increases with multiple transfusions.

(3) The use of leukopoor, irradiated packed RBCs in the laboratory or leukocyte-reduced filters can significantly reduce the chance of reactions in HSCT recipients.

  c) Risk of ABO incompatibility in the HSCT setting (see Table 6-7)
  d) Types of ABO incompatibility and potential adverse effects in the HSCT setting (see Figure 6-6)
6. Patient education: Educate patients and families about risk factors for anemia and the need for transfusions, possible causes of anemia, signs and symptoms of anemia, and the potential influence on ADL and self-management strategies to prevent increased fatigue related to anemia.
7. Nursing management
  a) Recipients of HSCT require multiple transfusions (platelets and RBCs) during the transplantation period until the cells have recovered.
  b) Transfusion decisions are guided by hematocrit and hemoglobin levels and the recipient's signs and symptoms.
  c) Risks of complications involved with transfusions include infectious diseases (e.g., hepatitis A, B, and C, HIV), alloimmunity, and febrile nonhemolytic transfusion reactions (an increase in temperature of 1°C [33.8°F] or more from baseline without known infection). Complications are grouped according to the following: acute or delayed; infec-

---

Table 6-7. ABO Incompatibility Chart for Hematopoietic Stem Cell Transplantation

Type of Incompatibility	Recipient ABO	Donor ABO
Major	O	A
		B
		AB
	A	AB
	B	AB
Minor	A	O
	B	O
	AB	A
		B
		O
Bidirectional	A	B
	B	A

Note. Based on information from Daniel-Johnson & Schwartz, 2011.

From "Hematologic Effects" (p. 167), by R.M. Rosselet in S.A. Ezzone (Ed.), *Hematopoietic Stem Cell Transplantation: A Manual for Nursing Practice* (2nd ed.), 2013, Pittsburgh, PA: Oncology Nursing Society. Copyright 2013 by Oncology Nursing Society. Reprinted with permission.

Figure 6-6. Types of ABO Incompatibility and Potential Adverse Effects in Stem Cell Transplantation

Major ABO Incompatibility
- Definition: recipient isoagglutinins (anti-A, anti-B, anti-AB) incompatible with donor red blood cells (RBCs)
- Donor–recipient ABO pairs
  - Group A, B, and AB donor and group O recipient
  - Group AB donor and group A and B recipient
- Potential adverse effects
  - Immediate hemolysis of the RBCs infused with donor marrow (acute hemolytic reaction)
  - Delayed hemolysis of RBCs produced by engrafted marrow
  - Delayed onset of erythropoiesis
  - Pure red cell aplasia

Minor ABO Incompatibility
- Definition: recipient RBCs incompatible with donor isoagglutinins
- Donor–recipient ABO pairs
  - Group O donor and group A, B, or AB recipient
- Potential adverse effects
  - Immediate hemolysis of recipient RBCs by infused marrow
  - Passenger lymphocyte syndrome causing delayed hemolysis

Major and Minor ABO Incompatibility (Bidirectional)
- Definition: combination of both incompatibilities
- Donor–recipient ABO pairs
  - Group A donor and B recipient
  - Group B donor and A recipient
- Potential adverse effects
  - Immediate hemolysis caused by recipient and/or donor
  - Passenger lymphocyte syndrome causing delayed hemolysis

Note. Based on information from Daniel-Johnson & Schwartz, 2011.

From "Hematologic Effects" (p. 168), by R.M. Rosselet in S.A. Ezzone (Ed.), *Hematopoietic Stem Cell Transplantation: A Manual for Nursing Practice* (2nd ed.), 2013, Pittsburgh, PA: Oncology Nursing Society. Copyright 2013 by Oncology Nursing Society. Reprinted with permission.

---

tious or noninfectious; mild, moderate, or severe; and immune related or non–immune related.

    F. Delayed engraftment (greater than 100 days following transplant)

        1. Definition (Chouinard & Finn, 2007; Rosselet, 2013; Wilson & Sylvanus, 2005)

            a) Several terms are used to describe delayed engraftment, such as graft failure, graft rejection, and primary and secondary graft failure.

            b) Primary graft failure for myeloablative bone marrow transplants is defined as a lack of functional hematopoiesis or neutrophil recovery of $500/mm^3$ or greater in recipients who survive more than 28 days following transplantation and who have not received a second transplant procedure.

            c) Secondary graft failure is defined as a decline in neutrophils to $500/mm^3$ or less after achieving engraftment that is unresponsive to growth factors, medications, or infection.

            d) In cord blood transplants, the cutoff point is 42 days.

        2. Pathophysiology

a) The causes of graft failure can be multifactorial. In autologous transplantation, it may be related to several factors such as inadequate volume or quality
of stem cells or damage during the collection procedure or the cryopreservation procedure. In allogeneic bone marrow transplantation, delayed engraftment may result with HLA-mismatched donor bone marrow or T-cell-
depleted marrow. This may be due to the donor's immune system decreasing host-versus-graft immunity.

b) Secondary graft failure occurs after transient hematopoiesis, which can be a
result of myelosuppression due to medications or infections; however, it usually is caused by rejection mediated by immunologic factors.

c) Recipients with an inherited nonmalignancy (i.e., aplastic anemia) have a 10%–
20% chance of developing primary graft failure. In contrast, less than 5% of
recipients with a hematologic malignancy will develop primary graft failure.

3. Management (Chouinard & Finn, 2007; Rosselet, 2013; Wilson & Sylvanus, 2005)

a) Discontinue potential immunosuppressive medications (e.g., ganciclovir,
TMP-SMX).

b) Treat underlying infection.

c) Complete second allogeneic transplant (with or without a conditioning regimen).

d) Administer G-CSFs.

4. Chimerism: Chimerism is a donor–recipient DNA assessment following both
myeloablative conditioning and RIC transplant. It can be performed on peripheral blood or bone marrow and can be predictive of engraftment, GVHD, and
potential for relapse (Riley et al., 2005; Rosselet, 2013).

a) After allogeneic bone marrow transplant with a myeloablative regimen, recovery is signified by CBC at normal levels without transfusions.

b) With nonmyeloablative regimens, it is difficult to distinguish between donor
and host cells by CBC after the allogeneic transplant. For this reason, detection of polymorphic differences between host and donor cells is important.

G. T-cell dysregulation

1. Definition (Mackall et al., 2009; Rosselet, 2013): T-lymphocyte recovery is prolonged from months to years following HSCT.

2. Physiology and pathophysiology (Mackall et al., 2009; Rosselet, 2013)

a) Normal

(1) T lymphocytes play an essential role in immunity. These functions
include inducing delayed-type hypersensitivity, directly killing foreign
invaders, eradicating cancer cells, and assisting B-cell immune response.

(2) T cells are derived from the bone marrow and are a cellular immune
response.

b) Abnormal

(1) Autologous transplant recipients do not develop GVHD because of
T-cell dysregulation. By day 14, circulating natural killer cells are further recovered to their cytotoxic function. In G-CSF–mobilized PBSC
recipients, lymphocytes are present in the graft, which contributes to
the rapid immune recovery. However, T-cell function remains depressed
because of monocyte-dependent T-cell inhibitory response.

(2) In allogeneic recipients following HSCT and the preparative regimen, T
cells increase apoptosis. The functional immune effector T cells recover

more slowly and are further complicated by the initiation of GVHD and the need for immune suppression to treat GVHD. The natural killer cells become the dominant lymphocyte at about four months following transplant. Additionally, the absolute T-cell counts recover gradually over the first 12 months and reach normal levels at approximately nine months following transplantation. Allogeneic recipients are at greater risk for late infections.

  (3) Umbilical cord transplants are associated with a delayed response of recovery, with suppression occurring within the immediate post-transplant period followed by rapid recovery in the next few weeks. However, the functional T lymphocytes may not recover for months to years following umbilical cord transplant.

H. Immune recovery following HSCT (Kang & Chao, 2015; Rosselet, 2013)
 1. The success of the HSCT depends on immune recovery.
 2. The type of graft is a risk factor for lack of immune reconstitution.
 3. Umbilical cord blood and T-cell-depleted haploidentical graft recipients are at greatest risk for lack of immune reconstitution.
 4. The absolute lymphocyte count (ALC) is the primary indicator for HSCT outcomes.
  a) An ALC of 200/mm^3 at day 29 following allogeneic HSCT predicts a relapse probability of 42%.
  b) An ALC of 500/mm^3 at day 17 following allogeneic HSCT predicts a one-year overall survival rate of 79%.
  c) A CD4+ T-cell count greater than the median of 8/mm^3 at day 35 predicts a decreased incidence of mortality related to infection.

V. GI complications
 A. Conditioning regimens used in the HSCT population can have major, acute toxic effects on the GI system. This is due to radiation and chemotherapy agents such as anthracyclines, paclitaxel, etoposide, cytarabine, melphalan, thiotepa, methotrexate, and busulfan. Severe GI effects include oral mucositis, esophagitis, salivary gland dysfunction, xerostomia, nausea and vomiting, diarrhea, abdominal pain, bloating, perineal-rectal skin changes, and altered nutrition. In allogeneic transplant patients, the late or chronic effects in the GI system are related to GVHD. During this time, recipients may experience poor appetite, pain and discomfort, decreased QOL, and a higher incidence of infection. Additionally, these toxic complications may result in increased length of hospital stay and resource needs.
 B. Oral mucositis and dental issues
  1. Definition (Harris, Eilers, Harriman, Cashavelly, & Maxwell, 2008; Lees & Keefe, 2015): Oral mucositis is an inflammatory process and biologic response that is caused by a physical and biologic trauma on the surface of the mucosal lining, oral cavity, or GI tract.
  2. Physiology and pathophysiology (Al-Dasooqi et al., 2013; Antunes et al., 2010; Cloutier, 2010; Dubberke et al., 2010; Ezzone, 2013; Feller et al., 2010; Fulton & Treon, 2007; Harris, Eilers, Cashavelly, Maxwell, & Harriman, 2009; Lees & Keefe, 2015; Nelson, 2015; Peterson, Bensadoun, & Roila, 2011; Polovich et al., 2014; Sonis, 2004, 2007; Stiff, 2001; Treister & Sonis, 2009; Vagliano et al., 2011; Vera-Llonch, Oster, Hagiwara, & Sonis, 2006)

a) Oral mucositis occurs as an inflammatory response of the epithelial cells located in the GI tract from the mouth to the anus. It has been attributed to oxidative stress causing DNA damage and cell death in which the oral mucosa breaks down to form large, painful ulcerations in the mouth. Mucositis can occur throughout the entire GI tract, resulting in esophagitis, nausea and vomiting, watery diarrhea, and abdominal pain. This can lead to electrolyte imbalances, dehydration, and hemorrhage. The loss of the mucosal barrier during the neutropenia period causes an increased risk for systemic infections, which includes streptococcal and enterococcal bacteremia. Chemotherapy-induced signs and symptoms typically begin four to five days following infusion and peak on day 12–14, with acute resolution in two to three weeks following completion of therapy. Severe mucositis lasts an average of seven days; however, the patient may report mouth pain that precedes the ulcerative phase and continues after the resolution of changes. Residual symptoms of xerostomia and anorexia may take weeks to resolve.

b) Five phases of oral mucositis (see Figure 6-7)

Figure 6-7. Pathobiology of Oral Mucositis

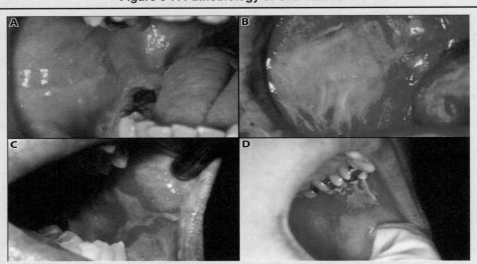

Although the cells and tissues of the submucosa and epithelium respond immediately and robustly to radiation and chemotherapy, the clinical appearance of the mucosa is deceivingly normal during the primary damage phase (**A**). Early superficial changes in the mucosa may be seen during the signaling and amplification phases, but the benign clinical appearance is in stark contrast to the biologic havoc that is taking place beneath the epithelium, which ultimately results in basal cell injury, apoptosis, and death (**B**). The toll of direct and indirect basal cell injury and death is most dramatically manifest by frank ulceration. This is the most symptomatic phase of mucositis and the one that is associated with the major significant adverse health and economic outcomes associated with the condition (**C**). In the majority of cases, signaling from the submucosa to the epithelium results in spontaneous healing (**D**).

Note. From "Pathobiology of Oral Mucositis: Novel Insights and Opportunities," by S.T. Sonis, 2007, *Journal of Supportive Oncology, 5*(9, Suppl. 4), p. 4. Copyright 2007 by Elsevier. Reprinted with permission.

(1) Initiation phase: Chemotherapy or radiation is administered, causing direct DNA damage.

(2) Primary damage response phase: Oral tissue and cells of the submucosa and epithelium respond to radiation and chemotherapy immediately; however, the mucosa appears normal.

(3) Signaling and amplification phase: Changes occur in the mucosa beneath the epithelium, which causes cellular injury and apoptosis (cell death), leading to the beginning of ulcerations.

(4) Ulcerative phase: Pain, edema, and bleeding result from pathogens colonizing oral submucosal tissues because of continued cytokine release from the oral and GI tract tissues. This reduces the normal amount of mucus and saliva, thus increasing permeability of the flow of pathogens into the blood and causing a greater risk for bacteremia infections.

(5) Healing phase: Healing begins with neutrophil recovery and epithelial repair of the mucosa. This phase occurs within two to three weeks after HSCT.

c) Several oral mucositis grading scales have been established and include the World Health Organization (WHO) scale, the Oral Assessment Guide, and the NCI Common Terminology Criteria for Adverse Events clinical scale and functional scale (see Table 6-8). An oral assessment tool assists with consistency in assessment, documentation, and evaluation of the oral cavity for treatment interventions and changes.

d) Mucositis of the GI mucosa can have the same acute complications as oral mucositis: nausea and vomiting, profuse diarrhea, and abdominal pain. Another complication is acute esophagitis, which can cause burning and retrosternal chest pain. During this period, recipients may have other associated causes of symptoms, which must be ruled out for other infectious agents (e.g., fungi, bacteria, protozoa). Additionally, there may be several pathogens evolving, which lead to fever, septicemia, and gastroenteritis.

(1) GI infections related to bacterial pathogens consist of *Giardia*, *Campylobacter*, *Escherichia (E.) coli*, *Pseudomonas*, nontoxigenic *C. difficile*, *Aeromonas*, and VRE. *C. difficile* is the most common pathogen reported. This is because antimicrobial treatment lowers recipients' normal GI flora, causing toxic inflammation of the colon and resulting in diarrhea.

(2) *Candida* occurs during myelosuppression and mucositis of the GI tract. It can be associated with GI yeast colonization, resulting in diarrhea. This may increase the recipient's risk for *Aspergillus* species infection.

(3) Viruses associated with gastroenteritis include pathogens such as adenovirus, rotavirus, and CMV.

(4) In recipients with severe neutropenia, neutropenic enterocolitis (also known as *necrotizing enterocolitis* or *typhlitis*) may lead to a higher risk for morbidity and mortality due to invasion of the mucosa by microorganisms. This diagnosis requires aggressive medical management with antibiotics and supportive care to decrease inflammation and manage symptoms.

3. Clinical features of GI mucositis (Al-Dasooqi et al., 2013; Antunes et al., 2010; Ezzone, 2013; Fulton & Treon, 2007; Lees & Keefe, 2015; Nelson, 2015; Sonis, 2004; Treister & Sonis, 2009; Vagliano et al., 2011)

Table 6-8. Grading Scales for Oral Mucositis	
Scale	**Grading System**
WHO scale	Grade 0—No changes Grade 1—Soreness with erythema Grade 2—Soreness with erythema and ulceration; ability to eat solid foods Grade 3—Soreness with erythema and ulceration; ability to eat liquids Grade 4—Soreness with erythema and ulceration; oral alimentation not possible
NCI CTCAE functional scale	Grade 1—Asymptomatic or mild symptoms; intervention not indicated Grade 2—Moderate pain; not interfering with oral intake; modified diet indicated Grade 3—Severe pain; interfering with oral intake Grade 4—Life-threatening consequences; urgent intervention indicated Grade 5—Death
Oral Assessment Guide	Examine each of the following: • Voice • Swallow • Lips • Tongue • Saliva • Mucous membranes • Gingiva • Teeth or dentures (or denture-bearing area) Assign each category a numeric value: 1 = normal findings; 2 = mild alterations without compromise; and 3 = severe alterations, and add all the scores. The potential total score can range from 8 (normal) to 24 (severe).

NCI CTCAE—National Cancer Institute Common Terminology Criteria for Adverse Events; WHO—World Health Organization

Note. Based on information from Knöös & Östman, 2010; National Cancer Institute Cancer Therapy Evaluation Program, 2010.

a) Etiology: All patients receiving high-dose chemotherapy conditioning regimens, radiation therapy, other myeloablative regimens in HSCT, and simultaneously experiencing myelosuppression

b) History: Risk factors are therapy and recipient related (e.g., chemotherapy agents, TBI, medications) (see Figure 6-8).

c) Signs and symptoms

    (1) Signs and symptoms include oral ulcerations, erythema, pain, edema, and bleeding in the oral cavity. Other symptoms include retrosternal chest pain, burning in the esophagus, nausea and vomiting, diarrhea, bloating, abdominal discomfort, and constipation.

    (2) In necrotizing enterocolitis or typhlitis, signs and symptoms may include nausea, vomiting, abdominal pain (which may progress to rigid abdomen), and fever. If GI perforation occurs, a surgical resection may be indicated if bleeding is uncontrollable.

d) Physical examination

    (1) Inspect the oral cavity for erythema, oral ulceration, and bleeding.

    (2) Assess the abdomen for bowel sounds and rebound tenderness.

e) Laboratory testing

Figure 6-8. Risk Factors for Oral Mucositis

Therapy-Related Risk Factors
- Chemotherapeutic agents—antimetabolites, antitumor antibiotics, alkylating agents, vinca alkaloids, taxanes, epipodophyllotoxins
- Total body irradiation—depending on type, field, total cumulative dose, and treatment schedules
- Graft-versus-host reactions
- Medications—opiates, sedatives, antihistamines, antidepressants, phenothiazines, diuretics
- Prolonged hospitalization—microfloral shift to gram-negative organisms
- Use of broad-spectrum antibiotics—predisposes patients to resistant bacterial and fungal infections
- Prolonged myelosuppression—low absolute granulocyte and platelet counts
- Vomiting—irritation to oral mucosa, loss of proteins and water-soluble vitamins
- Transplanted cell dose less than 3×10^8 nucleated cells/kg body weight

Patient-Related Risk Factors
- Age—younger than 20 years, older than 65 years
- Oral health—poor oral hygiene, history of oral lesions, periodontal disease, dental-related sources of trauma (ill-fitting prosthesis, sharp teeth), preexisting oral/dental infections, inadequate dental restorations, impacted wisdom teeth
- Xerostomia
- Herpes simplex virus (HSV)-positive serology—risk of reactivation is highest in patients with HSV IgG titer greater than 10,000 (ELISA)
- Hematologic malignancy
- Poor nutrition status
- Decreased renal function
- Tobacco use
- Alcohol consumption

ELISA—enzyme-linked immunosorbent assay; IgG—immunoglobulin G

Note. Based on information from Barker, 1999; Berendt & D'Agostino, 2005; Berger & Eilers, 1998; Heimdahl, 1999; Raber-Durlacher, 1999; Wojtaszek, 2000.

From "Gastrointestinal Complications" (p. 174), by S.A. Ezzone in S.A. Ezzone (Ed.), *Hematopoietic Stem Cell Transplantation: A Manual for Nursing Practice* (2nd ed.), 2013, Pittsburgh, PA: Oncology Nursing Society. Copyright 2013 by Oncology Nursing Society. Reprinted with permission.

---

    (1) Culture of oral mucosa

    (2) Stool specimen to rule out *C. difficile* or other infectious etiologies

    (3) Abdominal imaging with ultrasound with or without CT scan (if patient is experiencing severe abdominal pain that is unexplained by routine x-ray)

4. Differential diagnosis (Ezzone, 2013)

    a) HSV in recipients who are seropositive for HSV immunoglobulin G titer greater than 10,000 enzyme-linked immunosorbent assay, which increases the risk for reactivation

    b) Pathogens such as *C. difficile, Aspergillus, Candida, Giardia, Campylobacter, E. coli, Pseudomonas,* nontoxigenic *C. difficile, Aeromonas,* and neutropenic enterocolitis (typhlitis)

5. Treatment of GI mucositis (Antunes et al., 2010; Ezzone, 2013; Fulton & Treon, 2007; Harris et al., 2009; Lees & Keefe, 2015; McGuire et al., 2013; Mori & Kato, 2010; Nelson, 2015; Rodriguez & Gobel, 2011; Sonis, 2004, 2007; Tomblyn et al., 2009; Treister & Sonis, 2009; Vagliano et al., 2011)

    a) The mainstay of treatment is managing pain in HSCT recipients with GI mucositis. Esophageal mucositis may require additional medications, such as H_2 receptor blockers and proton pump inhibitors, to prevent pain and possible hemorrhage. Antibiotics may be indicated in recipients with fever, sepsis, or gastroenteritis.

  b) An oral care regimen is used to reduce mucosal biofilm accumulation, remove debris and microorganisms, decrease inflammation, and reduce pain. Other treatments include viscous lidocaine and magic mouthwash, which reduce pain and coat mucosal surfaces.

   (1) Generally, it is recommended that recipients with severe oral mucositis perform oral care more frequently throughout the day.

   (a) Pain management for oral mucositis includes frequent assessments using an appropriate grading scale for caregiver consistency and opioids (PO or IV).

   (b) Recipients with moderate to severe mucositis may require opioids as a continuous infusion and patient-controlled analgesia dosing for up to seven days or more depending on neutrophil recovery and resolution of inflammation, edema, and ulcerations.

   (2) Recipients may use a soft toothbrush to brush gently with mild tartar-control fluorinated toothpaste twice daily to remove gingival inflammation and decrease bacteria in the oral cavity.

   (3) Gentle flossing is encouraged to all recipients except those with thrombocytopenia.

   (4) Bland rinses such as normal saline, sodium bicarbonate, or both combined are encouraged in the oral care regimen.

   (5) It is recommended that all recipients receive a dental evaluation prior to their HSCT to treat existing and potential infections, if necessary. Dental cavities should be restored or extracted (if not restorable) with a minimum of 10–14 days for healing and infection to resolve prior to HSCT.

  c) Biopsy may be indicated to rule out other pathogens for lesions not responding to current therapy.

  d) Interventions

   (1) Monitor recipients' adherence to treatment.

   (2) Note changes in oral intake (hydration and nutrition).

   (3) Assess recipients' pattern and integrity of mucositis.

   (4) Assess the oral cavity frequently for changes.

   (5) Recommend cryotherapy in patients who receive melphalan to prevent mucositis.

 6. Patient education: Educate patients and their family members to report signs and symptoms promptly, such as increased temperature (greater than 38°C [100.4°F]), changes in nutritional intake, and pain not relieved by current measures. Patients and family members also should be educated on the oral care regimen and the importance of adequate hydration and high protein intake for mucosal repair.

C. Salivary gland dysfunction and xerostomia

 1. Definition (Davies & Hall, 2011; Ezzone, 2013; Furness, Bryan, McMillan, Birchenough, & Worthington, 2013; Hall, 2010; Macpherson, 2013; McMillian, 2013; Nelson, 2015; Radvansky, Pace, & Siddiqui, 2013; Rieger, 2012): Xerostomia is the subjective report of dry mouth in recipients receiving conditioning regimens with chemotherapy agents or radiation therapy, thus compromising the composition and flow of saliva.

2. Physiology and pathophysiology (Ezzone, 2013; Furness et al., 2013; Hall, 2010; Macpherson, 2013; McMillian, 2013; Nelson, 2015; Radvansky et al., 2013; Rieger, 2012)
   a) Normal
      (1) Salivary glands produce approximately one liter of fluid in the oral cavity per day to enhance speech, remove food residue from teeth and gingiva, enhance taste, and lubricate the mouth.
      (2) Other substances in saliva promote wound healing, tissue growth, and epidermal growth factors, such as antibacterial, antifungal, and antiviral agents, to balance oral flora and prevent infections.
   b) The toxicities of chemotherapy or radiation therapy cause saliva volume, consistency, and pH levels to become altered and secretions to become thick, tenacious, and more acidic. These changes increase mouth bacteria that adhere to the teeth, leading to tooth caries.
   c) Recipients are at increased risk for *Candida* infections, and antifungal prophylaxis should be initiated.
3. Clinical features (Ezzone, 2013; Furness et al., 2013; Hall, 2010; Macpherson, 2013; McMillian, 2013; Nelson, 2015; Radvansky et al., 2013; Rieger, 2012)
   a) Etiology
      (1) Salivary gland dysfunction and xerostomia are generally treatment related in HSCT recipients.
      (2) Other drugs contributing to altered salivary function and xerostomia are antihistamines, decongestants, anticholinergics, diuretics, antidepressants, and opioids.
      (3) Several factors may contribute to the severity (e.g., mouth breathing, GVHD).
      (4) Xerostomia occurs 7–10 days following the conditioning regimen treatment and may continue for up to several months in transplant recipients.
   b) History
      (1) Previous chemotherapy or radiation therapy
      (2) Prescription and nonprescription medications
      (3) Previous or current history of xerostomia
      (4) Effect on recipient's taste, intake, or swallowing
   c) Signs and symptoms
      (1) Mouth dryness or mouth pain
      (2) Difficulty talking, swallowing, or eating
      (3) Dysgeusia or altered taste
      (4) Halitosis
   d) Physical examination
      (1) Assess for the following:
         (a) Dry, shiny mucous membranes in the mouth
         (b) Erythema
         (c) Presence of thick, ropy saliva
         (d) Debris on teeth, gums, mucosa, and tongue
         (e) Bleeding
         (f) Fever
         (g) Ability to swallow

(2) Assess nutritional status.

(3) Ascertain the patient's level of pain using an organization-approved scale.

4. Diagnostic tests (Schelenz et al., 2011): Culture any oral lesions if present.

5. Treatment (Ezzone, 2013; Furness et al., 2013; Hall, 2010; Macpherson, 2013; McMillian, 2013; Nelson, 2015; Radvansky et al., 2013; Rieger, 2012): The mainstay of treatment for altered salivary gland function and xerostomia is alleviation of symptoms with strategies such as frequent self-suctioning, bland mouth rinses, frequent sips of fluid, and artificial saliva substitutes.

6. Patient education

a) Educate recipients on performing oral hygiene at least four times daily: after each meal and at bedtime. For example, brushing with a soft toothbrush or rinsing dentures after each meal, using fluorinated toothpaste, and flossing (if not thrombocytopenic).

b) Educate recipients on promoting mucous membrane moisture by using a bland rinse, keeping water at the bedside, applying a lip moisturizer, and sucking on ice chips.

c) Educate recipients on avoiding food or liquids with high sugar content. Provide recipients with a list of high-protein foods to enhance nutrition and healing.

D. Taste changes

1. Definition (Boer, Correa, Miranda, & de Souza, 2010; Ezzone, 2013): An actual or recipient-perceived change in taste sensation. Taste change can be defined as any of the following:

a) Hypogeusia: A decrease in the acuity of taste sensation experience

b) Dysgeusia: An unusual perception in taste, which is perceived as unpleasant

c) Ageusia: An absence of the entire taste sensation experience

2. Physiology and pathophysiology (Boer et al., 2010; Ezzone, 2013)

a) Taste changes occur in association with conditioning regimens (i.e., chemotherapy, radiation therapy), stomatitis, xerostomia, malnutrition (i.e., deficiencies in zinc, copper, niacin, vitamin A), and myelosuppression.

b) Toxicity can occur in recipients' taste receptors, causing hypogeusia, dysgeusia, or ageusia.

c) In HSCT recipients, taste alterations may persist for up to three years and may not be associated with GVHD.

3. Clinical features (Boer et al., 2010; Cope, 2015; Ezzone, 2013)

a) Etiology: Specific chemotherapy drugs may affect taste more frequently than others, such as cisplatin, cyclophosphamide, dactinomycin, methotrexate, vincristine, and 5-fluorouracil.

b) History

(1) Recipient complaints of changes in taste

(2) Presence of hypogeusia, dysgeusia, or ageusia

c) Signs and symptoms

(1) Poor oral intake

(2) Weight loss

(3) Poor appetite

d) Physical examination

(1) Perform an oral assessment to evaluate oral cavity for presence of dryness, erythema, or ulcerations.

(2) Examine for signs and symptoms of secondary oral infection.

(3) Monitor for weight changes.

(4) Assess for altered food and liquid intake.

4. Diagnostic tests (Cope, 2015; Ezzone, 2013): Evaluate for abnormal laboratory values such as decreased albumin, zinc, niacin, and vitamin A levels.

5. Treatment (Cope, 2015; Ezzone, 2013): The mainstay of treatment for symptom management includes performing frequent oral care; using saliva substitutes; sucking on hard candy; eating small, frequent meals; and avoiding foods high in fat and with unpleasant sight and smell factors.

6. Patient education: Educate recipients to perform diligent oral care and inspection of the oral cavity.

E. Nausea and vomiting

1. Definition (Ezzone, 2013; Hawkins & Grunberg, 2009; Hesketh, 2008; Lees & Keefe, 2015; Nelson, 2015)

a) Nausea is a subjective, unobservable phenomenon that stems from an unpleasant feeling in the throat, esophagus, or abdomen with an inclination to vomit. Other symptoms associated with nausea include increased salivation, tachycardia, and swallowing.

b) Vomiting is a somatic experience performed by the muscles of the respiratory tract, which causes a forceful oral explosion of gastric contents through the mouth.

c) Nausea and vomiting may occur with high-dose chemotherapy regimens in conjunction with or without TBI prior to HSCT.

2. Pathophysiology (Ezzone, 2013; Hawkins & Grunberg, 2009; Hesketh, 2008; Lees & Keefe, 2015; Nelson, 2015)

a) The mechanism involved is due to the effects on the midbrain vomiting center and direct toxicity to the GI mucosa.

b) Several proposed mechanisms for acute, delayed, and anticipatory chemotherapy-induced nausea and vomiting (CINV) are as follows (see Table 6-9):

Table 6-9. Patterns and Mechanisms of Chemotherapy-Induced Vomiting

Type of Emesis	Onset and Duration	Proposed Mechanisms
Acute	0–24 hours after chemotherapy	Release of $5\text{-}HT_3$ from enterochromaffin cells in gastrointestinal tract (and probably areas in the brain)
Delayed	From about 24 hours after chemotherapy lasting up to 7 or more days	Substance P thought to be involved
Anticipatory	Before chemotherapy	A conditioned response to poor emetic control with prior chemotherapy

$5\text{-}HT_3$—5-hydroxytryptamine-3

Note. From "Gastrointestinal Complications of Hematopoietic Stem Cell Transplantation" (p. 482), by J. Lees and D.M. Keefe in J.R. Wingard, D.A. Gastineau, H.L. Leather, E.L. Snyder, and Z.M. Szczepiorkowski (Eds.), *Hematopoietic Stem Cell Transplantation: A Handbook for Clinicians* (2nd ed.), 2015, Bethesda, MD: AABB. Copyright 2015 by AABB. Reprinted with permission.

(1) Acute CINV occurs 0–24 hours after the beginning the conditioning regimen with the release of 5-HT$_3$ from enterochromaffin cells in the GI mucosa and areas of the brain.

(2) Delayed CINV occurs from 24 hours up to one week following the conditioning regimen and is related to substance P.

(3) Anticipatory CINV occurs prior to chemotherapy administration and is a conditioned response to poor emetic control from past chemotherapy experiences.

(4) Acute nausea and vomiting peaks during the first 48 hours following fractionated TBI and declines as treatment proceeds.

(5) Nausea and vomiting in HSCT recipients sometimes will occur with a delayed onset. It also can occur weeks later and may be a result of the rate of gastric emptying.

(6) GVHD must be considered in allogeneic transplant recipients.

3. Clinical features (Ezzone, 2013; Hawkins & Grunberg, 2009; Hesketh, 2008; Lees & Keefe, 2015; Nelson, 2015)

  a) Etiology

  (1) In recipients receiving high-dose conditioning regimens prior to HSCT, the toxic effects activate the vomiting center located in the lateral reticular formation of the medulla. This triggers the visceral and vagal nerve pathways from the GI tract, the chemoreceptor zone, the vestibular apparatus, and the cerebral cortex (see Table 6-10).

  (2) As a result of the toxic effects damaging the enterochromaffin cells in the GI mucosa, 5-HT$_3$ receptors are activated, causing impulses to increase heart rate, respiratory rate, and saliva to cause CINV.

  b) History

  (1) Presence of risk factors for vomiting include age, gender, alcohol intake, motion sickness, and anxiety.

  (2) Current symptoms

  (3) Patterns of nausea and vomiting (onset, frequency, precipitating factors, aggravating factors, and alleviating factors)

  c) Signs and symptoms

  (1) Sweating

  (2) Tachycardia

  (3) Increased respiratory rate

  (4) Dizziness

  (5) Pallor

  (6) Excessive salivation

  (7) Increased blood pressure

  d) Physical examination

  (1) Assess for the following:

     (a) Diaphoresis

     (b) Tachycardia

     (c) Pallor

     (d) Increased salivation

     (e) Dizziness

     (f) Weakness

  (2) Assess nutritional status, including hydration.

Table 6-10. Emetic Risk for Single Intravenous Chemotherapy Agents of Potential Use in Hematopoietic Stem Cell Transplantation Setting

Emetic Risk	Chemotherapeutic Agent
High (> 90% of patients)	Carmustine Cyclophosphamide ≥ 1,500 mg/m² Dacarbazine
Moderate (30%–90% of patients)	Busulfan (> 4 mg/day) Carboplatin Cyclophosphamide < 1,500 mg/m² Cytarabine > 1,000 mg/m² Ifosfamide Melphalan*
Low (10%–30% of patients)	Cytarabine < 1,000 mg/m² Etoposide Paclitaxel
Minimal (< 10% of patients)	Busulfan (< 4 mg/day) Fludarabine Rituximab

* High-dose melphalan usually is considered highly emetogenic.

Note. From "Gastrointestinal Complications of Hematopoietic Stem Cell Transplantation" (p. 483), by J. Lees and D.M. Keefe in J.R. Wingard, D.A. Gastineau, H.L. Leather, E.L. Snyder, and Z.M. Szczepiorkowski (Eds.), *Hematopoietic Stem Cell Transplantation: A Handbook for Clinicians* (2nd ed.), 2015, Bethesda, MD: AABB. Copyright 2015 by AABB. Reprinted with permission.

    (3) Assess intake and output.

    (4) Monitor blood pressure, which includes orthostatic readings.

    (5) Additional assessments include skin turgor, vital signs, cardiac regularity, blood in emesis secondary to thrombocytopenia, and aspiration pneumonia.

4. Diagnostic tests (Ezzone, 2013; Nelson, 2015): Assess electrolyte levels and kidney function studies frequently, such as potassium, magnesium, chloride, blood urea nitrogen, creatinine, and hydrogen.

5. Differential diagnosis (Nelson, 2015; Sonis, Treister, Lees, & Keefe, 2009)

    a) Intracranial bleeding

    b) Infection

    c) Obstruction (bowel, bladder, gallbladder)

    d) Medications

6. Treatment (Ezzone, 2013; Hawkins & Grunberg, 2009; Hesketh, 2008; Nelson, 2015; Sonis et al., 2009)

    a) The mainstay of treatment includes prophylactic antiemetics, acid-reducing agents, and anxiolytics prescribed based on the recipient's previous experiences and conditioning regimen.

    b) Treatment for acute, delayed, and anticipatory nausea or vomiting includes a variety of antiemetic medications.

    c) Assess the recipient's ongoing responses to therapy—pharmacologic and nonpharmacologic—which may need to be modified.

    d) Dietary modifications are helpful in recipients with delayed nausea and vomiting.

7. Patient education

    a) Educate recipients on specific side effects of antiemetic medications.

    b) Advise recipients to avoid spicy, greasy, or fatty foods and concentrated sweets.

    c) Explain to recipients that cold foods and dry toast may be more tolerable.

    d) Educate recipients to notify caregiver immediately if experiencing nausea or vomiting and presence of coffee-ground vomitus or blood in vomit.

    e) Emphasize the need for adequate hydration to prevent nausea and vomiting and replace fluid loss (to prevent dehydration).

F. Diarrhea

1. Definition (Coleman, 2010; Ezzone, 2013; Kuck & Ricciardi, 2005; Muehlbauer et al., 2009; Nelson, 2015; Shaw & Taylor, 2012; Sonis et al., 2009): Diarrhea is the presence of an increase of four or more loose or watery stools than normal, with or without nocturnal bowel movements or abdominal cramping.

2. Physiology and pathophysiology (Ezzone, 2013; Muehlbauer et al., 2009; Nelson, 2015; Shaw & Taylor, 2012; Sonis et al., 2009)

    a) Normal

        (1) Bowel movements constitute a balance between oral intake, GI secretions, metabolism, and fluid reabsorption.

        (2) Normality of bowel movements can vary between three times daily to once every three days.

        (3) Diarrhea or abdominal bloating and discomfort are common side effects following the conditioning regimen in HSCT recipients and generally resolve approximately three weeks following transplantation.

    b) The most common types of diarrhea following the conditioning regimen include secretory, osmotic, and infectious components and are directly related to villous atrophy, excessive mucous secretion, and alteration in functioning of the gut brush border enzymes (see Table 6-11).

    c) Diarrhea mechanisms related to HSCT

        (1) Early-onset diarrhea is due to the underlying villous atrophy, excess mucous secretions, and an alteration in functioning of the gut brush border enzymes, which is known as *regimen-related diarrhea*.

        (2) Delayed-onset diarrhea is related to leaky tight junctions allowing bacterial translocation and is associated with *C. difficile* or *E. coli*.

        (3) Targeted therapies, such as interferon and interleukin-2, inhibit epidermal growth factor receptors and also may cause diarrhea. Other drugs associated with the development of diarrhea include antacids, laxatives, and antibiotics.

        (4) Radiation therapy also contributes to severe diarrhea in transplant recipients.

3. Clinical features (Coleman, 2010; Ezzone, 2013; Hall, 2010; Muehlbauer et al., 2009; NCI CTEP, 2010; Nelson, 2015; Shaw & Taylor, 2012; Sonis et al., 2009)

    a) Etiology: Disease or treatment related

    b) History

        (1) Previous and current chemotherapy conditioning regimen or radiation therapy

Table 6-11. Types and Causes of Diarrhea	
Type of Diarrhea	**Causes**
Secretory	• Inhibition of mucosal absorption or overstimulation of secretion of fluid and electrolytes • Intestinal inflammation or bacterial enterotoxins • Mucositis • Graft-versus-host disease
Exudative	• Excessive blood, serum protein, and mucus in the intestine from inflammation, ulceration, and a loss of functional intestinal mucosa • Radiation therapy • Neutropenic enterocolitis • Infections
Osmotic	• Excessive amount of water entering the bowel because of the ingestion of nonabsorbable solutes or hyperosmolar substances, such as blood, enteral feedings, or sorbitol that retard fluid absorption
Malabsorptive	• Malabsorption of solutes • Lactose insufficiency
Dysmotility	• Caused from dysfunctional intestinal motility resulting in an abnormally rapid transit time • Peristaltic stimulants • Fecal impaction or ileus

Note. Based on information from Coleman, 2010; Engelking, 1998; Hogan, 1998; Ippoliti, 1998.

From "Gastrointestinal Complications" (p. 182), by S.A. Ezzone in S.A. Ezzone (Ed.), *Hematopoietic Stem Cell Transplantation: A Manual for Nursing Practice* (2nd ed.), 2013, Pittsburgh, PA: Oncology Nursing Society. Copyright 2013 by Oncology Nursing Society. Reprinted with permission.

    (2) Usual bowel pattern
    (3) Known food or medication intolerances
    (4) Dietary changes that may increase bowel frequency (e.g., high-fiber foods, fruit juices, coffee, alcohol, fried or fatty foods)
  c) Signs and symptoms: NCI has developed a toxicity scale for grading the severity of the diarrhea (see Table 6-12).
  d) Physical examination
    (1) Assess for hyperactive bowel sounds and perineal skin irritation.
    (2) Monitor for the following and document the information in the medical record:
      (a) Vital signs
      (b) Skin turgor
      (c) Dry mucous membranes
      (d) Blood pressure
      (e) Orthostatic hypotension
      (f) Tachycardia
      (g) Number and consistency of diarrhea stools per day
      (h) Elevated temperature (infection)
    (3) Monitor for signs and symptoms of blood loss and hemorrhage.

Table 6-12. Common Terminology Criteria for Adverse Events Grading of Diarrhea	
Grade	**Description**
1	Increase of < 4 stools per day over baseline; mild increase in ostomy output compared to baseline
2	Increase of 4–6 stools per day over baseline; moderate increase in ostomy output compared to baseline
3	Increase of ≥ 7 stools per day over baseline; incontinence; hospitalization indicated; severe increase in ostomy output compared to baseline; limiting self-care ADL
4	Life-threatening consequences; urgent intervention indicated
5	Death

ADL—activities of daily living

Note. From *Common Terminology Criteria for Adverse Events* [v.4.03], by National Cancer Institute Cancer Therapy Evaluation Program, 2010. Retrieved from http://evs.nci.nih.gov/ftp1/CTCAE/CTCAE_4.03_2010-06-14_QuickReference_5x7.pdf.

4. Diagnostic tests (Ezzone, 2013; Nelson, 2015)
    a) Laboratory
        (1) Serum chemistry panels, including creatinine, to identify electrolyte abnormalities such as potassium, magnesium, sodium, and calcium alterations.
        (2) Albumin levels to assess protein loss, which may affect therapeutic levels of certain medications
        (3) CBC to evaluate presence of neutropenia, hematocrit, and platelet levels
        (4) Stool analysis for electrolytes, infectious pathogens (i.e., bacterial, viral, or fungi), and occult blood
    b) Diagnostic
        (1) Endoscopic procedure and examination to include biopsies, brushings, and cultures, if necessary, to determine differential diagnosis
        (2) CT scans to evaluate for possible bowel perforation, obstruction, paralytic ileus, and neutropenic enterocolitis
5. Differential diagnosis
    a) Chemotherapy-induced neutropenic enterocolitis or typhlitis
    b) GVHD
    c) Irritable bowel syndrome or Crohn disease
6. Treatment (Ezzone, 2013; Muehlbauer et al., 2009; NCI CTEP, 2010; Nelson, 2015; Shaw & Taylor, 2012; Sonis et al., 2009): The mainstay of treatment is adequate assessments and fluid and electrolyte replacements as needed.
    a) Antidiarrheal medications such as loperamide
    b) Possible modification of therapy if severe diarrhea
    c) Treatment associated with *C. difficile*, *E. coli*, or GVHD
    d) Bowel rest encouraged with severe diarrhea
7. Patient education
    a) Educate recipients to report number of diarrhea stools per day.
    b) Educate recipients on dietary modifications to minimize diarrhea.

      c) Educate recipients on signs and symptoms related to complications of diarrhea, such as weakness, dizziness, or heart palpitations.

      d) Educate recipients on the importance of a perineal hygiene program, which includes cleaning the perineal area and applying a barrier cream.

      e) Educate recipients on the importance of prompt reporting of diarrhea, especially if severe, frothy, or foul-smelling, as the diarrhea may be infectious.

      f) Educate recipients on the importance of checking stools for *C. difficile* before taking antidiarrheal medications and not exceeding the recommended amount of antidiarrheal medications per day.

G. Perineal-rectal skin alterations

  1. Definition (Coleman, 2010; Ezzone, 2013; Haas, 2011; Haisfield-Wolfe & Rund, 2000): The skin provides a protective barrier and is the first line of defense from infectious organisms. The perineal-rectal skin region is considered the area between the vulva and anus in females and between the scrotum and anus in males.

  2. Physiology and pathophysiology (Coleman, 2010; Ezzone, 2013; Haas, 2011; Haisfield-Wolfe & Rund, 2000)

      a) HSCT recipients may experience perineal-rectal skin alterations as a direct result of the toxic effects of the high-dose conditioning regimen and associated diarrhea.

      b) High-dose chemotherapy and radiation therapy from the conditioning regimen causes interference of the mitotic reproduction in the basal membrane, resulting in epidermal thinning, changes to skin pigmentation, fibrosis of skin dermis, and hypersensitivity of the skin area.

      c) Diarrhea associated with the conditioning regimen and the frequent use of cleansing agents may lead to skin integrity impairment.

      d) Because of the anatomic environment in which moisture resides, the risk is increased for skin friction, permeability, and infectious pathogens.

  3. Clinical features (Coleman, 2010; Ezzone, 2013; Haas, 2011; Haisfield-Wolfe & Rund, 2000)

      a) Etiology

        (1) Increased moisture, cleansing agents, chemotherapy agents, and radiation therapy

        (2) Baseline hemorrhoids are an important component of the physical assessment, as hemorrhoids place patients at significant risk for infection, bleeding, and pain.

      b) History: Recent conditioning regimen for HSCT and associated diarrhea

      c) Signs and symptoms

        (1) Erythema: Warm pink or red skin and swelling (initial symptom)

        (2) Dry, flaking, and peeling of skin with accompanying pruritus as erythema resolves

        (3) Moist desquamation in which the entire epithelium is destroyed, exposing nerve endings in the dermis and causing increased pain and discomfort (final symptom)

      d) Physical examination: Assess for dry and moist desquamation.

        (1) Dry desquamation: Scaling, flaking, pruritus, and increased reports of pain and discomfort

        (2) Moist desquamation: Increased erythema, sloughing of the skin, exudate on the skin surface

4. Diagnostic tests (Ezzone, 2013): Obtain cultures to evaluate for the presence of HSV infection.

5. Treatment (Coleman, 2010; Ezzone, 2013; Haas, 2011; Haisfield-Wolfe & Rund, 2000): Treatment of perineal-rectal skin impairment is targeted to routine skin care management and infection prevention following HSCT conditioning regimens and during diarrheal episodes.

   a) Dry desquamation

      (1) Cleanse area with tepid water or mild soap.

      (2) Apply barrier cream.

      (3) For pruritus symptoms, apply antihistamine cream.

      (4) Consider pain medications or antihistamines.

      (5) Assess for fungal infection and provide antifungal medications if needed.

      (6) Provide perineal-rectal area care at least twice daily or after each bowel movement.

   b) Moist desquamation

      (1) Consider warm baths or showers.

      (2) Cleanse area with mild soap or wound cleanser.

      (3) Apply moisture barrier.

      (4) Consider pain medications.

      (5) If area worsens, notify physician, obtain wound consult, or apply hydrogel.

      (6) Provide perineal-rectal area care at least twice daily or after each bowel movement.

6. Patient education

   a) Educate recipients on the importance of routine skin care management and infection prevention measures.

   b) Educate recipients to notify the nurse of any worsening symptoms or increased pain.

VI. Disease relapse and advance care planning

   A. HSCT is an established curative treatment modality in many malignant and nonmalignant hematologic disorders. The intent of HSCT is to eradicate disease, but the disease will sometimes relapse or secondary malignancies will develop. Numerous approaches have been employed to treat relapse and secondary malignancies; however, patient prognosis is poor if this occurs (Shannon, 2013). Given the substantial risks of life-threatening short- and intermediate-term complications of relapse and secondary malignancies, practitioners should consider exploring options and strategies for advance care planning (ACP) and end-of-life (EOL) decision making and palliative care. Examples of these might include designation of a healthcare proxy, completion of a living will, preparation of an estate will, and conversations with loved ones and healthcare providers about the patient's wishes in various circumstances (Joffe, Mello, Cook, & Lee, 2007).

   B. Disease relapse and secondary malignancies: HSCT has established itself as an effective therapy for malignant and nonmalignant hematologic diseases. In some cases, such as mantle cell lymphoma and multiple myeloma, the purpose of AHSCT is to lengthen the period of remission and postpone relapse (Shannon, 2013). In other conditions, AHSCT has a curative intent. Unfortunately, relapse continues to be the most common cause of failure following AHSCT. For those who do relapse, approximately 75% relapse within one year and more than 95% relapse within the first three years after AHSCT. The prognosis for patients who relapse following AHSCT is poor (Freytes & Lazarus, 2009), and several approaches have been investigated to improve outcomes following disease relapse.

1. Relapse following AHSCT
   a) Approaches to decrease rate of relapse and improve results following AHSCT (Shannon, 2013)
      (1) Recognizing patients who are eligible for AHSCT and executing AHSCT earlier in the course of the disease could possibly reduce drug resistance and diminish stem cell exposure to changes associated with prior therapies.
      (2) Patients with chemosensitive and minimal residual disease demonstrate the most favorable responses.
      (3) Superior and intensified preparative regimens improve the likelihood that high-dose chemotherapy will eliminate the disease; therefore, stem cells should be harvested when a matched related donor is available.
      (4) In vivo and ex vivo purging may reduce the likelihood of stem cell product contamination with tumor cells.
   b) Clinical trials investigating approaches to avoid relapse following AHSCT are ongoing. Areas being explored include the following:
      (1) Novel conditioning agents such as radioimmunoconjugates
      (2) In vivo and ex vivo autograft purging
      (3) Post-AHSCT maintenance therapy
      (4) Involved-field radiation therapy
      (5) Immunologic interventions employing cytokines and cellular therapy (Laport & Negrin, 2009)
   c) Freytes and Lazarus (2009) conducted a literature review of patients with lymphoma who relapsed more than one year following AHSCT. They concluded that these patients may derive benefit from a reduced-intensity allo-HSCT if they meet the following criteria:
      (1) Availability of donors who are HLA compatible
      (2) Good performance status
      (3) Chemosensitive disease
2. Relapse following allo-HSCT
   a) Disease and disease stage are strong predictors for relapse following allo-HSCT.
   b) When relapse occurs, disease is present in host cells. This may be a result of an inadequate conditioning therapy, graft failure, or the absence of GVHD.
   c) Treatment strategies for relapsed disease (Freytes & Lazarus, 2009)
      (1) Withdrawal of immunosuppression to elicit a graft-versus-tumor effect
         (a) Although high response rates using this approach have been reported in chronic-phase chronic myeloid leukemia (CML), this tactic has been less successful in advanced CML and acute leukemias.
         (b) The chance of patients developing severe GVHD is increased.
      (2) DLI
         (a) DLI is studied extensively in CML.
         (b) Long-term survival rates of 60%–90% have been reported.

(3) Second myeloablative or reduced-intensity HSCT followed by second allo-HSCT bears a considerable possibility of treatment-related mortality and should be executed in the setting of a clinical trial.

(4) Clinical trials examining cellular adoptive immunotherapy, ex vivo–activated T cells (activated DLI), cytokine-induced killer cells, natural killer cells, and antigen-specific cytotoxic T lymphocytes are ongoing. These interventions strive to exploit the potent therapeutic benefits of the donor's immune system to eradicate residual host tumor (Laport & Negrin, 2009).

(5) Patients who relapse and are ineligible for a clinical trial may decline further therapy. In these circumstances, supportive and palliative care alternatives should be provided so that patients and their families may make informed decisions regarding EOL care.

3. Secondary malignancies
   a) Receiving cancer therapy is associated with the development of secondary malignancies.
   b) Bhatia et al. (2005) reported that AHSCT survivors have a 12-fold chance for late deaths related to development of secondary malignancies when compared to the general population. A later report from the same study noted that allo-HSCT survivors have a 3.5-fold increased threat for late deaths caused by development of secondary malignancies, when compared to the general population (Bhatia et al., 2007).
   c) Secondary malignancies are classified into three distinct groups.
      (1) MDS and AML
      (2) PTLDs
      (3) Second solid malignancies

4. MDS and AML (Bhatia et al., 2005)
   a) Therapy-related MDS (t-MDS) and AML (t-AML) occur in 5%–15% of AHSCT survivors and usually develop within two to five years following transplant.
   b) T-MDS and t-AML are rare in the allo-HSCT setting.
   c) WHO describes two classifications of t-MDS and t-AML (Swerdlow et al., 2008).
      (1) Alkylating agent/radiation-related MDS and AML typically occur four to seven years following exposure. Approximately two-thirds of the affected population present with MDS, whereas the rest develop AML with myelodysplastic features. A high incidence of abnormalities involving chromosomes 5 (–5/del[5q]) and 7 (–7/del[7q]) has been demonstrated.
      (2) Topoisomerase II inhibitor–related AML usually appears two to three years after exposure. It does not have a preceding myelodysplastic phase and presents as overt acute leukemia, often with a prominent monocytic component. This often is associated with balanced translocations involving chromosome bands 11q23 or 21q22.
   d) Post-AHSCT t-MDS has a poor prognosis. When patients are treated with conventional chemotherapy, median survival is predicted at six months.

5. PTLDs (Bhatia et al., 2005)

a) PTLDs are an aggressive and potentially fatal proliferation of lymphoid cells of donor origin that usually occur within the first year after allo-HSCT. They are strongly associated with EBV.

b) WHO (Swerdlow et al., 2008) has identified four basic histologic categories of PTLD and has classified them into distinct categories.

   (1) Early lesions, such as reactive lymphoplasmacytic hyperplasia and infectious mononucleosis–like lesions

   (2) Polymorphic PTLD (P-PTLD)

   (3) Monomorphic PTLD (M-PTLD)

   (4) Classical Hodgkin lymphoma

c) Treatment for PTLDs (Bhatia et al., 2005)

   (1) Type 1 PTLDs often require no intervention and are self-limiting. Withdrawal of immunosuppression may be considered.

   (2) Type 2 P-PTLDs typically arise within the first six months following allo-HSCT. Reduction of immunosuppression often is required but has demonstrated variable responses.

   (3) Type 3 M-PTLDs may continue to develop five or more years following transplant. The most common type is diffuse large B-cell lymphoma. Treatment includes reduction of immunosuppression and, often, chemotherapy.

   (4) Type 4 PTLDs, or classical Hodgkin lymphoma, develop at least 2.5 years post-transplant and have a fairly good prognosis if treated with aggressive chemotherapy.

d) For allo-HSCT recipients who are at risk for developing PTLD, sequential blood samples should be obtained for measurement of EBV load by quantitative polymerase chain reaction–based assays for at least the first six months following transplant.

e) If EBV titers rise above a certain level, preemptive therapy is initiated with the anti-CD20 monoclonal antibody rituximab. Clinical trials are needed to identify and refine treatment options for HSCT recipients.

6. Second solid malignancies (Bhatia et al., 2005)

  a) Described in both the AHSCT and allo-HSCT setting

  b) Risk is higher among those surviving 10 years or more, with a reported incidence 8.3 times higher than in the general population. This may be reduced in the setting of RIC regimens or in those that use very little or no radiation.

  c) Squamous cell carcinomas occur most frequently and are associated with chronic GVHD and male sex.

  d) Nonsquamous cell carcinomas are strongly linked to radiation-containing conditioning regimens received at an early age. Other solid tumors often associated with radiation include melanoma and cancers of the oral cavity, salivary glands, brain, liver, uterine cervix, thyroid, breast, bone, and connective tissue.

  e) Treatment should consist of the best available therapy for that tumor.

C. ACP and EOL considerations

1. The assertive nature of hematologic malignancies and HSCT has a powerful effect on patients and families (Kasberg, Brister, & Barnard, 2011).

2. The field of HSCT has made promising improvements in recent years, and overall success rates have been steadily rising, as novel therapies emerge and advances in supportive care improve overall survival and cure rates.

3. Nevertheless, high-dose therapy is associated with mortality risk (Chung, Lyckholm, & Smith, 2009). The need for ACP and EOL care becomes more apparent when treatment focus shifts from cure to palliation.

4. Given the considerable risks of serious short- and intermediate-term complications, ACP is particularly pertinent for patients contemplating HSCT (Joffe et al., 2007).

5. Fundamentals of ACP
   a) Designation of a healthcare proxy
   b) Completion of a living will
   c) Preparation of an estate will
   d) Conversations with loved ones and healthcare providers regarding patients' wishes in a variety of situations

6. Besides the sizable risks from both underlying disease and high-dose therapy, situations may occur that promote the need for ACP in patients considering HSCT.
   a) The elective nature of transplant (Typically, weeks to months pass between initial consultation and admission for HSCT.)
   b) Predictability of potentially fatal post-HSCT complications: Generally associated with loss of decision-making capacity, resultant of critical illness
   c) The reality that many patients undergoing HSCT have lived with life-threatening illness for some time

7. Notwithstanding these reasons for promoting ACP prior to HSCT, some patients might prefer to defer planning or discussion of EOL scenarios.
   a) Patients may have underlying psychological impulses to avoid dwelling on the substantial risks.
   b) Living wills may be problematic tools for extending patients' autonomy through times of decision-making incapacity; their deficiencies are somewhat mitigated when complications are predictable.
   c) Patients and clinicians might not deem formal designation of a healthcare proxy as essential if a patient's preferred proxy (e.g., spouse) already receives priority under state laws regarding surrogate decision making for medical care.

8. Few systematic data exist regarding ACP in patients undergoing HSCT. Suggested questions that clinicians may ask regarding ACP preparedness include the following:
   a) Have you designated a healthcare proxy (i.e., someone to make medical decisions on your behalf)?
   b) Have you prepared a will?
   c) Have you completed a living will?
   d) Have you discussed your wishes regarding life support with your family and friends?
   e) Have you discussed your wishes regarding life support with your doctor or nurse?

9. A considerable minority of patients have not taken these steps. Research has shown the following:
   a) ACP is more common in older, college-educated, and allogeneic transplant patients.
   b) Patient-reported and documented discussions between patients and clinicians about most elements of ACP are rare.

     c) Although a sizable number of patients had written advance directives available in their hospital charts, most did not.

     d) Other factors that might be expected to predict completion of ACP, such as being married, having children, disease risk group, perceived mortality risk, and performance status or physical functioning before HSCT, were not associated with ACP.

10. Limited evidence supports that advance directives significantly modify the trajectory of EOL care, although some studies suggest improved psychological outcomes in survivors who had previously discussed their EOL preferences.

     a) Proxies also have been found to be poor judges of patients' preferences regarding EOL decisions; however, this finding may simply highlight the need for more frank conversations between patients and proxies.

     b) Even with these limitations, a consensus exists that an inclusive approach to ACP, including the use of written advance directives as well as candid discussion between patients, their loved ones, and clinicians, is an essential component of high-quality care for patients with life-threatening illness.

D. Transitions in level of care

  1. Transfer to the intensive care unit (ICU) (Kasberg et al., 2011)

     a) The transfer of an HSCT patient to the ICU can be a crisis for the patient, family, and transplant team. The patient is confronted with a perilous situation and also may suffer loss of control and autonomy.

     b) Transition to this higher level of care also indicates a shift in what is the most critical threat to recovery. A transfer from a singular focus on the blood and marrow to the body or body systems in failure is necessary. This change may be difficult for patients and families who are used to HSCT routines such as daily monitoring of neutrophil counts. It is common for families to request transplant team involvement in treatment decisions in the ICU, especially when futility of continued life support becomes apparent.

     c) Because most HSCT patients are incapacitated and unable to participate in decisions to withhold or withdraw life-sustaining treatments at this point, it is essential that a multidisciplinary approach between family decision makers and the ICU and HSCT teams be carried out using a communication strategy that will lessen the family onus of life-and-death decisions.

  2. Palliative care (Button, Gavin, & Keogh, 2014; Chung et al., 2009)

     a) Definition: As stated by the National Consensus Project for Quality Palliative Care (2009), "The goal of palliative care is to prevent and relieve suffering and to support the best quality of life for patients and their families, regardless of the stage of the disease or the need for other therapies" (p. 6).

     b) WHO recommends that palliative care be incorporated in all cancer settings to maximize quality of life for patients and families facing physical, psychosocial, and spiritual obstacles brought on by serious illness.

     c) Research is limited on the assimilation of palliative care in the HSCT process. Recently published literature indicates that palliative care is poorly understood and has not been adequately integrated into the HSCT setting.

     d) Transplant clinicians may not realize that palliative care is not the same as hospice care. Palliative care is care administered to seriously ill patients alongside usual medical and surgical care; the two fields should be complementary.

e) Allo-HSCT recipients who relapse have a poor prognosis. When combined with factors such as the physical and psychosocial consequences of previous treatment, limited therapeutic options, and potential for high symptom burden, these issues increase the likelihood of the need for palliative care services.

3. Symptom management: Satisfactory evidence exists that palliative care is effective in decreasing cancer symptoms, thus increasing QOL and survival. Areas where palliative care has demonstrated improvement include the following:
   a) Pain relief
   b) Mucositis prevention to reduce pain, infection risk, altered nutritional status, and GVHD by decreasing epithelial disruption
   c) Nausea and vomiting
   d) Nutrition, anorexia, and weight loss
   e) Diarrhea

4. Effect of palliative care and HSCT on family
   a) To aid in the discussion of palliative care during the process of HSCT with the patient, it is helpful to gain insight into the relationships with the significant other, family members, and friends.
   b) Data show that patients and caregivers want factual information but often do not know where to go for answers.
   c) Factors that may affect caregivers and family members include diagnosis, prognosis, the process of transplantation and its risks and benefits, the possibility of moving to another city or state, and potential changes in family roles and dynamics.

5. Barriers to palliative care (Cooke, Gemmill, & Grant, 2011)
   a) Unpredictability of the illness trajectory with acute exacerbation requiring highly technical therapies
   b) Variability of prognostication
   c) Ambiguous goals of care
   d) Concentration on cure that precludes palliative care
   e) Unawareness of palliative care
   f) Intricate configuration of the healthcare system

6. A challenge that HSCT patients may face is an inability to leave the hospital without the consequence of decreased life expectancy caused by severe infections, GVHD, or transfusion dependence. These situations, particularly GVHD, can be quite debilitating and exceed the capacity of family members and even inpatient hospice units.
   a) It is imperative that the transplant unit and unit staff are equipped to care for those patients who cannot leave the hospital and are unable to be cared for elsewhere. In these circumstances, the goals of care must be adjusted from driving assertively onward to providing the best comfort measures possible for the dying patient.
   b) Unit staff may require significant assistance in fine-tuning their own goals of care for the patient, as that transition can be confusing and create moral and psychological anguish among the nursing and other patient care staff.

7. Problems specific to HSCT that make transition to hospice difficult (Button et al., 2014; Chung et al., 2009)
   a) Palliative care and EOL care are not synonymous.

b) The question of when does comfort rather than longevity become the primary goal of medical care often is difficult to answer.

c) Palliative care is provided at all times, both in tandem with very aggressive medical care and, particularly, at EOL.

8. EOL care (Adams, Bailey, Anderson, & Docherty, 2011; Ganti et al., 2007; Keating et al., 2010; Perry, Rivlin, & Goldstone, 1999)

a) EOL choices, such as when to end therapy aimed at treating the disease process and when to concentrate on palliative care, are universal concerns of patients undergoing HSCT.

b) Reports in the literature and clinical observations suggest that conversations regarding ineffectual treatment options can be challenging for some healthcare providers and often are not initiated prior to transplantation, but rather only after a patient's clinical status deteriorates.

c) Futile treatment is commonly referred to as "treatment that is unable to reverse the course of the disease and that offers no hope of benefit" (Coveney, 2007, p. 68).

d) Research indicates physicians may defer EOL discussions because they fear that discussions early in a patient's terminal course may be linked with decreased hope and inferior outcomes. Studies also suggest that physicians postpone talking about EOL options while patients still feel well and may instead wait for the onset of symptoms or until no further curative options are available.

e) In this situation, it is optimal that advance care directives be finalized while the patient is competent to ensure that care is congruent with the patient's wishes. The virtues of having advance directives include autonomy in decision making, consistency between personal values and EOL actions, a diminished burden on family and healthcare providers because wishes are known, and a possible reduction in costs.

9. Nurses' roles in promoting EOL care (Murray, Wilson, Kryworuchko, Stacey, & O'Connor, 2009; Rolland & Kalman, 2007; Tee, Balmaceda, Granada, Fowler, & Payne, 2013)

a) EOL care is a field in which nurses are well positioned to take the lead in developing patient- and family-centered interventions aimed at improving care during this significant part of their patients' lives.

b) Nursing research suggests that nurses believe assisting patients in their decision-making process is a critical element of patient-centered care, yet many nurses report feeling that they lack the skills, confidence, and tools to provide the necessary support.

c) Some studies also indicate that nurses believe that patients should be involved in the decision-making process. However, nurses also specified that they continue to be uncomfortable discussing EOL care with patients and identified their primary knowledge deficit as not knowing how to speak with dying patients.

d) Although most patients die while hospitalized rather than at home, many terminally ill patients and their families describe disappointment with EOL care.

e) Rolland and Kalman (2007) observed that patients and families have an overall greater perception of EOL care when healthcare efforts are attentive to QOL and the goals of palliative and hospice care. Unfortunately, few people profit from this service because of delayed referrals.

　　　f) Rolland and Kalman (2007) also demonstrated that numerous patients were referred too late to use hospice services successfully: A large percentage of patients died within one week of hospice admission.

　　　g) Early hospice or palliative care referral is crucial to improve dying patients' QOL and their role in EOL care.

　　　h) Rolland and Kalman's (2007) research on evaluating clinician attitudes regarding how EOL care can help patients understand and accept their situation, assess interventions, and enrich care for the dying was based on three concepts: professional responsibility, efficacy of hospice, and clinician–patient communication.

　10. The nurse is the primary healthcare professional to bring about supported self-care (Johnston et al., 2009).

　　　a) Topics depicted in clinical instruction, symptom-motivated interventions, and arrangements for dying support can be adopted, employing nominal resources and time.

　　　b) Self-care approaches for patients with terminal illness should be associated with supporting patients with the following:

　　　　(1) Symptom and pain management that affects QOL

　　　　(2) Psychological and emotional adaptation to their illness

　　　　(3) Stress relief with symptoms that cannot easily be altered

Key Points

- Nurses caring for hematopoietic stem cell transplantation (HSCT) survivors must be knowledgeable of long-term, treatment-related complications. Proper assessment, monitoring, and interventions are critical to ensure the best possible outcomes.

- Ocular adverse events following HSCT are common. Most events are treatable and do not typically lead to long-term visual sequelae.

- Baseline pretransplant and frequent post-transplant ophthalmologic examinations are recommended throughout the transplant continuum.

- Patients should be monitored closely in the setting of neutropenia, immunosuppression, graft-versus-host disease (GVHD), and systemic viral reactivation.

- Patient education should include reporting of symptoms, adherence to anti-infective prophylaxis and immunosuppression regimen, and liberal use of lubricants and emollients when warranted.

- The skeletal system is an area at risk for long-term complications. Knowledge of etiologies, risk factors, diagnoses, and treatment options associated with these problems will help nurses identify patients at risk and ensure appropriate monitoring for skeletal complications, thereby guaranteeing the best possible skeletal structure and function for survivors (Ruble, 2008).

- Psychological distress has been linked not only with various aspects regarding the HSCT process, but also with poor treatment outcomes.

- Potential complications cross the range of quality-of-life domains and represent a spectrum of physical, functional, emotional, and social complexities.

- Delayed effects, including difficulties with fatigue, alterations in sleep patterns, disturbance of cognitive abilities, sexual dysfunction, and psychological and interpersonal issues, have been identified.

- Assessment of psychological distress may be particularly useful at critical points in the HSCT trajectory (e.g., at the beginning, middle, and end of the transplant process) (Andrykowski et al., 1999; Trask et al., 2002). Nurses play a pivotal role in identifying psychosocial complications and implementing effective therapeutic interventions.

- Bone marrow or poor hematologic function following allogeneic HSCT can be a factor that contributes to increased post-transplant mortality as well as complicated and prolonged hospitalizations (Weisdorf et al., 1995). Restoring hematopoiesis and durable engraftment of donor progenitor cells is essential to survival.

- Graft composition is an important aspect in predicting the short- and long-term engraftment performance and degree of rejection (Ricci, Medin, & Foley, 2014).

- Although other mechanisms may exist, graft rejection is primarily caused by immunized T cells.

- Rejection may be overcome by augmenting cell dose or intensifying immunosuppression and conditioning prior to transplant.

- The expansive use of human leukocyte antigen–mismatched grafts and reduced-intensity conditioning regimens has contributed to the incidence of graft failure (Mattsson et al., 2008).

- Routine chimerism analysis during the first month following HSCT may help to distinguish graft failure from delayed engraftment.

- The risk for cardiac complications is increased with the use of high-dose chemotherapy. Therefore, adequate cardiac function is generally a prerequisite for transplantation.

- Care of patients undergoing transplantation requires knowledge of common causes of infection.

- Prevention of infection is key and begins with patient and caregiver education.

- Immunizations should be administered after transplant per institutional policy.

- Hydration is a state in which the body survives and maintains all bodily functions, such as maintaining temperature, regulating wastes, and lubricating joints.

- Hydration is one of the most important factors in HSCT supportive care management.

- Fluid and electrolyte imbalances occur in the majority of transplant recipients as a result of the conditioning regimens, medical interventions, and complications following HSCT.

- Fluid status in HSCT recipients requires close monitoring because of the constant flux, especially in the early transplant period. Endothelial cell injury can result in capillary leak syndrome.

- The goal of maintaining adequate fluid balance is to maintain baseline weight by aggressive diuresis and to prevent fluid overload.

- The most common electrolyte imbalances in HSCT recipients are hypokalemia, hypophosphatemia, hypomagnesemia, and hypocalcemia.

- Recipients should be monitored closely when receiving cyclophosphamide for hyponatremia resulting in syndrome of inappropriate antidiuretic hormone secretion.

- During tacrolimus and cyclosporine administration, nurses should continuously monitor for decreased magnesium levels.

- Amphotericin B potentiates the development of hypokalemia and hypomagnesemia.

- Foscarnet can affect the renal tubules and cause electrolyte imbalances such as hypocalcemia, hypomagnesemia, hypokalemia, hypophosphatemia, and hyperphosphatemia. Prehydration is essential prior to foscarnet administration.

- Transplant recipients are at greatest risk for opportunistic infections during the neutropenic period, which is a common cause of morbidity and mortality.
- Key factors related to the duration of neutropenia are chemotherapy, radiation therapy, amount of stem cells infused, use of growth factors, steroidal medication, and occurrence of HSCT complications.
- Gram-positive and gram-negative bacteria account for 90% of infections in the neutropenic period and are associated with disruptions in the skin, mucous membranes, and indwelling catheters.
- Gram-negative pathogens are caused by *Escherichia coli*, *Klebsiella pneumoniae*, and *Pseudomonas aeruginosa*.
- Three critical phases in HSCT pose a high risk for opportunistic infections: pre-engraftment, postengraftment, and late phase.
- During the pre-engraftment phase, viral reactivation of herpes simplex virus, herpes zoster virus, and cytomegalovirus (CMV) may occur because of prior exposure.
- Vancomycin-resistant *Enterococcus* is a common cause of infection in HSCT recipients.
- Fungal infections, such as *Candida*, affect the oral mucosa, and *Aspergillus* affects the sinuses and lungs during the HSCT period.
- The Foundation for the Accreditation of Cellular Therapy standards recommend to use HEPA filters in positive-pressure, private rooms for recipients.
- Allogeneic HSCT recipients are at increased risk for CMV compared to autologous recipients, especially those recipients who are seropositive prior to transplant.
- Adenovirus infection is a common concern and may cause hemorrhagic cystitis and pneumonitis.
- Neutrophil engraftment, also known as *homing*, generally results in 14–21 days with an absolute neutrophil count of 500/mm³ for three consecutive days.
- Engraftment syndrome may develop in the pre-engraftment phase with absence of infectious source.
- Infection in the postengraftment period for allogeneic transplant recipients is a result of immunosuppressive agents and GVHD.
- Delayed engraftment is a result of graft failure, graft rejection, or secondary graft failure.
- T-cell dysregulation is prolonged recovery of T lymphocytes from months to years following HSCT.
- Patient education about infectious complications, medications, and care planning is essential in the late phase for ongoing follow-up.
- Conditioning regimens with high-dose chemotherapy and radiation therapy in HSCT can have major, acute toxic effects on the gastrointestinal (GI) system.
- Severe GI effects include oral mucositis, esophagitis, salivary gland dysfunction, xerostomia, taste changes, nausea and vomiting, diarrhea, abdominal pain, bloating, perineal-rectal skin changes, and altered nutrition.
- Establishing an oral care regimen is essential for recipients at risk for oral mucositis.
- Oral herpes simplex virus reactivation is an early viral infection and may appear on the soft palate, lip, or gingiva as one or multiple painful vesicles.
- Recipients often experience one or more causes of GI symptoms—for example, *Clostridium difficile* colitis, which is the most common bacterial infection.

- Xerostomia may appear 7–10 days following the conditioning regimen and can persist for months.
- Recipients experiencing xerostomia are at increased risk for *Candida* infections. Antifungals should be started prophylactically.
- Many preparative regimens are highly emetogenic with or without radiation therapy.
- Common types of diarrhea occurring in transplant recipients include secretory and exudative.
- Infectious diarrhea should be considered in transplant recipients with concurrent neutropenia.
- Daily nursing assessments of the perineal-rectal skin area should be performed in recipients with diarrhea and at times of myelosuppression because of mechanical and chemical trauma to the dermis and epidermis.
- Transplant survivors have a high risk for relapse and secondary malignancies. The likelihood of developing a second neoplasm is related to previous chemotherapy, radiation, and immunosuppression.
- Nurses must educate patients on the importance of routine health maintenance and health promotion. Patients should be cognizant to minimize exposure to tobacco, ultraviolet light, and other environmental carcinogens.
- Patient adherence to routine follow-up care with their transplant team is critical to monitor for late toxicities of treatment.
- Blood tests, restaging scans, or bone marrow biopsies are necessary to evaluate for engraftment and relapse.
- Although the notions of advance care planning, palliative care, and end-of-life considerations for patients undergoing HSCT may remain controversial to some healthcare providers, evidence points to a need for modifications in the transition from cure to palliation (Tee et al., 2013).
- Useful and empathetic communication is the basis of effective palliative nursing care (Malloy, Virani, Kelly, & Munévar, 2010). Nonetheless, communication is a skill resulting from education and experience rather than something that occurs organically.
- Nurses are a constant fixture in the clinical setting and frequently spend considerable amounts of time with patients and families.
- Nursing staff may be able to enhance the palliative and end-of-life care of relapsed allogeneic HSCT recipients through nurse-led education sessions, advance care planning, and nurse-initiated referrals to palliative care services (Button et al., 2014; Chung et al., 2009).

References

Adams, J.A., Bailey, D.E., Jr., Anderson, R.A., & Docherty, S.L. (2011). Nursing roles and strategies in end-of-life decision making in acute care: A systematic review of the literature. *Nursing Research and Practice, 2011,* Article 527834. doi:10.1155/2011/527834

Agarwal, N., & Burkart, T.A. (2013). Transient, high-grade atrioventricular block from high-dose cyclophosphamide. *Texas Heart Institute Journal, 40,* 626–627.

Al-Dasooqi, N., Sonis, S.T., Bowen, J.M., Bateman, E., Blijlevens, N., Gibson, R.J., ... Lalla, R.V. (2013). Emerging evidence on the pathobiology of mucositis. *Supportive Care in Cancer, 21,* 2075–2083. doi:10.1007/s00520-013-1810-y

Aleman, B.M.P., van den Belt-Dusebout, A.W., De Bruin, M.L., van't Veer, M.B., Baaijens, M.H.A., de Boer, J.P., ... van Leeuwen, F.E. (2007). Late cardiotoxicity after treatment for Hodgkin lymphoma. *Blood, 109,* 1878–1886. doi:10.1182/blood-2006-07-034405

Allan, E.J., Flowers, M.E.D., Lin, M.P., Bensinger, R.E., Martin, P.J., & Wu, M.C. (2011). Visual acuity and anterior segment findings in chronic graft-versus-host disease. *Cornea, 30,* 1392–1397. doi:10.1097/ICO.0b013e31820ce6d0

Andrykowski, M.A. (1994). Psychosocial factors in bone marrow transplantation: A review and recommendations for research. *Bone Marrow Transplantation, 13,* 357–375.

Andrykowski, M.A., Cordova, M.J., Hann, D.M., Jacobsen, P.B., Fields, K.K., & Phillips, G. (1999). Patients' psychosocial concerns following stem cell transplantation. *Bone Marrow Transplantation, 24,* 1121–1129. doi:10.1038/sj.bmt.1702022

Angarone, M., & Ison, M.G. (2008). Prevention and early treatment of opportunistic viral infections in patients with leukemia and allogeneic stem cell transplantation recipients. *Journal of the National Comprehensive Cancer Network, 6,* 191–201. Retrieved from http://www.jnccn.org/content/6/2/191.abstract

Antin, J.H., & Raley, D.Y. (2013). *Manual of stem cell and bone marrow transplantation* (2nd ed.). New York, NY: Cambridge University Press.

Antunes, H.S., de Sá Ferreira, E.M., de Faria, L.M.D., Schirmer, M., Rodrigues, P.C., Small, I.Á., … Ferreira, C.G. (2010). Streptococcal bacteremia in patients submitted to hematopoietic stem cell transplantation: The role of tooth brushing and use of chlorhexidine. *Medicina Oral Patología Oral y Cirugía Bucal, 15,* e303–e309. doi:10.4317/medoral.15.e303

Antunes, H.S., Pereira, A., & Cunha, I. (2013). Chediak-Higashi syndrome: Pathognomonic feature. *Lancet, 382,* 1514. doi:10.1016/S0140-6736(13)60020-3

Armstrong, L.E. (2007). Assessing hydration status: The elusive gold standard. *Journal of the American College of Nutrition, 26*(Suppl. 5), 575S–584S. doi:10.1080/07315724.2007.10719661

Ayuso, V.K., Hettinga, Y., van der Does, P., Boelens, J.J., Rothova, A., & de Boer, J. (2013). Ocular complications in children within 1 year after hematopoietic stem cell transplantation. *JAMA Ophthalmology, 131,* 470–475. doi:10.1001/jamaophthalmol.2013.2500

Bachanova, V., Brunstein, C.G., Burns, L.J., Miller, J.S., Luo, X., Defor, T., … Tomblyn, M. (2009). Fewer infections and lower infection-related mortality following non-myeloablative versus myeloablative conditioning for allo-transplantation of patients with lymphoma. *Bone Marrow Transplantation, 43,* 237–244. doi:10.1038/bmt.2008.313

Baker, W.F., Jr. (2000). Approach to diagnosis. In H.R. Schumacher, W.A. Rock, Jr., & S.A. Stass (Eds.), *Handbook of hematologic pathology* (pp. 275–292). New York, NY: Marcel Dekker.

Balasubramaniam, S.C., Raja, H., Nau, C.B., Shen, J.F., & Schornack, M.M. (2015). Ocular graft-versus-host disease: A review. *Eye and Contact Lens, 41,* 256–261. doi:10.1097/ICL.0000000000000150

Barker, G.J. (1999). Current practices in the oral management of the patient undergoing chemotherapy or bone marrow transplantation. *Supportive Care in Cancer, 7,* 17–20.

Berendt, M., & D'Agostino, S. (2005). Alterations in nutrition. In J.K. Itano & K.N. Taoka (Eds.), *Core curriculum for oncology nursing* (4th ed., pp. 277–317). Philadelphia, PA: Elsevier Saunders.

Berger, A.M., & Eilers, J. (1998). Factors influencing oral cavity status during high-dose antineoplastic therapy: A secondary data analysis. *Oncology Nursing Forum, 25,* 1623–1626.

Beyer, J., Schwella, N., Zingsem, J., Strohscheer, I., Schwaner, I., Oettle, H., … Stieger, W. (1995). Hematopoietic rescue after high-dose chemotherapy using autologous peripheral-blood progenitor cells or bone marrow: A randomized comparison. *Journal of Clinical Oncology, 13,* 1328–1335.

Bhatia, S., Francisco, L., Carter, A., Sun, C.-L., Baker, K.S., Gurney, J.G., … Weisdorf, D.J. (2007). Late mortality after allogeneic hematopoietic cell transplantation and functional status of long-term survivors: Report from the Bone Marrow Transplant Survivor Study. *Blood, 110,* 3784–3792. doi:10.1182/blood-2007-03-082933

Bhatia, S., Robison, L.L., Francisco, L., Carter, A., Liu, Y., Grant, M., … Forman, S.J. (2005). Late mortality in survivors of autologous hematopoietic-cell transplantation: Report from the Bone Marrow Transplant Survivor Study. *Blood, 105,* 4215–4222. doi:10.1182/blood-2005-01-0035

Blennow, O., Fjaertoft, G., Winiarski, J., Ljungman, P., Mattsson, J., & Remberger, M. (2014). Varicella-zoster reactivation after allogeneic stem cell transplantation without routine prophylaxis—The incidence remains high. *Biology of Blood and Marrow Transplantation, 20,* 1646–1649. doi:10.1016/j.bbmt.2014.06.002

Boer, C.C., Correa, M.E.P., Miranda, E.C.M., & de Souza, C.A. (2010). Taste disorders and oral evaluation in patients undergoing allogeneic hematopoietic SCT. *Bone Marrow Transplantation, 45,* 705–711. doi:10.1038/bmt.2009.237

Broadway-Duren, J.B., & Klaassen, H. (2013). Anemias. *Critical Care Nursing Clinics of North America, 25,* 411–426. doi:10.1016/j.ccell.2013.09.004

Burgunder, M.R. (2007). Pulmonary and cardiac effects. In S. Ezzone & K. Schmit-Pokorny (Eds.), *Blood and marrow stem cell transplantation: Principles, practice, and nursing insights* (3rd ed., pp. 245–262). Burlington, MA: Jones & Bartlett Learning.

Button, E.B., Gavin, N.C., & Keogh, S.J. (2014). Exploring palliative care provision for recipients of allogeneic hematopoietic stem cell transplantation who relapsed. *Oncology Nursing Forum, 41,* 370–381. doi:10.1188/14.ONF.370-381

Campbell, S., Sun, C.-L., Kurian, S., Francisco, L., Carter, A., Kulkarni, S., … Bhatia, S. (2009). Predictors of avascular necrosis of bone in long-term survivors of hematopoietic cell transplantation. *Cancer, 115,* 4127–4135. doi:10.1002/cncr.24474

Camp-Sorrell, D. (2005). Myelosuppression. In J.K. Itano & K.N. Taoka (Eds.), *Core curriculum for oncology nursing* (4th ed., pp. 259–264). Philadelphia, PA: Elsevier Saunders.

Camp-Sorrell, D. (2011). Chemotherapy toxicities and management. In C.H. Yarbro, D. Wujcik, & B.H. Gobel (Eds.), *Cancer nursing: Principles and practice* (7th ed., pp. 458–503). Burlington, MA: Jones & Bartlett Learning.

Camus, P., & Costabel, U. (2005). Drug-induced respiratory disease in patients with hematological diseases. *Seminars in Respiratory and Critical Care Medicine, 26,* 458–481. doi:10.1055/s-2005-922030

Centers for Disease Control and Prevention. (2011). General recommendations on immunization: Recommendations of the Advisory Committee on Immunization Practices. *Morbidity and Mortality Weekly Report, 60*(RR02), 1–60. Retrieved from http://www.cdc.gov/mmwr/preview/mmwrhtml/rr6002a1.htm

Chemaly, R.F., Shah, D.P., & Boeckh, M.J. (2014). Management of respiratory viral infections in hematopoietic cell transplant recipients and patients with hematologic malignancies. *Clinical Infectious Diseases, 59*(Suppl. 5), S344–S351. doi:10.1093/cid/ciu623

Chouinard, M.S., & Finn, K.T. (2007). Understanding hematopoiesis. In S. Ezzone & K. Schmit-Pokorny (Eds.), *Blood and marrow stem cell transplantation: Principles, practice, and nursing insights* (3rd ed., pp. 29–58). Burlington, MA: Jones & Bartlett Learning.

Chow, E.J., Mueller, B.A., Baker, K.S., Cushing-Haugen, K.L., Flowers, M.E.D., Martin, P.J., … Lee, S.J.L. (2011). Cardiovascular hospitalizations and mortality among recipients of hematopoietic stem cell transplantation. *Annals of Internal Medicine, 155,* 21–32. doi:10.7326/0003-4819-155-1-201107050-00004

Chung, H.M., Lyckholm, L.J., & Smith, T.J. (2009). Palliative care in BMT. *Bone Marrow Transplantation, 43,* 265–273. doi:10.1038/bmt.2008.436

Cloutier, R.L. (2010). Neutropenic enterocolitis. *Hematology/Oncology Clinics of North America, 24,* 577–584. doi:10.1016/j.hoc.2010.03.005

Coleman, J. (2010). Diarrhea. In C.G. Brown (Ed.), *A guide to oncology symptom management* (pp. 173–198). Pittsburgh, PA: Oncology Nursing Society.

Cooke, L.D., Gemmill, R., & Grant, M.L. (2011). Creating a palliative educational session for hematopoietic stem cell transplantation recipients at relapse. *Clinical Journal of Oncology Nursing, 15,* 411–417. doi:10.1188/11.CJON.411-417

Cooke, L.D., Gemmill, R., Kravits, K., & Grant, M. (2009). Psychological consequences of hematopoietic stem cell transplant. *Seminars in Oncology Nursing, 25,* 139–150. doi:10.1016/j.soncn.2009.03.008

Coomes, S.M., Hubbard, L.L.N., & Moore, B.B. (2011). Impaired pulmonary immunity post-bone marrow transplant. *Immunologic Research, 50,* 78–86. doi:10.1007/s12026-010-8200-z

Cope, D.G. (2015). Alterations in nutrition. In J.K. Itano (Vol. ed.), *Core curriculum for oncology nursing* (5th ed., pp. 406–411). Philadelphia, PA: Elsevier Saunders.

Coveney, A. (2007). Ethical issues surrounding advanced disease. In K.K. Kuebler, D.E. Heidrich, & P. Esper (Eds.), *Palliative and end-of-life care: Clinical practice guidelines* (2nd ed., pp. 63–74). St. Louis, MO: Elsevier Saunders.

Dahi, P.B., Perales, M.A., Devlin, S.M., Olson, A., Lubin, M., Gonzales, A.M., … Barker, J.N. (2015). Incidence, nature and mortality of cytomegalovirus infection after double-unit cord blood transplant. *Leukemia and Lymphoma, 56,* 1799–1805. doi:10.3109/10428194.2014.963079

Daniel-Johnson, J., & Schwartz, J. (2011). How do I approach ABO-incompatible hematopoietic progenitor cell transplantation? *Transfusion, 51,* 1143–1149. doi:10.1111/j.1537-2995.2011.03069.x

Davies, A., & Hall, S. (2011). Salivary gland dysfunction (dry mouth) in patients with advanced cancer. *International Journal of Palliative Nursing, 17,* 477–482. doi:10.12968/ijpn.2011.17.10.477

De Pas, T.D., Curigliano, L., Franceschelli, L., Catania, C., Spaggiari, L., & de Braud, F. (2001). Gemcitabine-induced systemic capillary leak syndrome. *Annals of Oncology, 12,* 1651–1652. doi:10.1023/A:1013163831194

Despotis, G.J., Zhang, L., & Lublin, D.M. (2007). Transfusion risks and transfusion-related pro-inflammatory responses. *Hematology/Oncology Clinics of North America, 21,* 147–161. doi:10.1016/j.hoc.2006.11.002

Doig, A.K., & Huether, S.E. (2014). The cellular environment: Fluids and electrolytes, acids and bases. In K.L. McCance, S.E. Huether, V.L. Brashers, & N.S. Rote (Eds.), *Pathophysiology: The biologic basis for disease in adults and children* (7th ed., pp. 103–126). St. Louis, MO: Elsevier.

Douglas, T.T., & Shelton, B.K. (2007). Renal and hepatic effects. In S. Ezzone & K. Schmit-Pokorny (Eds.), *Blood and marrow stem cell transplantation: Principles, practice, and nursing insights* (3rd ed., pp. 263–296). Burlington, MA: Jones & Bartlett Learning.

Dubberke, E.R., Reske, K.A., Srivastava, A., Sadhu, J., Gatti, R., Young, R.M., … Fraser, V.J. (2010). *Clostridium difficile*-associated disease in allogeneic hematopoietic stem-cell transplant recipients: Risk associations, protective associations, and outcomes. *Clinical Transplantation, 24*, 192–198. doi:10.1111/j.1399-0012.2009.01035.x

Eldredge, D.H., Nail, L.M., Maziarz, R.T., Hansen, L.K., Ewing, D., & Archbold P.G. (2006). Explaining family caregiver role strain following autologous blood and marrow transplantation. *Journal of Psychosocial Oncology, 24*, 53–74. doi:10.1300/J077v24n03_03

Engelking, C. (1998). Cancer-related diarrhea: A neglected cause of cancer-related symptom distress: Introduction. *Oncology Nursing Forum, 25*, 859–860.

Erard, V., Wald, A., Corey, L., Leisenring, W.M., & Boeckh, M. (2007). Use of long-term suppressive acyclovir after hematopoietic stem-cell transplantation: Impact on herpes simplex virus (HSV) disease and drug-resistant HSV disease. *Journal of Infectious Diseases, 196*, 266–270. doi:10.1086/518938

Ezzone, S.A. (2009). Blood and marrow stem cell transplantation. In B.H. Gobel, S. Triest-Robertson, & W.H. Vogel (Eds.), *Advanced oncology nursing certification review and resource manual* (pp. 261–303). Pittsburgh, PA: Oncology Nursing Society.

Ezzone, S.A. (2013). Gastrointestinal complications. In S.A. Ezzone (Ed.), *Hematopoietic stem cell transplantation: A manual for nursing practice* (2nd ed., pp. 173–190). Pittsburgh, PA: Oncology Nursing Society.

Feller, L., Essop, R., Wood, N.H., Khammissa, R.A., Chikte, U.M., Meyerov, R., & Lemmer, J. (2010). Chemotherapy- and radiotherapy-induced oral mucositis: Pathobiology, epidemiology and management. *Journal of the South African Dental Association, 65*, 372–374.

Filipovich, A.H., Weisdorf, D., Pavletic, S., Socie, G., Wingard, J.R., Lee, S.J., … Flowers, M.E.D. (2005). National Institutes of Health consensus development project on criteria for clinical trials in chronic graft-versus-host disease: I. Diagnosis and staging working group report. *Biology of Blood and Marrow Transplantation, 11*, 945–956. doi:10.1016/j.bbmt.2005.09.004

Flores, F.X., Brophy, P.D., Symons, J.M., Fortenberry, J.D., Chua, A.N., Alexander, S.R., … Goldstein, S.L. (2008). Continuous renal replacement therapy (CRRT) after stem cell transplantation. A report from the prospective pediatric CRRT Registry Group. *Pediatric Nephrology, 23*, 625–630. doi:10.1007/s00467-007-0672-2

Freytes, C.O., & Lazarus, H.M. (2009). Second hematopoietic SCT for lymphoma patients who relapse after auto-transplantation: Another autograft or switch to allograft? *Bone Marrow Transplantation, 44*, 559–569. doi:10.1038/bmt.2009.214

Frick, E., Ramm, G., Bumeder, I., Schulz-Kindermann, F., Tyroller, M., Fischer, N., & Hasenbring, M. (2006). Social support and quality of life of patients prior to stem cell or bone marrow transplantation. *British Journal of Health Psychology, 11*, 451–462. doi:10.1348/135910705X53849

Fulton, J.S., & Treon, M.L. (2007). Oral mucositis. In M.E. Langhorne, J.E. Fulton, & S.E. Otto (Eds.), *Oncology nursing* (5th ed., pp. 505–523). Maryland Heights, MO: Elsevier Mosby.

Furness, S., Bryan, G., McMillan, R., Birchenough, S., & Worthington, H.V. (2013). Interventions for the management of dry mouth: Non-pharmacological interventions. *Cochrane Database of Systematic Reviews, 2013*(9). doi:10.1002/14651858.CD009603.pub3

Ganti, A.K., Lee, S.J., Vose, J.M., Devetten, M.P., Bociek, R.G., Armitage, J.O., … Loberiza, F.R., Jr. (2007). Outcomes after hematopoietic stem-cell transplantation for hematologic malignancies in patients with or without advance care planning. *Journal of Clinical Oncology, 25*, 5643–5648. doi:10.1200/JCO.2007.11.1914

Gea-Banacloche, J., Masur, H., Arns da Cuhna, C., Chiller, T., Kirchhoff, L., Shaw, P., … Cordonnier, C. (2009). Regionally limited or rare infections: Prevention after hematopoietic cell transplantation. *Bone Marrow Transplantation, 44*, 489–494. doi:10.1038/bmt.2009.260

Girmenia, C., Barosi, G., Piciocchi, A., Arcese, W., Aversa, F., Bacigalupo, A., … Rambaldi, A. (2014). Primary prophylaxis of invasive fungal diseases in allogeneic stem cell transplantation: Revised recommendations from a consensus process by Gruppo Italiano Trapianto Midollo Osseo (GITMO). *Biology of Blood and Marrow Transplantation, 20*, 1080–1088. doi:10.1016/j.bbmt.2014.02.018

Gobel, B.H., & O'Leary, C. (2007). Bone marrow suppression. In M.E. Langhorne, J.S. Fulton, & S.E. Otto (Eds.), *Oncology nursing* (5th ed., pp. 488–504). Maryland Heights, MO: Elsevier Mosby.

Gobel, B.H., Peterson, G.J., & Hoffner, B. (2013). Sepsis and septic shock. In M. Kaplan (Ed.), *Understanding and managing oncologic emergencies: A resource for nurses* (2nd ed., pp. 287–335). Pittsburgh, PA: Oncology Nursing Society.

Goldman, L., & Schafer, A.I. (Eds.). (2012). *Goldman's Cecil medicine* (24th ed.). Maryland Heights, MO: Elsevier Saunders.

Haas, M.L. (2011). Radiation therapy: Toxicities and management. In C.H. Yarbro, D. Wujcik, & B.H. Gobel (Eds.), *Cancer nursing: Principles and practice* (7th ed., pp. 312–351). Burlington, MA: Jones & Bartlett Learning.

Haisfield-Wolfe, M.E., & Rund, C. (2000). A nursing protocol for the management of perineal-rectal skin alterations. *Clinical Journal of Oncology Nursing, 4,* 15–21.

Hakki, M., Limaye, A.P., Kim, H.W., Kirby, K.A., Corey, L., & Boeckh, M. (2007). Invasive *Pseudomonas aeruginosa* infections: High rate of recurrence and mortality after hematopoietic cell transplantation. *Bone Marrow Transplantation, 39,* 687–693. doi:10.1038/sj.bmt.1705653

Hall, D. (2010). Catching on to *C. difficile. American Nurse Today, 5*(7), 12–14.

Hannon, M.J., & Thompson, C.J. (2010). The syndrome of inappropriate antidiuretic hormone: Prevalence, causes and consequences. *European Journal of Endocrinology, 162*(Suppl. 1), S5–S12. doi:10.1530/EJE-09-1063

Harris, D.J., Eilers, J.G., Cashavelly, B.J., Maxwell, C.L., & Harriman, A. (2009). ONS PEP resource: Mucositis. In L.H. Eaton & J.M. Tipton (Eds.), *Putting evidence into practice: Improving oncology patient outcomes* (pp. 201–213). Pittsburgh, PA: Oncology Nursing Society.

Harris, D.J., Eilers, J., Harriman, A., Cashavelly, B.J., & Maxwell, C. (2008). Putting evidence into practice: Evidence-based interventions for the management of oral mucositis. *Clinical Journal of Oncology Nursing, 12,* 141–152. doi:10.1188/08.CJON.141-152

Hartung, H.D., Olson, T.S., & Bessler, M. (2013). Acquired aplastic anemia in children. *Pediatric Clinics of North America, 60,* 1311–1336. doi:10.1016/j.pcl.2013.08.011

Hawkins, R., & Grunberg, S. (2009). Chemotherapy-induced nausea and vomiting: Challenges and opportunities for improved patient outcomes. *Clinical Journal of Oncology Nursing, 13,* 54–64. doi:10.1188/09.CJON.54-64

Heimdahl, A. (1999). Prevention and management of oral infections in cancer patients. *Supportive Care in Cancer, 7,* 224–228.

Helbig, G., Stella-Holowiecka, B., Wojnar, J., Krawczyk, M., Krzemien, S., Wojciechowska-Sadus, M., ... Holowiecki, J. (2007). Pure red-cell aplasia following major and bi-directional ABO-incompatible allogeneic stem-cell transplantation: Recovery of donor-derived erythropoiesis after long-term treatment using different therapeutic strategies. *Annals of Hematology, 86,* 677–683. doi:10.1007/s00277-007-0304-8

Hesketh, P. (2008). Chemotherapy-induced nausea and vomiting. *New England Journal of Medicine, 358,* 2482–2494. doi:10.1056/NEJMra0706547

Hessen, M., & Akpek, E.K. (2012). Ocular graft-versus-host disease. *Current Opinion in Allergy and Clinical Immunology, 12,* 540–547. doi:10.1097/ACI.0b013e328357b4b9

Hillman, R.S., Ault, K.A., Leporrier, M., & Rinder, H.M. (2011). *Hematology in clinical practice* (5th ed.). New York, NY: McGraw-Hill Medical.

Hirst, L.W., Jabs, D.A., Tutschka, P.J., Green, W.R., & Santos, G.W. (1983). The eye in bone marrow transplantation. I: Clinical study. *Archives of Ophthalmology, 101,* 580–584. doi:10.1001/archopht.1983.01040010580010

Hogan, C.M. (1998). The nurse's role in diarrhea management. *Oncology Nursing Forum, 25,* 879–886.

Hovinga, J.A.K., & Lämmle, B. (2012). Role of ADAMTS13 in the pathogenesis, diagnosis, and treatment of thrombotic thrombocytopenic purpura. *ASH Education Book, 2012,* 610–616. doi:10.1182/asheducation-2012.1.610

Ippoliti, C. (1998). Antidiarrheal agents for the management of treatment-related diarrhea in cancer patients. *American Journal of Health-System Pharmacy, 55,* 1573–1580.

Jabbour, E., Rondon, G., Anderlini, P., Giralt, S.A., Couriel, D.R., Champlin, R.E., & Khouri, I.F. (2007). Treatment of donor graft failure with nonmyeloablative conditioning of fludarabine, antithymocyte globulin, and a second allogeneic hematopoietic transplantation. *Bone Marrow Transplantation, 40,* 431–435. doi:10.1038/sj.bmt.1705760

Jacobsen, P.B., Sadler, I.J., Booth-Jones, M., Soety, E., Weitzner, M.A., & Fields, K.K. (2002). Predictors of posttraumatic stress disorder symptomatology following bone marrow transplantation for cancer. *Journal of Consulting and Clinical Psychology, 70,* 235–240. doi:10.1037/0022-006X.70.1.235

Joffe, S., Mello, M.M., Cook, E.F., & Lee, S.J. (2007). Advance care planning in patients undergoing hematopoietic cell transplantation. *Biology of Blood and Marrow Transplantation, 13,* 65–73. doi:10.1016/j.bbmt.2006.08.042

Johnson, D.W., Cagnoni, P.J., Schossau, T.M., Stemmer, S.M., Grayeb, D.E.M., Baron, A.E., ... Jones, R.B. (1999). Optic disc and retinal microvasculopathy after high-dose chemotherapy and autologous hematopoietic progenitor cell support. *Bone Marrow Transplantation, 24,* 785–792. doi:10.1038/sj.bmt.1701913

Johnston, B., McGill, M., Milligan, S., McElroy, D., Foster, C., & Kearney, N. (2009). Self care and end of life care in advanced cancer: Literature review. *European Journal of Oncology Nursing, 13,* 386–398. doi:10.1016/j.ejon.2009.04.003

Jubelirer, S.J. (2011). The benefit of the neutropenic diet: Fact or fiction? *Oncologist, 16,* 704–707. doi:10.1634/theoncologist.2011-0001

Kamboj, M., Chung, D., Seo, S.K., Pamer, E.G., Sepkowitz, K.A., Jakubowski, A.A., & Papanicolaou, G. (2010). The changing epidemiology of vancomycin-resistant enterococcus (VRE) bacteremia in allogeneic hematopoietic stem cell transplant (HSCT) recipients. *Biology of Blood and Marrow Transplantation, 16,* 1576–1581. doi:10.1016/j.bbmt.2010.05.008

Kang, Y., & Chao, N.J. (2015). Immune reconstitution. In J.R. Wingard, D.A. Gastineau, H.L. Leather, Z.M. Szczepiorkowski, & E.L. Snyder (Eds.), *Hematopoietic stem cell transplantation: A handbook for clinicians* (2nd ed., pp. 181–196). Bethesda, MD: AABB.

Kasberg, H., Brister, L., & Barnard, B. (2011). Aggressive disease, aggressive treatment: The adult hematopoietic stem cell transplant patient in the intensive care unit. *AACN Advanced Critical Care, 22,* 349–364. doi:10.1097/NCI.0b013e318232c690

Keating, N.L., Landrum, M.B., Rogers, S.O., Jr., Baum, S.K., Virnig, B.A., Huskamp, H.A., ... Kahn, K.L. (2010). Physician factors associated with discussions about end-of-life care. *Cancer, 116,* 998–1006. doi:10.1002/cncr.24761

Khan, H., Belsher, J., Yilmaz, M., Afessa, B., Winters, J.L., Moore, S.B., ... Gajic, O. (2007). Fresh-frozen plasma and platelet transfusions are associated with development of acute lung injury in critically ill medical patients. *Chest, 131,* 1308–1314. doi:10.1378/chest.06-3048

Khan, R.S. (2015). Fluid and electrolyte management. In J.R. Wingard, D.A. Gastineau, H.L. Leather, Z.M. Szczepiorkowski, & E.L. Snyder (Eds.), *Hematopoietic stem cell transplantation: A handbook for clinicians* (2nd ed., pp. 356–362). Bethesda, MD: AABB.

Khanal, S., & Tomlinson, A. (2012). Tear physiology in dry eye associated with chronic GVHD. *Bone Marrow Transplantation, 47,* 115–119. doi:10.1038/bmt.2011.36

Kim, S.K. (2005). Ocular graft vs. host disease. *Ocular Surface, 3,* S177–S179. doi:10.1016/s1542-0124(12)70250-1

Kim, S.K. (2006). Update on ocular graft-versus-host disease. *Current Opinion in Ophthalmology, 17,* 334–338. doi:10.1097/01.icu.0000233952.09595.d8

Knöös, M., & Östman, M. (2010). Oral Assessment Guide—Test of reliability and validity for patients receiving radiotherapy to the head and neck region. *European Journal of Cancer Care, 19,* 53–60. doi:10.1111/j.1365-2354.2008.00958.x

Kontoyiannis, D.P., Marr, K.A., Park, B.J., Alexander, B.D., Anaissie, E.J., Walsh, T.J., ... Pappas, F.G. (2010). Prospective surveillance for invasive fungal infections in hematopoietic stem cell transplant recipients, 2001–2006: Overview of the Transplant-Associated Infection Surveillance Network (TRANSNET) Database. *Clinical Infectious Diseases, 50,* 1091–1100. doi:10.1086/651263

Kuck, A.W., & Ricciardi, E. (2005). Alterations in elimination. In J.K. Itano & K.N. Taoka (Eds.), *Core curriculum for oncology nursing* (4th ed., pp. 327–331). Philadelphia, PA: Elsevier Saunders.

Kumar, G., Ahmad, S., Taneja, A., Patel, J., Guddati, A.K., Nanchal, R., & Milwaukee Initiative in Critical Care Outcomes Research Group of Investigators. (2015). Severe sepsis in hematopoietic stem cell transplant recipients. *Critical Care Medicine, 43,* 411–421. doi:10.1097/CCM.0000000000000714

Laport, G.G., & Negrin, R.S. (2009). Management of relapse after hematopoietic cell transplantation. In F.R. Appelbaum, S.J. Forman, R.S. Negrin, & K.G. Blume (Eds.), *Thomas' hematopoietic cell transplantation: Stem cell transplantation* (4th ed., pp. 1059–1075). doi:10.1002/9781444303537

Lassiter, M., & Schneider, S.M. (2015). A pilot study comparing the neutropenic diet to a non-neutropenic diet in the allogeneic hematopoietic stem cell transplantation population. *Clinical Journal of Oncology Nursing, 19,* 273–278. doi:10.1188/15.CJON.19-03AP

Leather, H.L., & Wingard, J.R. (2001). Infections following hematopoietic stem cell transplantation. *Infectious Disease Clinics of North America, 15,* 483–520. doi:10.1016/S0891-5520(05)70157-4

Lees, J., & Keefe, D.M. (2015). Gastrointestinal complications in hematopoietic stem cell transplantation. In J.R. Wingard, D.A. Gastineau, H.L. Leather, E.L. Snyder, & Z.M. Szczepiorkowski (Eds.), *Hematopoietic stem cell transplantation: A handbook for clinicians* (2nd ed., pp. 481–492). Bethesda, MD: AABB.

Lemoine, C., & Gobel, B.H. (2011). Hematopoietic therapy. In C.H. Yarbro, D. Wujcik, & B.H. Gobel (Eds.), *Cancer nursing: Principles and practice* (7th ed., pp. 600–625). Burlington, MA: Jones & Bartlett Learning.

Ljungman, P. (2014). The role of cytomegalovirus serostatus on outcome of hematopoietic stem cell transplantation. *Current Opinion in Hematology, 21,* 466–469. doi:10.1097/MOH.0000000000000085

Ljungman, P., Cordonnier, C., Einsele, H., Englund, J., Machado, C.M., Storek, J., ... Centers for Disease Control and Prevention. (2009). Vaccination of the hematopoietic cell transplant recipients. *Bone Marrow Transplantation, 44,* 521–526. doi:10.1038/bmt.2009.263

Mackall, C., Fry, T., Gress, R., Peggs, K., Storek, J., Toubert, A., ... Centers for Disease Control and Prevention. (2009). Background to hematopoietic cell transplantation, including post transplant immune recovery. *Bone Marrow Transplantation, 44,* 457–462. doi:10.1038/bmt.2009.255

Mackenzie, I. (2002). Assessment and management of fluid and electrolyte balance. *Surgery, 20,* 121–126. doi:10.1383/surg.20.6.121.14633

Macpherson, P. (2013). Dry mouth management in palliative and cancer care. *Dental Nursing, 9*, 68–74. doi:10.12968/denn.2013.9.2.68

Majhail, N.S., Rizzo, J.D., Lee, S.J., Aljurf, M., Atsuta, Y., Bonfim, C., … Tichelli, A. (2012). Recommended screening and preventive practices for long-term survivors after hematopoietic cell transplantation. *Bone Marrow Transplantation, 47*, 337–341. doi:10.1038/bmt.2012.5

Malloy, P., Virani, R., Kelly, K., & Munévar, C. (2010). Beyond bad news: Communication skills of nurses in palliative care. *Journal of Hospice and Palliative Nursing, 12*, 166–174. doi:10.1097/NJH.0b013e3181d99fee

Marchesi, F., Mengarelli, A., Giannotti, F., Tendas, A., Anaclerico, B., Porrini, R., … Rome Transplant Network. (2014). High incidence of post-transplant cytomegalovirus reactivations in myeloma patients undergoing autologous stem cell transplantation after treatment with bortezomib-based regimens: A survey from the Rome Transplant Network. *Transplant Infectious Disease, 16*, 158–164. doi:10.1111/tid.12162

Marini, B.L., Choi, S.W., Byersdorfer, C.A., Cronin, S., & Frame, D.G. (2015). Treatment of dyslipidemia in allogeneic hematopoietic stem cell transplant patients. *Biology of Blood and Marrow Transplantation, 21*, 809–820. doi:10.1016/j.bbmt.2014.10.027

Marks, P.W., & Glader, B. (2009). Approach to anemia in the adult and child. In R. Hoffman, E.J. Benz Jr., S.J. Shattil, B. Furie, L.E. Silberstein, P. McGlave, & H. Heslop (Eds.), *Hematology: Basic principles and practice* (5th ed., pp. 439–446). Philadelphia, PA: Elsevier Churchill Livingstone.

Marr, K.A. (2012). Delayed opportunistic infections in hematopoietic stem cell transplantation patients: A surmountable challenge. *ASH Education Book, 2012*, 265–270. doi:10.1182/asheducation-2012.1.265

Marr, K.A., Bow, E., Chiller, T., Maschmeyer, G., Ribaud, P., Segal, B., … Centers for Disease Control and Prevention. (2009). Fungal infection prevention after hematopoietic cell transplantation. *Bone Marrow Transplantation, 44*, 483–487. doi:10.1038/bmt.2009.259

Marrs, J.A. (2006). Care of patients with neutropenia. *Clinical Journal of Oncology Nursing, 10*, 164–166.

Martin, P.J., Counts, G.W., Jr., Appelbaum, F.R., Lee, S.J., Sanders, J.E., Deeg, H.J., … Storer, B.E. (2010). Life expectancy in patients surviving more than 5 years after hematopoietic cell transplantation. *Journal of Clinical Oncology, 28*, 1011–1016. doi:10.1200/JCO.2009.25.6693

Martín-Peña, A., Aguilar-Guisado, M., Espigado, I., Parody, R., & Cisneros, J.M. (2011). Prospective study of infectious complications in allogeneic hematopoietic stem cell transplant recipients. *Clinical Transplantation, 25*, 468–474. doi:10.1111/j.1399-0012.2010.01286.x

Mattsson, J., Ringdén, O., & Storb, R. (2008). Graft failure after allogeneic hematopoietic cell transplantation. *Biology of Blood and Marrow Transplantation, 14*, 165–170. doi:10.1016/j.bbmt.2007.10.025

McGuire, D.B., Fulton, J.S., Park, J., Brown, C.G., Correa, M.E., Eilers, J., … Lalla, R.V. (2013). Systematic review of basic oral care for the management of oral mucositis in cancer patients. *Supportive Care in Cancer, 21*, 3165–3177. doi:10.1007/s00520-013-1942-0

McMillan, R. (2013). Dry mouth—A review of this common oral problem. *Dental Nursing, 9*, 638–644. doi:10.12968/denn.2013.9.11.638

Mehta, A.B., & Hoffbrand, A.V. (2013). *Hematology at a glance* (4th ed.). Malden, MA: Blackwell Science.

Miceli, T., Lilleby, K., Noonan, K., Kurtin, S., Faiman, B., & Mangan, P.A. (2013). Autologous hematopoietic stem cell transplantation for patients with multiple myeloma: An overview for nurses in community practice. *Clinical Journal of Oncology Nursing, 17*(Suppl. 6), 13–24. doi:10.1188/13.CJON.S2.13-24

Mikulska, M., Del Bono, V., & Viscoli, C. (2014). Bacterial infections in hematopoietic stem cell transplantation recipients. *Current Opinion in Hematology, 21*, 451–458. doi:10.1097/MOH.0000000000000088

Mitchell, S.A. (2009). Hematopoietic stem cell transplantation. In S. Newton, M. Hickey, & J. Marrs (Eds.), *Mosby's oncology nursing advisor: A comprehensive guide to clinical practice* (pp. 142–159). St. Louis, MO: Elsevier Mosby.

Mitchell, S.A. (2013). Acute and chronic graft-versus-host disease. In S.A. Ezzone (Ed.), *Hematopoietic stem cell transplantation: A manual for nursing practice* (2nd ed., pp. 103–142). Pittsburgh, PA: Oncology Nursing Society.

Mori, T., & Kato, J. (2010). Cytomegalovirus infection/disease after hematopoietic stem cell transplantation. *International Journal of Hematology, 91*, 588–595. doi:10.1007/s12185-010-0569-x

Mount, D.B. (2012). Fluid and electrolyte disturbances. In D.L. Longo, A.S. Fauci, D.L. Kasper, S.L. Hauser, J.L. Jameson, & J. Loscalzo (Eds.), *Harrison's principles of internal medicine* (18th ed., pp. 341–359). New York, NY: McGraw-Hill.

Muehlbauer, P.M., Thorpe, D., Davis, A., Drabot, R., Rawlings, B.L., & Kiker, E. (2009). Putting evidence into practice: Evidence-based interventions to prevent, manage, and treat chemotherapy- and radiotherapy-induced diarrhea. *Clinical Journal of Oncology Nursing, 13*, 336–341. doi:10.1188/09.CJON.336-341

Munker, R., Hiller, E., & Paquette, R. (2007). *Modern hematology: Biology and clinical management* (2nd ed.). Totowa, NJ: Humana.

Murray, M.A., Wilson, K., Kryworuchko, J., Stacey, D., & O'Connor, A. (2009). Nurses' perceptions of factors influencing patient decision support for place of care at the end of life. *American Journal of Hospice and Palliative Medicine, 26*, 254–263. doi:10.1177/1049909108331316

Muto, T., Takeuchi, M., Kawaguchi, T., Tanaka, S., Tsukamoto, S., Sakai, S., … Nakaseko, C. (2011). Low-dose trimethoprim–sulfamethoxazole for *Pneumocystis jiroveci* pneumonia prophylaxis after allogeneic hematopoietic SCT. *Bone Marrow Transplantation, 46*, 1573–1575. doi:10.1038/bmt.2010.335

Nassar, A., Tabbara, K.F., & Aljurf, M. (2013). Ocular manifestations of graft-versus-host disease. *Saudi Journal of Ophthalmology, 27*, 215–222. doi:10.1016/j.sjopt.2013.06.007

Nassiri, N., Eslani, M., Panahi, N., Mehravaran, S., Ziaei, A., & Djalilian, A.R. (2013). Ocular graft versus host disease following allogeneic stem cell transplantation: A review of current knowledge and recommendations. *Journal of Ophthalmic and Vision Research, 8*, 351–358.

National Cancer Institute Cancer Therapy Evaluation Program. (2010). *Common terminology criteria for adverse events* [v.4.03]. Retrieved from http://evs.nci.nih.gov/ftp1/CTCAE/CTCAE_4.03_2010-06-14_QuickReference_5x7.pdf

National Consensus Project for Quality Palliative Care. (2009). *Clinical practice guidelines for quality palliative care* (2nd ed.). Retrieved from http://www.nationalconsensusproject.org/guideline.pdf

Nelson, L. (2015). Alterations in gastrointestinal functions. In J.K. Itano (Vol. ed.), *Core curriculum for oncology nursing* (5th ed., pp. 340–351). Philadelphia, PA: Elsevier Saunders.

Novartis Pharmaceuticals. (2013). *Sandimmune® (cyclosporine)* [Package insert]. East Hanover, NJ: Author.

O'Donnell, P.V. (2009). Engraftment. In J.R. Wingard, D.A. Gastineau, H.L. Leather, Z.M. Zczepiorkowski, & E.L. Snyder (Eds.), *Hematopoietic stem cell transplantation: A handbook for clinicians* (pp. 163–180). Bethesda, MD: AABB.

Ogawa, Y., Okamoto, S., Wakui, M., Watanabe, R., Yamada, M., Yoshino, M., … Tsubota, K. (1999). Dry eye after haematopoietic stem cell transplantation. *British Journal of Ophthalmology, 83*, 1125–1130. doi:10.1136/bjo.83.10.1125

Pandey, T., Maximin, S., & Bhargava, P. (2014). Imaging complications from hematopoietic stem cell transplant. *Indian Journal of Radiology and Imaging, 24*, 327–338. doi:10.4103/0971-3026.143895

Park, G.R., & Roe, P.G. (2000). *Fluid balance and volume resuscitation for beginners.* London, England: Greenwich Medical Media.

Parody, R., Martino, R., de la Cámara, R., García-Noblejas, A., Esquirol, A., Garcia-Cadenas, I., … Vazquez, L. (2015). Fungal and viral infections after allogeneic hematopoietic transplantation from unrelated donors in adults: Improving outcomes over time. *Bone Marrow Transplantation, 50*, 274–281. doi:10.1038/bmt.2014.229

Patel, S.R., & Zimring, J.C. (2013). Transfusion-induced bone marrow transplant rejection due to minor histocompatibility antigens. *Transfusion Medicine Reviews, 27*, 241–208. doi:10.1016/j.tmrv.2013.08.002

Perry, A.R., Rivlin, M.M., & Goldstone, A.H. (1999). Bone marrow transplant patients with life-threatening organ failure: When should treatment stop? *Journal of Clinical Oncology, 17*, 298–303.

Peterson, D.E., Bensadoun, R.-J., & Roila, F. (2011). Management of oral and gastrointestinal mucositis: ESMO clinical practice guidelines. *Annals of Oncology, 22*(Suppl. 6), S78–S84. doi:10.1093/annonc/mdr391

Philibert, D., Desmeules, S., Filion, A., Poirier, M., & Agharazii, M. (2008). Incidence and severity of early electrolyte abnormalities following autologous hematopoietic stem cell transplantation. *Nephrology Dialysis Transplantation, 23*, 359–363. doi:10.1093/ndt/gfm571

Phillips, K.M., McGinty, H.L., Cessna, J., Asvat, Y., Gonzalez, B., Cases, M.G., … Jim, H.S.L. (2013). A systematic review and meta-analysis of changes in cognitive functioning in adults undergoing hematopoietic stem cell transplantation. *Bone Marrow Transplantation, 48*, 1350–1357. doi:10.1038/bmt.2013.61

Pillay, B., Lee, S.J., Katona, L., Burney, S., & Avery, S. (2014). Psychosocial factors associated with quality of life in allogeneic stem cell transplant patients prior to transplant. *Psycho-Oncology, 23*, 642–649. doi:10.1002/pon.3462

Polovich, M., Olsen, M., & LeFebvre, K.B. (Eds.). (2014). *Chemotherapy and biotherapy guidelines and recommendations for practice* (4th ed.). Pittsburgh, PA: Oncology Nursing Society.

Porth, C.M. (2014). *Essentials of pathophysiology: Concepts of altered health states* (4th ed.). Philadelphia, PA: Lippincott Williams & Wilkins.

Pulsipher, M.A., Skinner, R., McDonald, G.B., Hingorani, S., Armenian, S.H., Cooke, K.R., … Baker, S. (2012). National Cancer Institute, National Heart, Lung, and Blood Institute/Pediatric Blood and Marrow Transplantation Consortium First International Consensus Conference on late effects after pediatric hematopoietic cell transplantation: The need for pediatric-specific long-term follow-up guidelines. *Biology of Blood and Marrow Transplantation, 18*, 334–347. doi:10.1016/j.bbmt.2012.01.003

Raber-Durlacher, J.E. (1999). Current practices for management of oral mucositis in cancer patients. *Supportive Care in Cancer, 7*, 71–74.

Radvansky, L.J., Pace, M.B., & Siddiqui, A. (2013). Prevention and management of radiation-induced dermatitis, mucositis, and xerostomia. *American Journal of Health-System Pharmacy, 70,* 1025–1032. doi:10.2146/ajhp120467

Reiner, S.L. (2008). Peripheral T lymphocytes and function. In W.E. Paul (Ed.), *Fundamental immunology* (6th ed., pp. 407–426). Philadelphia, PA: Lippincott Williams & Wilkins.

Ricci, M.J., Medin, J.A., & Foley, R.S. (2014). Advances in haploidentical stem cell transplantation in adults with high-risk hematological malignancies. *World Journal of Stem Cells, 6,* 380–390. doi:10.4252/wjsc.v6.i4.380

Rieger, J.M. (2012). Recent advances in the prevention and treatment of xerostomia: A review of the literature. *Canadian Journal of Dental Hygiene, 46,* 159–165. Retrieved from https://www.cdha.ca/pdfs/Profession/Journal/v46n3.pdf

Riley, R.S., Idowu, M., Chesney, A., Zhao, S., McCarty, J., Lamb, L.S., & Ben-Ezra, J.M. (2005). Hematologic aspects of myeloablative therapy and bone marrow transplantation. *Journal of Clinical Laboratory Analysis, 19,* 47–79. doi:10.1002/jcla.20055

Rimkus, C. (2009). Acute complications of stem cell transplant. *Seminars in Oncology Nursing, 25,* 129–138. doi:10.1016/j.soncn.2009.03.007

Ritchie, R.F., Ledue, T.B., & Craig, W.Y. (2007). Patient hydration: A major source of laboratory uncertainty. *Clinical Chemistry and Laboratory Medicine, 45,* 158–166. doi:10.1515/cclm.2007.052

Rodrigue, J.R., Pearman, T.P., & Moreb, J. (1999). Morbidity and mortality following bone marrow transplantation: Predictive utility of pre-BMT affective function, compliance, and social support stability. *International Journal of Behavioral Medicine, 6,* 241–254. doi:10.1207/s15327558ijbm0603_3

Rodriguez, A.L., & Gobel, B.H. (2011). Bleeding. In C.H. Yarbro, D. Wujcik, & B.H. Gobel (Eds.), *Cancer nursing: Principles and practice* (7th ed., pp. 745–772). Burlington, MA: Jones & Bartlett Learning.

Rolland, R.A., & Kalman, M. (2007). Nurses' attitudes about end-of-life referrals. *Journal of the New York State Nurses Association, 38*(2), 10–12.

Rosselet, R.M. (2013). Hematologic effects. In S.A. Ezzone (Ed.), *Hematopoietic stem cell transplantation: A manual for nursing practice* (2nd ed., pp. 155–172). Pittsburgh, PA: Oncology Nursing Society.

Rothaermel, J.M., & Baum, B. (2009). Biological response modifier agents. In S. Newton, M. Hickey, & J. Marrs (Eds.), *Mosby's oncology nursing advisor: A comprehensive guide to clinical practice* (pp. 173–182). St. Louis, MO: Elsevier Mosby.

Roy, C.N. (2010). Anemia of inflammation. *ASH Education Book, 2010,* 276–280. doi:10.1182/asheducation-2010.1.276

Rubin, L.G., Levin, M.J., Ljungman, P., Davies, E.G., Avery, R., Tomblyn, M., … Kang, I. (2014). 2013 IDSA clinical practice guideline for vaccination of the immunocompromised host. *Clinical Infectious Diseases, 58,* 309–318. doi:10.1093/cid/cit816

Ruble, K. (2008). Skeletal complications after bone marrow transplant in childhood. *Journal of Pediatric Oncology Nursing, 25,* 79–85. doi:10.1177/1043454207313322

Saleh, U.S., & Brockopp, D.Y. (2001). Quality of life one year following bone marrow transplantation: Psychometric evaluation of the quality of life in bone marrow transplant survivors' tool. *Oncology Nursing Forum, 28,* 1457–1464.

Schelenz, S., Abdallah, S., Gray, G., Stubbings, H., Gow, I., Baker, P., & Hunter, P.R. (2011). Epidemiology of oral yeast colonization and infection in patients with hematological malignancies, head neck and solid tumors. *Journal of Oral Pathology and Medicine, 40,* 83–89. doi:10.1111/j.1600-0714.2010.00937

Seely, A.J.E., Pascual, J.L., & Christou, N.V. (2003). Science review: Cell membrane expression (connectivity) regulates neutrophil delivery, function and clearance. *Critical Care, 7,* 291–307. doi:10.1186/cc1853

Sekhon, S.S., & Roy, V. (2006). Thrombocytopenia in adults: A practical approach to evaluation and management. *Southern Medical Journal, 99,* 491–498. doi:10.1097/01.smj.0000209275.75045.d4

Serio, B., Pezzullo, L., Fontana, R., Annunziata, S., Roamilio, R., Sessa, M., … Selleri, C. (2013). Accelerated bone mass senescence after hematopoietic stem cell transplantation. *Translational Medicine at UniSa, 5*(4), 7–13.

Shannon, S.P. (2013). Relapse and secondary malignancies. In S.A. Ezzone (Ed.), *Hematopoietic stem cell transplantation: A manual for nursing practice* (2nd ed., pp. 245–249). Pittsburgh, PA: Oncology Nursing Society.

Shaw, C., & Taylor, L. (2012). Treatment-related diarrhea in patients with cancer. *Clinical Journal of Oncology Nursing, 16,* 413–417. doi:10.1188/12.CJON.413-417

Shelton, B.K. (2016). Myelosuppression and second malignancies. In B.H. Gobel, S. Triest-Robertson, & W.H. Vogel (Eds.), *Advanced oncology nursing certification review and resource manual* (2nd ed., pp. 451–490). Pittsburgh, PA: Oncology Nursing Society.

Sherman, R.S., Cooke, E., & Grant, M. (2005). Dialogue among survivors of hematopoietic cell transplantation. *Journal of Psychosocial Oncology, 23,* 1–24. doi:10.1300/J077v23n01_01

Sonis, S.T. (2004). The pathobiology of mucositis. *Nature Reviews Cancer, 4,* 277–284. doi:10.1038/nrc1318

Sonis, S.T. (2007). Pathobiology of oral mucositis: Novel insights and opportunities. *Journal of Supportive Oncology, 5*(Suppl. 4), 3–11.

Sonis, S.T., Treister, N.S., Lees, J., & Keefe, D.M. (2009). Gastrointestinal complications of hematopoietic stem cell transplantation. In J.R. Wingard, D.A. Gastineau, H.L. Leather, Z.M. Szczepiorkowski, & E.L. Snyder (Eds.), *Hematopoietic stem cell transplantation: A handbook for clinicians* (pp. 163–180). Bethesda, MD: AABB.

Soubani, A.O., & Pandya, C.M. (2010). The spectrum of noninfectious pulmonary complications following hematopoietic stem cell transplantation. *Hematology/Oncology and Stem Cell Therapy, 3,* 143–157. doi:10.1016/S1658-3876(10)50025-6

Stiff, P. (2001). Mucositis associated with stem cell transplantation: Current status and innovative approaches to management. *Bone Marrow Transplantation, 27*(Suppl. 2), 3–11. doi:10.1038/sj.bmt.1702863

Swerdlow, S.H., Campo, E., Harris, N.L., Jaffe, E.S., Pileri, S.A., Stein, H., … Vardiman, J.W. (Eds.). (2008). *WHO classification of tumours of haematopoietic and lymphoid tissues* (4th ed.). Lyon, France: IARC Press.

Syrjala, K.L., Langer, S.L., Abrams, J.R., Storer, B.E., & Martin, P.J. (2005). Late effects of hematopoietic cell transplantation among 10-year adult survivors compared with case-matched controls. *Journal of Clinical Oncology, 23,* 6596–6606. doi:10.1200/JCO.2005.12.674

Tabarra, K.F., Al-Ghamdi, A., Al-Mohareb, F., Ayas, M., Chaudhri, N., Al-Sharif, F., … Aljurf, M. (2009). Ocular findings after allogeneic hematopoietic stem cell transplantation. *Ophthalmology, 116,* 1624–1629. doi:10.1016/j.ophtha.2009.04.054

Tang, B.L., Zhu, X.Y., Zheng, C.C., Liu, H.L., Geng, L.Q., Wang, X.B., … Sun, Z.M. (2014). Successful early unmanipulated haploidentical transplantation with reduced-intensity conditioning for primary graft failure after cord blood transplantation in hematologic malignancy patients. *Bone Marrow Transplantation, 50,* 1–5. doi:10.1038/bmt.2014.250

Tauchmanovà, L., De Rosa, G., Serio, B., Fazioli, F., Mainolfi, C., Lombardi, G., … Selleri, C. (2003). Avascular necrosis in long-term survivors after allogeneic or autologous stem cell transplantation. *Cancer, 97,* 2453–2461. doi:10.1002/cncr.11373

Tee, M.E., Balmaceda, G.Z., Granada, M.A., Fowler, C.S., & Payne, J.K. (2013). End-of-life decision making in hematopoietic cell transplantation recipients. *Clinical Journal of Oncology Nursing, 17,* 640–646. doi:10.1188/13.CJON.640-646

Thompson, A.M. (2002). Anesthesia. In L. Shields & H. Werder (Eds.), *Perioperative nursing* (pp. 92–93). London, England: Greenwich Medical Media.

Tichelli, A., Bucher, C., Rovó, A., Stussen, G., Stern, M., Paulussen, M., … Gratwohl, A. (2007). Premature cardiovascular disease after allogeneic hematopoietic stem-cell transplantation. *Blood, 110,* 3463–3471. doi:10.1182/blood-2006-10-054080

Tomblyn, M., Chiller, T., Einsele, H., Gress, R., Sepkowitz, K., Storek, J., … Boeckh, M.J. (2009). Guidelines for preventing infectious complications among hematopoietic cell transplantation recipients: A global perspective. *Biology of Blood and Marrow Transplantation, 15,* 1143–1238. doi:10.1016/j.bbmt.2009.06.019

Trask, P.C., Paterson, A., Riba, M., Brines, B., Griffith, K., Parker, P., … Ferrara, J. (2002). Assessment of psychological distress in prospective bone marrow transplant patients. *Bone Marrow Transplantation, 29,* 917–925. doi:10.1038/sj.bmt.1703557

Treister, N.S., & Sonis, S.T. (2009). Oral complications in hematopoietic stem cell transplantation. In J.R. Wingard, D.A. Gastineau, H.L. Leather, Z.M. Szczepiorkowski, & E.L. Snyder (Eds.), *Hematopoietic stem cell transplantation: A handbook for clinicians* (pp. 397–410). Bethesda, MD: AABB.

Vachon, M. (2006). Psychosocial distress and coping after cancer treatment: How clinicians can assess distress and which interventions are appropriate—What we know and what we don't. *American Journal of Nursing, 106*(Suppl. 3), 26–31. doi:10.1097/00000446-200603003-00011

Vagliano, L., Feraut, C., Gobetto, G., Trunfio, A., Errico, A., Campani, V., … Dimonte, V. (2011). Incidence and severity of oral mucositis in patients undergoing hematopoietic SCT—Results of a multicentre study. *Bone Marrow Transplantation, 46,* 727–732. doi:10.1038/bmt.2010.184

Vaidya, C., Ho, W., & Freda, B.J. (2010). Management of hyponatremia: Providing treatment and avoiding harm. *Cleveland Clinic Journal of Medicine, 77,* 715–726. doi:10.3949/ccjm.77a.08051

Vera-Llonch, M., Oster, G., Hagiwara, M., & Sonis, S. (2006). Oral mucositis in patients undergoing radiation treatment for head and neck carcinoma. *Cancer, 106,* 329–336. doi:10.1002/cncr.21622

Vermont, C.L., Jol-van der Zijde, E.C.M., Muller, P.H., Ball, L.M., Bredius, R.G.M., Vossen, A.C., & Lankester, A.C. (2014). Varicella zoster reactivation after hematopoietic stem cell transplant in children strongly correlated with leukemia treatment and suppression of host T-lymphocyte immunity. *Transplant Infectious Disease, 16,* 188–194. doi:10.1111/tid.12180

Wagner, J.E., Jr., Eapen, M., Carter, S., Wang, Y., Schultz, K.R., Wall, D.A., … Kurtzberg, J. (2014). One-unit versus two-unit cord-blood transplantation for hematologic cancers. *New England Journal of Medicine, 371,* 1685–1694. doi:10.1056/NEJMoa1405584

Wang, Y., Ogawa, Y., Dogru, M., Tatematsu, Y., Uchino, M., Kamoi, M., ... Tsubota, K. (2010). Baseline profiles of ocular surface and tear dynamics after allogeneic hematopoietic stem cell transplantation in patients with or without chronic GVHD-related dry eye. *Bone Marrow Transplantation, 45,* 1077–1083. doi:10.1038/bmt.2009.312

Weisdorf, D.J., Verfaillie, C.M., Davies, S.M., Filipovich, A.H., Wagner, J.E., Jr., Miller, J.S., ... McGlave, P.B. (1995). Hematopoietic growth factors for graft failure after bone marrow transplantation: A randomized trial of granulocyte-macrophage colony-stimulating factor (GM-CSF) versus sequential GM-CSF plus granulocyte-CSF. *Blood, 85,* 3452–3456.

Widows, M.R., Jacobsen, P.B., Booth-Jones, M., & Fields, K.K. (2005). Predictors of posttraumatic growth following bone marrow transplantation for cancer. *Health Psychology, 24,* 266–273. doi:10.1037/0278-6133.24.3.266

Wiesmann, A., Pereira, P., Böhm, P., Faul, C., Kanz, L., & Einsele, H. (1998). Avascular necrosis of bone following allogeneic stem cell transplantation: MR screening and therapeutic options. *Bone Marrow Transplantation, 22,* 565–569. doi:10.1038/sj.bmt.1701374

Wilkes, G.M. (2016). Chemotherapy, targeted biotherapy, and molecular therapy. In B.H. Gobel, S. Triest-Robertson, & W.H. Vogel (Eds.), *Advanced oncology nursing certification review and resource manual* (2nd ed., pp. 141–222). Pittsburgh, PA: Oncology Nursing Society.

Willems, L., Porcher, R., Lafaurie, M., Casin, I., Robin, M., Xhaard, A., ... Peffault de Latour, R. (2012). *Clostridium difficile* infection after allogeneic hematopoietic stem cell transplantation: Incidence, risk factors, and outcome. *Biology of Blood and Marrow Transplantation, 18,* 1295–1301. doi:10.1016/j.bbmt.2012.02.010

Wilson, C., & Sylvanus, T. (2005). Graft failure following allogeneic blood and marrow transplant: Evidence-based nursing case study review. *Clinical Journal of Oncology Nursing, 9,* 151–159. doi:10.1188/05.CJON.151-159

Wojtaszek, C. (2000). Management of chemotherapy-induced stomatitis. *Clinical Journal of Oncology Nursing, 4,* 263–270.

Wolff, S.N. (2002). Second hematopoietic stem cell transplantation for the treatment of graft failure, graft rejection or relapse after allogeneic transplantation. *Bone Marrow Transplantation, 29,* 545–552.

Woodard, P., Tong, X., Richardson, S., Srivastava, D.K., Horwitz, E.M., Benaim, E., ... Handgretinger, R. (2003). Etiology and outcome of graft failure in pediatric hematopoietic stem cell transplant recipients. *Journal of Pediatric Hematology/Oncology, 25,* 955–959.

Worel, N., Greinix, H.T., Leitner, G., Mitterbauer, M., Rabitsch, W., Rosenmayr, A., ... Kalhs, P. (2007). ABO-incompatible allogeneic hematopoietic stem cell transplantation following reduced-intensity conditioning: Close association with transplant-associated microangiopathy. *Transfusion and Apheresis Science, 36,* 297–304. doi:10.1016/j.transci.2007.03.004

Wyeth Pharmaceuticals, Inc. (2011). *Rapamune® (sirolimus)* [Package insert]. Philadelphia, PA: Author.

Yldrm, A.T., Güneş, B.T., Oymak, Y., Yaman, Y., Özek, G., Cart, O., ... Vergin, C. (2015). Congenital amegakaryocytic thrombocytopenia: Three case reports from patients with different clinical diagnoses and somatic abnormalities. *Blood Coagulation and Fibrinolysis, 26,* 337–341. doi:10.1097/MBC.0000000000000192

Yoshihara, S., Ikegame, K., Taniguchi, K., Kaida, K., Kim, E.H., Nakata, J., ... Ogawa, H. (2012). Salvage haploidentical transplantation for graft failure using reduced-intensity conditioning. *Bone Marrow Transplantation, 47,* 369–373. doi:10.1038/bmt.2011.84

Zuckerman, R.A. (2009). Infectious hepatitis in hematopoietic stem cell transplantation. In J.R. Wingard, D.A. Gastineau, H.L. Leather, Z.M. Szczepiorkowski, & E.L. Snyder (Eds.), *Hematopoietic stem cell transplantation: A handbook for clinicians* (pp. 394–395). Bethesda, MD: AABB.

Study Questions

1. Which of the following is NOT an identified risk factor associated with infection?
   A. Personal history of infection
   B. Type of transplantation (autologous or allogeneic)
   C. Myeloablative transplant
   D. None of the above

2. *Clostridium difficile* is not a common infection in the post-transplant setting.
   A. True
   B. False

3. A cord blood transplantation is associated with all of the following EXCEPT:
   A. Prolonged neutrophil and immune recovery
   B. Increase in viral infections
   C. Decrease in bacterial infections
   D. Decrease in graft-versus-host disease (GVHD)

4. Which of the following is true when considering bacterial infections in patients after transplant?
   A. Patients are at a significant risk for encapsulated bacterial infections.
   B. Multidrug-resistant organisms are not a major concern.
   C. *Streptococcus pneumoniae* is not a common post-transplant bacterial infection.
   D. Immunizations are not effective in controlling post-transplant bacterial or viral infections.

5. The following strategies should be considered in an effort to prevent post-transplant infectious complications.
   (1) Immunizations should begin immediately following transplant discharge.
   (2) Antiviral and antifungal prophylaxis medications should be considered in the post-transplant setting.
   (3) Lifestyle restrictions vary in each transplant center and often are enforced to decrease post-transplant infections. It is important to communicate lifestyle expectations and restrictions to patients and their families.
   (4) Measles, mumps, and rubella immunization should be administered at 12 months.
   A. 1, 2, 3, 4
   B. 2 and 3
   C. 2 and 4
   D. 2, 3, 4

6. Cardiovascular disease may be underreported in hematopoietic stem cell transplant (HSCT) recipients because symptoms may occur several months to several years following HSCT.
   A. True
   B. False

7. Which risk factors are associated with post-HSCT cardiovascular disease?
   (1) Hypertension, (2) Gender, (3) Certain immunosuppressive medications, (4) Previous anthracycline chemotherapy
   A. 1, 2, 3, 4
   B. 1, 3, 4
   C. 2, 3, 4
   D. 1, 2, 3

8. The following strategies are used to manage cardiovascular disease in post-HSCT patients EXCEPT:
   A. Antihypertensive medications
   B. Statin therapy
   C. Dietary counseling
   D. Prophylactic antifungal medications

9. Patients should be monitored for the clinical signs and symptoms of cardiac disease post-HSCT by which of the following?
   A. Annual clinical assessment that includes baseline vital signs, review of symptoms, and physical examination
   B. Careful attention to travel over the last year
   C. Lifestyle counseling about smoking cessation, weight management, and stress reduction
   D. All of the above except B
   E. All of the above except C

10. Which of the following chemotherapy agents is associated with patients with cardiac disease in the post-HSCT setting?
    A. Bendamustine
    B. Melphalan
    C. Doxorubicin
    D. Methotrexate

11. Graft failure or graft rejection is associated with all of the following EXCEPT:
    A. Incidence of 1%–20%
    B. Favorable prognosis
    C. Loss of donor cells after initial engraftment
    D. Potential for marrow aplasia and pancytopenia

12. Graft failure may result from which of the following?
    A. Type of primary disease
    B. Human leukocyte antigen (HLA) disparity
    C. Immunosuppression
    D. GVHD
    E. All of the above

13. Strategies to prevent graft failure may include all of the following EXCEPT:
    A. Using a nonmyeloablative conditioning regimen
    B. Employing antithymocyte globulin in combination with cyclophosphamide for aplastic anemia
    C. Augmenting cell dose by giving donor buffy coat transfusion
    D. Administering granulocyte–colony-stimulating factor–mobilized peripheral blood stem cells as an alternative to bone marrow
    E. Reducing the frequency of pretransplant blood transfusions

14. Early and late transplant-related musculoskeletal complications include all of the following EXCEPT:
    A. Avascular necrosis (AVN)
    B. Improved exercise tolerance
    C. Osteoporosis
    D. Fracture
    E. Osteomyelitis

15. Which of the following is a risk factor for AVN?
    A. Steroid therapy
    B. Younger age
    C. Absence of GVHD
    D. Primary diagnosis of multiple myeloma

16. Which of the following is a treatment for diminished bone mineral density?
    A. Nutritional supplementation with calcium and vitamin D
    B. Correction of possible endocrinopathies
    C. Correction of renal dysfunction
    D. Use of bisphosphonates
    E. All of the above

17. Which of the following is true of post-HSCT ocular damage?
    A. It can involve all parts of the eye.
    B. It may be a consequence of immunosuppression.
    C. It may be influenced by conditioning regimens (chemotherapy, radiation, or both).
    D. It may be a result of underlying disease.
    E. All of the above

18. Manifestations of ocular GVHD include all of the following EXCEPT:
    A. Dry, gritty, or painful eyes
    B. Cicatricial conjunctivitis
    C. Keratoconjunctivitis sicca
    D. Absence of early morning mucoid secretions
    E. Confluent areas of punctate keratopathy

19. Which of the following is true of cataract formation?
    A. It can be attributed to radiation and steroid therapy and is not a direct result of GVHD itself.
    B. It is an uncommon cause of visual acuity loss.
    C. The risk is decreased with total body irradiation.
    D. It does not lead to increased incidence of cataract surgery.

20. Risk factors that can predict a poorer overall psychological outcome include all of the following EXCEPT:
    A. Prior psychiatric morbidity or history
    B. Pretransplant nonadherence
    C. Lack of stable social support
    D. History of considerable regimen-related toxicity
    E. Male sex

21. What effect might higher levels of depression have on transplant patients?
    A. Influence post-transplant physical health systems
    B. Increase symptom-related distress
    C. Contribute to a higher suicide rate
    D. Decrease survival
    E. All of the above

22. In a study by Widows et al. (2005), patients who exhibited higher incidences of post-traumatic stress disorder symptoms had all of the following EXCEPT:
    A. Positive assessment of the transplant experience
    B. Larger use of avoidance-based coping strategies
    C. Decreased social support
    D. Increased social constraint
    E. Decreased assessment of general well-being

23. An HSCT recipient diagnosed with herpes simplex virus (HSV) is scheduled to receive foscarnet intravenously. The nurse anticipates an order for which of the following?
    A. Echocardiogram
    B. Urine sodium
    C. Pulmonary function tests
    D. Prehydration fluids

24. Which of the following is a major cause of electrolyte imbalances in HSCT recipients?
    A. Decreased oral intake
    B. Fluctuation in body weight
    C. Altered gastrointestinal absorption
    D. Restriction of fresh fruits

25. An HSCT recipient is complaining of increased weakness and numbness around the mouth. This symptom may be related to which of the following?
    A. Hyperkalemia
    B. Hypocalcemia
    C. Hyperphosphatemia
    D. Hyponatremia

26. A patient with acute myeloid leukemia is receiving a myeloablative conditioning regimen with cyclophosphamide. The nurse would closely monitor for which electrolyte imbalance?
    A. Hypercalcemia
    B. Hypokalemia
    C. Hyperphosphatemia
    D. Hyponatremia

27. Amphotericin B and corticosteroids can result in which of the following electrolyte imbalances?
    A. Hypernatremia
    B. Hypocalcemia
    C. Hypokalemia
    D. Hypercalcemia

28. The nurse is caring for an HSCT recipient with acute lymphoblastic leukemia and has drawn and sent laboratory samples for the morning. The recipient's laboratory report shows a corrected calcium level of 7.6 mg/dl and the patient is symptomatic. The nurse would anticipate an order to administer:
    A. Calcium gluconate IV
    B. Zoledronate acid IV
    C. Sodium bicarbonate IV
    D. Insulin/glucose IV

29. A patient is receiving tacrolimus IV following allogeneic HSCT. The patient is at greatest risk for developing which electrolyte imbalance?
    A. Hyponatremia
    B. Hyperkalemia
    C. Hypomagnesemia
    D. Hypernatremia

30. A patient with multiple myeloma is complaining of increased weakness seven days following HSCT. Morning laboratory results reveal the following: potassium + 3.8, magnesium + 2.2, phosphorus + 1.9, and corrected calcium 10.2 mg/dl. The nursing priority would be to obtain an order to administer which of the following medications?
    A. Sodium bicarbonate IV
    B. Potassium phosphate IV
    C. Magnesium sulfate IV
    D. Calcium gluconate IV

31. A patient is receiving cisplatin as part of the conditioning regimen prior to HSCT. Which of the following metabolic alterations would the nurse expect?
    A. Hypomagnesemia
    B. Hypokalemia
    C. Hyperkalemia
    D. Hypocalcemia

32. A recipient is being admitted for an allogeneic HSCT. One of the most important assessments during admission is to establish which of the following?
    A. Favorite foods
    B. Anxiety level
    C. Baseline weight
    D. Learning preference

33. A recipient has received an autologous HSCT. When does the nurse anticipate neutrophil engraftment?
    A. 26–28 days following HSCT
    B. 14–21 days following HSCT
    C. 7–9 days following HSCT
    D. 30–42 days following HSCT

34. A recipient is 15 days post–allogeneic HSCT with high-dose chemotherapy and is complaining of mouth sores. On assessment, the nurse observes erythema and ulcerations in the oral cavity. History includes seropositivity for HSV, cytomegalovirus (CMV), and Epstein-Barr virus (EBV). What is the possible reactivation?
    A. EBV
    B. CMV
    C. HSV
    D. Varicella-zoster virus (VZV)

35. Which of the following is a common fungal pathogen in the late transplant phase?
    A. Aspergillus
    B. HSV
    C. CMV
    D. Streptococcus

36. A post-HSCT recipient has a decreased platelet count of 32,000/mm^3. Which grade of thrombocytopenia is the patient experiencing?
    A. Grade 1
    B. Grade 2
    C. Grade 3
    D. Grade 4

37. A recipient is more than 100 days post-autologous HSCT transplant and is relocating to another state. What is the most important nursing intervention in this situation?
    A. Provide care planning.
    B. Monitor current medications.
    C. Ensure adequate diet.
    D. Assess dry weight.

38. Late transplant infections are directly related to which of the following?
    A. Radiation therapy
    B. Neutrophil engraftment
    C. Hepatitis B infection
    D. T-cell impairment

39. A recipient is seven days post-autologous HSCT and is complaining of chills, rash, and difficulty breathing. Current temperature is 38.5°C (101.3°F), rash is noted on anterior and posterior torso, and oxygen saturation is 89% on room air. The nurse should suspect which of the following?
    A. Community-acquired pneumonia
    B. Deep vein thrombosis
    C. Acute GVHD
    D. Engraftment syndrome

40. A patient is 28 days post-allogeneic HSCT with the following laboratory values: white blood cells = 2,100; hematocrit = 25.9; neutrophils (polys) = 22%; and bands = 4%. What is the patient's absolute neutrophil count?
    A. 546
    B. 795
    C. 1,848
    D. 378

41. An HSCT recipient is more likely to have a febrile nonhemolytic reaction from which of the following transfusions?
    A. Red blood cells
    B. Fresh frozen plasma
    C. Platelets
    D. Cryoprecipitate

42. A recipient is 14 days post-autologous HSCT and is experiencing pallor, shortness of breath with exertion, fatigue, tachycardia, and dizziness. Which of the following could these symptoms be indicating?
    A. Anemia
    B. Thrombocytopenia
    C. Pulmonary edema
    D. Acute cutaneous GVHD

43. A patient is on day 14 after undergoing an allogeneic HSCT and has continued to experience poor appetite and severe, watery diarrhea. A several-day history includes neutropenic fever with antibiotics and antiemetics. A priority nursing intervention would include which of the following?
    A. Obtaining a stool sample for culture
    B. Applying a barrier cream to the rectal area
    C. Planning a diet with bland foods
    D. Providing small, frequent meals

44. On day 9 following the conditioning regimen, a transplant recipient reports inability to swallow with dry mouth. On examination of the oral mucosa, the nurse observes debris on the teeth and gums. What is the most likely complication?
    A. *Candida*
    B. Dysphagia
    C. Mucositis
    D. Xerostomia

45. A recipient reports a decrease in taste sensation with decreased intake of breakfast and lunch. What is this symptom called?
    A. Stomatitis
    B. Xerostomia
    C. Hypogeusia
    D. Infection

46. An HSCT recipient is complaining of diarrhea for the past three days consisting of five episodes in the last 24 hours. According to the National Cancer Institute Common Terminology Criteria for Adverse Events, this indicates which grade of diarrhea?
    A. Grade 2
    B. Grade 3
    C. Grade 4
    D. Grade 5

47. A transplant recipient has received a myeloablative conditioning regimen over the past two days, which is now complete. On the beginning of day 4, the recipient develops nausea and vomiting. The recipient is experiencing which type of chemotherapy-induced nausea and vomiting?
    A. Acute
    B. Delayed
    C. Chronic
    D. Anticipatory

48. A recipient has developed oral mucositis following the start of an intense conditioning regimen. When does oral mucositis peak?
    A. 8–10 days
    B. 3–5 days
    C. 1–2 days
    D. 12–14 days

49. What is the mainstay for treatment of severe oral mucositis?
    A. Pain management
    B. Magic mouthwash
    C. Viscous lidocaine
    D. Bland rinses

50. Which of the following is a chemotherapy agent with a high emetic risk?
    A. Paclitaxel
    B. Cyclophosphamide
    C. Bleomycin
    D. Vinorelbine

51. A recipient is experiencing signs and symptoms of xerostomia. The recipient is at highest risk to develop what infection?
    A. EBV
    B. HSV
    C. Candidiasis
    D. CMV

52. A recipient who has diarrhea over the past two days is complaining of discomfort and itching in the perineal-rectal area. On assessment, the nurse observes dry, flaking, and peeling skin. This symptom is a result of which of the following?
    A. Chronic dryness
    B. Dry desquamation
    C. Vesicle formation
    D. Sloughing presentation

53. What treatment strategy might be included for relapsed disease?
    A. Withdrawal of immunosuppression to elicit a graft-versus-tumor effect
    B. Donor lymphocyte infusion
    C. Second myeloablative or reduced-intensity HSCT followed by second allogeneic HSCT outside the setting of a clinical trial
    D. Exploration of clinical trials examining cellular adoptive immunotherapy, ex vivo–activated T cells, cytokine-induced killer cells, natural killer cells, and antigen-specific cytotoxic T lymphocytes
    E. None of the above

54. Patient characteristics that may predict benefit from a reduced-intensity allogeneic HSCT include all of the following EXCEPT:
    A. Availability of a donor who is HLA compatible
    B. Good performance status
    C. Large tumor burden
    D. Chemosensitive disease
    E. None of the above

55. Post-transplant lymphoproliferative disorders are strongly associated with which of the following?
    A. HSV
    B. VZV
    C. EBV
    D. BK virus
    E. CMV

56. What is a fundamental component of advance care planning?
    A. Designation of a healthcare proxy
    B. Completion of a living will
    C. Preparation of an estate will
    D. Conversations with loved ones and healthcare providers regarding patient wishes in a variety of situations
    E. All of the above

57. Which of the following is a barrier to palliative care?
    A. Unpredictability of the illness trajectory with acute exacerbation requiring highly technical therapies
    B. The patient and family asking for information regarding palliative care services
    C. Social work
    D. Discussing options with the patient and family at a time when the patient can make an informed, autonomous decision

58. Self-care approaches for patients with terminal illness should include all of the following EXCEPT:
    A. Symptom and pain management that affects quality of life
    B. Psychological and emotional adaptation to their illness
    C. Stress relief with symptoms that cannot easily be altered
    D. Self-titration of pain medication by patients

CHAPTER 7

Survivorship Issues

Lisa A. Pinner, RN, MSN, CPON®, BMTCN®, and
D. Kathryn Tierney, RN, PhD, BMTCN®

I. Introduction: The number of hematopoietic stem cell transplantation (HSCT) survivors is increasing because of improvements in outcomes, expanding indications for transplantation, treatment of older recipients with reduced-intensity conditioning (RIC), and an increased number of available donors.
   A. An estimated 250,000 HSCT survivors are more than five years post-HSCT; it is projected that this number will rapidly increase (Horowitz, 2016).
   B. The goals of HSCT are to cure the underlying disease and return survivors to an optimal state of health and well-being. Therefore, healthcare providers must address the issues survivors face, including secondary malignancies, quality-of-life (QOL) impairments, psychosocial distress, altered sexuality, and infertility.
   C. Pediatric HSCT survivors face unique challenges related to growth and development, cognitive development, and school reentry.
   D. Additionally, available data indicate that caregivers experience significant short- and long-term stressors that negatively affect well-being. As the understanding of these stressors evolves, HSCT providers need to intervene to reduce emotional distress in HSCT caregivers.

II. Secondary malignancies
   A. Secondary malignancies are cancers caused by prior treatment with radiation or chemotherapy or long-term immunosuppression (CancerConnect, 2014).
   B. Second primary cancer is a new primary cancer in a person with a history of cancer (National Cancer Institute, n.d.).
   C. Categories of second malignancies (American Cancer Society, 2014; Bhatia et al., 1996)
      1. Acute leukemia and myelodysplastic syndrome (MDS)
      2. Lymphoma including post-transplant lymphoproliferative disorders (PTLDs)
      3. Solid tumors
      4. Skin cancers such as dermal squamous cell carcinoma
   D. Incidence
      1. Compared to the general population, autologous HSCT recipients have a 12-fold increased risk of death due to second malignancies (Bhatia et al., 2005).
      2. A recent systematic review and meta-analysis indicated a higher rate of MDS and acute myeloid leukemia in patients following autologous transplantation com-

pared to other therapies (relative risk = 1.71 [1.18–2.48], I^2 = 0%, 8,778 patients) (Vaxman et al., 2015).

3. Compared to the general population, allogeneic HSCT recipients were 3.6 times more likely to die of a second malignancy (Bhatia et al., 2007).

4. Across a number of large studies, the cumulative incidence of solid cancers after allogeneic transplant was 1.2%–1.6% at 5 years and 3.8%–14.9% at 15 years (Baker et al., 2003; Bhatia et al., 1996, 2001; Curtis et al., 1997; Gallagher & Forrest, 2007; Kolb et al., 1999; Rizzo et al., 2009; Shimada et al., 2005).

5. PTLD is the most common second malignancy in the first year following allogeneic HSCT using a T-cell-depleted graft (Bhatia & Bhatia, 2009).

6. Compared to the general population, survivors who are more than 15 years post-allogeneic HSCT have a threefold higher risk of developing a solid malignancy compared to the general population (Rizzo et al., 2009).

7. Incidence of solid tumors in post-HSCT pediatric survivors (Socié & Rizzo, 2012)
    a) 1.2%–1.6% at 5 years
    b) 2.2%–6.1% at 10 years
    c) 3.5%–14.9% at 15 years

E. Risk factors: Therapy-related acute leukemia and MDS is associated with alkylating agents, radiation, and topoisomerase II inhibitors (Vardiman, Harris, & Brunning, 2002).

1. Certain genetic predispositions increase the risk of primary and secondary cancers, including neurofibromatosis type 1 and Fanconi anemia (Jans, Schomerus, & Bygum, 2015; Malric et al., 2015).

2. Risk factors for PTLD fall into three categories (Bhatia et al., 1996; Curtis et al., 1999).
    a) Characteristics of the graft: T-cell depletion of donor marrow or mismatched related or unrelated donor transplant
    b) Agents in the preparative regimen or used for prevention or treatment of graft-versus-host disease (GVHD): Busulfan, antithymocyte globulin, anti-CD3 monoclonal antibody (mAb), and total body irradiation (TBI)
    c) Patient characteristics: Primary immunodeficiency and acute or extensive chronic GVHD, or Epstein-Barr virus (EBV)

3. Risk factors for solid tumors (Bhatia et al., 1996, 2001; Curtis et al., 1997; Majhail, 2008; Rizzo et al., 2009)
    a) Younger age at HSCT
    b) TBI
        (1) Higher doses associated with a higher risk
        (2) Younger age at the time of radiation associated with a higher risk
    c) Chronic GVHD
    d) Increasing time from transplant
    e) Genetic predisposition
    f) Infections
    g) Lifestyle factors (e.g., use of tobacco products, exposure of skin to ultraviolet light)

F. Pathophysiology

1. Because of their ability to form cross-links and transfer alkyl groups, alkylating agents cause secondary malignancies (Bhatia & Bhatia, 2009).

2. Topoisomerase II inhibitors cause chromosomal breakage; the repair of these breaks leads to translocations associated with the development of leukemia (Felix et al., 1998; Lovett et al., 2001; Megonigal et al., 2000).

3. In the setting of EBV infection, incompetent T cells lead to a loss of EBV control, resulting in PTLD (Bhatia & Bhatia, 2009).

4. Radiation damages DNA, resulting in mutations that may lead to the development of secondary malignancies (American Cancer Society, 2014).

G. Screening (Majhail & Rizzo, 2013; Majhail et al., 2012; Rizzo et al., 2006)

1. General cancer screening guidelines

   a) Screening should begin 12 months post-HSCT and repeated annually.

   b) Colonoscopies should begin at age 50 and then every 10 years. For pediatric survivors who received greater than 30 Gy of radiation to the abdomen, pelvis, or spine, screening should begin at age 35 (Carlson, 2014).

   c) Mammogram screening in women who have received radiation therapy should begin at age 25 or eight years after exposure, but no later than age 40.

   d) Pap smears should be performed every one to three years in women older than age 21 or within three years of becoming sexually active.

   e) EBV titers should be monitored for at least six months after allogeneic HSCT for recipients at high risk for PTLD (Shannon, 2013).

2. Health maintenance and counseling

   a) Review the risks of secondary malignancies.

   b) Perform self-examinations as appropriate: skin, breast, testicles, and oral cavity.

   c) Practice meticulous oral hygiene.

   d) Avoid use of tobacco products.

   e) Use sunscreen and protective clothing.

   f) Follow basic health maintenance.

      (1) Maintain a healthy weight.

      (2) Exercise regularly.

      (3) Reduce stress.

      (4) Eat a nutritious diet.

      (5) Practice modest alcohol intake and avoid illicit drug use.

H. Treatment

1. Options for MDS or acute leukemia include conventional chemotherapy or allogeneic transplantation. Outcomes are generally poor, secondary to disease relapse or high treatment-related mortality (Bhatia & Bhatia, 2009; Friedberg et al., 1999; Radich et al., 2000).

2. Options for PTLD include EBV-specific cytotoxic T cells, mAbs targeted to B cells, such as rituximab, and combination chemotherapy (Fox et al., 2014; Gerdemann et al., 2013; Kuehnle et al., 2000; Kuriyama, Kawano, Yamashita, & Ueda, 2014).

3. Options for solid malignancies consist of the best available therapy for the specific malignancy (Bhatia & Bhatia, 2009).

III. QOL

A. Definition

1. QOL is a multidimensional and multifactorial construct that defines an individual's sense of well-being.

2. The World Health Organization (WHO) defines health as "a state of complete physical, mental, and social well-being and not merely the absence of disease or infirmity" (WHO, 1946).

3. WHO's definition of health contains three of the broad domains examined in QOL research: physical, mental, and social.

4. QOL is subjective and includes the individual's assessment on his or her health and well-being (Syrjala & Artherholt, 2009).

B. Measurement (Kiviat, 2013)

1. Many validated instruments with established psychometric properties are available.

2. Commonly used instruments

   a) Functional Assessment of Cancer Therapy (FACT) and a version specific to patients undergoing bone marrow transplantation, the FACT-BMT

   b) European Organisation for Research and Treatment of Cancer Quality of Life Questionnaire (EORTC QLQ-C30)

   c) Medical Outcomes Study 36-Item Short Form (SF-36®)

C. QOL domains (Ferrell et al., 1992; Kiviat, 2013)

1. Physical

2. Functional

3. Psychological

4. Social

5. Spiritual or existential

6. Multiple interactions between domains

D. Domain impairments and recovery

1. Physical domain impairments

   a) Musculoskeletal pain and stiffness (Syrjala, Langer, Abrams, Storer, & Martin, 2005)

   b) Fatigue

      (1) Fatigue or low energy is common and can persist for many years (Andrykowski et al., 1997, 1999; Hjermstad et al., 2004).

      (2) Fatigue interferes with activities related to reintegration into preillness activities, roles, and lifestyle (McQuellon et al., 1998).

   c) Altered sexual health (Tierney, 2009)

   d) Chronic GVHD (Fraser et al., 2006; Lee et al., 2006; Pidala, Anasetti, & Jim, 2009): With resolution of chronic GVHD, the physical health of individuals improves.

   e) Neurocognitive changes affect 10%–60% of HSCT survivors (Andrykowski et al., 1999; Harder et al., 2002; Jim, Syrjala, & Rizzo, 2012). Alterations can occur in the following:

      (1) Attention

      (2) Concentration

      (3) Learning

      (4) Memory

      (5) Processing speed

      (6) Executive function

      (7) Fine motor control

   f) Survivors who are more than three years post-HSCT with the highest physical distress reported an average of 12–14 symptoms (Bevans et al., 2014).

2. Psychological domain impairments

        a) Depression

        b) Anxiety

        c) Poor self-image and self-esteem

        d) Body image changes

        e) Fear of recurrence

        f) Worries about family and the future

        g) Survivor guilt including guilt about causing family distress

        h) Ongoing physical symptom distress exerts a negative effect on emotional well-being (Bevans et al., 2014).

        i) Social support and less social constraint are predictive of improved mental health (Wingard et al., 2010).

        j) Adolescents and young adults may rebel against medical advice as they strive toward independence (Tewari et al., 2014).

    3. Social domain impairments

        a) Altered sexual health

            (1) Infertility may be a concern for some individuals—in particular, those younger than 40 years and those without children prior to undergoing HSCT (Hammond, Abrams, & Syrjala, 2007).

            (2) Pediatric survivors may be unaware of the infertility risk at the time of treatment, but as they transition to adulthood, infertility becomes a concern (Klassen et al., 2015).

        b) Reduced or limited social interactions and activity

        c) Ability to work

            (1) By one year post-HSCT, approximately 60% of autologous and allogeneic HSCT recipients have returned to work, including those who maintain their home or attend school (Lee et al., 2001).

            (2) The proportion continues to increase by five years (Syrjala et al., 2004).

        d) Strained personal relationships

        e) Insurance concerns and financial issues: Denials for health insurance were reported by 24% of 10-year HSCT survivors, and 27% were denied life insurance (Syrjala et al., 2005).

    4. Spiritual or existential domain impairments

        a) Loss of hope

        b) Spiritual crisis with a loss of faith

        c) Loss of life purpose or meaning

E. Interventions to improve QOL (Kiviat, 2013)

    1. Healthy living

        a) Nutritious diet

        b) Exercise and physical therapy (Carlson, Smith, Russell, Fibich, & Whittaker, 2006; Wilson, Jacobsen, & Fields, 2005)

        c) Restful and adequate sleep

        d) Stress management

    2. Social support

    3. Counseling and therapy

F. Physical recovery (Bevans et al., 2014; Duell et al., 1997; Heinonen et al., 2001; Hjermstad et al., 2004; Kiss et al., 2002; Pidala et al., 2009; Syrjala et al., 2004)

    1. Factors associated with slower recovery or diminished QOL

        a) Poor physical health

        b) Younger age

        c) Depression

        d) Lack of social support

        e) Lower education level

        f) Ongoing physical symptoms (particularly fatigue)

        g) Immunosuppressive therapy

        h) Chronic GVHD

2. The pace of physical recovery after transplant is variable but begins about three months following HSCT. Physical recovery can take between one and five years (Bevans et al., 2014; McQuellon et al., 1998; Syrjala et al., 2004).

IV. Psychosocial issues

  A. Psychological distress (Chang, Orav, McNamara, Tong, & Antin, 2005; Kurtz & Abrams, 2010; Lee et al., 2005; Syrjala et al., 2004, 2005)

    1. Anxiety and depression have been identified in up to 44% of adult survivors and 7%–32% of pediatric survivors.

      a) Individuals with chronic GVHD report more adverse effects on mental health (Fraser et al., 2006).

      b) Depression is associated with a higher level of physical restrictions and chronic GVHD (Syrjala et al., 2004).

    2. Anxiety and depression are 2.7 times more frequent in children who have undergone HSCT than in those who have not (Gerson & Rappaport, 2013; Sun et al., 2013).

      a) Triggers may include the anniversary of diagnosis or transplant, health concerns, fear of relapse, school or peer issues, and survivor guilt.

      b) Adjustment in pediatric survivors depends on multiple factors, including the following (Carlson, 2014):

        (1) Age

        (2) Developmental stage at the time of HSCT

        (3) Coping styles of both survivor and family

        (4) Ability to assimilate the experience

    3. Symptoms of depression

      a) Persistent feelings of sadness, anxiety, or emptiness

      b) Feelings of hopelessness

      c) Decreased energy or fatigue

      d) Restlessness and irritability

      e) Risky behavior

  B. Learning and cognitive development

    1. Pediatric survivors should have neuropsychological testing prior to undergoing HSCT and routinely as part of long-term follow-up, especially recipients of TBI. Evaluation should include the following (Baileys, 2013; Cooke, Chung, & Grant, 2011):

      a) Memory and learning

      b) Executive function

      c) Intelligence quotient

    2. Testing and early interventions can decrease difficulties in school, work, and daily life.

      a) Testing should begin one year following HSCT and be repeated every year or every other year.

b) Pediatric HSCT survivors experiencing difficulties in school should be tested.

c) Testing also may be needed during transitions from junior high to high school and high school to college.

C. School reentry

1. Children who have been treated for or continue to battle a chronic illness may experience neurocognitive delays.

2. Young children are at highest risk for neurocognitive damage, particularly children who received treatment at younger than age 3 (Nathan et al., 2007).

3. Gaps in education present challenges to both knowledge acquisition and social function.

4. Learning challenges can happen at any time but especially during transitions from junior high to high school and high school to college.

5. Difficulties include impairments in the following (Nathan et al., 2007):

a) Attention and concentration

b) Processing

c) Visual perception skills

d) Executive function

e) Memory

6. Survivors often feel isolated from peers because of prolonged absences from school and different life experiences, creating barriers to establishing friendships. Risk factors include the following:

a) TBI and cranial spinal boosts

b) Chemotherapies including methotrexate, cytarabine, and corticosteroids (Nathan et al., 2007)

c) Lower socioeconomic status (Children's Oncology Group, 2007; Patel, Lo, Dennis, & Bhatia, 2013)

7. The right to an education is guaranteed by a number of federal laws (Children's Oncology Group, 2007).

a) The Individuals With Disabilities Education Act requires all school districts to identify children with special education needs and provide appropriate programs and services through an Individual Educational Program (American Psychological Association, n.d.).

b) The Rehabilitation Act of 1973 (Section 504) requires schools and universities with federal funding to provide reasonable accommodation to students who are "perceived to have an impairment," including childhood cancer survivors (U.S. Department of Education, 2015).

c) The Americans With Disabilities Act prohibits discrimination against people with disabilities in employment, transportation, public accommodation, communications, and government activities (U.S. Department of Labor, 2009).

D. Psychological growth (Andrykowski et al., 2005; Fromm, Andrykowski, & Hunt, 1996; Widows, Jacobsen, Booth-Jones, & Fields, 2005)

1. Improved self-esteem

2. Greater inner strength

3. Enhanced appreciation for life

4. Reordering of priorities

5. Stronger sense of compassion

6. Improved interpersonal relationships

    7. Enhanced spirituality

E. Recovery themes (Bevans et al., 2014; McQuellon & Andrykowski, 2009)

    1. Reestablishing primary identity

    2. Leaving the role of patient

    3. Reengagement in valued personal, professional, and community roles

    4. Acknowledgment and acceptance of losses secondary to HSCT

    5. Acceptance of any potential or actual long-term effects of transplantation

F. Caregiver and sibling distress

    1. Caregiving is associated with significant physical and emotional stress that often extends past the acute phase of HSCT (Bishop et al., 2007; Norberg, Mellgren, Winiarski, & Forinder, 2014).

    2. Compared to HSCT survivors, caregivers experienced significantly more problems with the following (Bishop et al., 2007):

        a) Alertness and fatigue

        b) Support

        c) Loneliness

        d) Spiritual well-being

        e) Post-traumatic growth

    3. Caregivers may experience long-lasting QOL impairments (Bishop et al., 2007; Langer, Abrams, & Syrjala, 2003).

    4. Siblings may experience the following (Alderfer et al., 2010; Long, Marsland, Wright, & Hinds, 2015):

        a) Decreased QOL

        b) Increased emotional strain

        c) Post-traumatic stress disorder (PTSD) with feelings of sadness and helplessness

        d) Grief related to sibling's diagnosis

        e) Loss of parental attention

G. Assessment

    1. Psychosocial distress after transplant can be predicted based on pre-HSCT assessment of distress (Andorsky, Loberiza, & Lee, 2006; Lee et al., 2005).

    2. Screening for late psychosocial distress is imperative to identify HSCT survivors who are suffering and to intervene to reduce distress.

    3. Guidelines developed by the Center for International Blood and Marrow Transplant Research, American Society for Blood and Marrow Transplantation, and the European Society for Blood and Marrow Transplantation have incorporated assessment for psychosocial distress. Screening should occur at 6 and 12 months and annually thereafter (Rizzo et al., 2006).

    4. The National Comprehensive Cancer Network® (NCCN®) Distress Thermometer is one tool that can be used to assess distress.

        a) The Distress Thermometer asks patients to circle a number between 0 and 10, with 10 representing extreme distress.

        b) Current NCCN distress management guidelines recommend that those who score 4 or above be referred for treatment (NCCN, 2015).

H. Interventions

    1. Nonpharmacologic interventions

        a) Exercise has been shown to have a positive effect on reducing psychological distress (Carlson et al., 2006; Wilson et al., 2005).

> > *b)* Interventions focus on changing specific thoughts or behaviors or learning coping skills (Fulcher, Kim, Smith, & Sherner, 2014; Pidala et al., 2009; Smith, Cope, Sherner, & Walker, 2014).
> > > (1) Relaxation training
> > > (2) Deep breathing exercises
> > > (3) Guided imagery
> > > (4) Meditation (Horton-Deutsch, Day, Haight, & Babin-Nelson, 2007)
> > > (5) Behavior modification or reinforcement
> > > (6) Cognitive therapy
> > 2. Pharmacologic interventions
> > > *a)* Antidepressants (Fulcher et al., 2014)
> > > *b)* Stimulants
> > > *c)* Anxiolytics
> > 3. Education (Fulcher et al., 2014; Smith et al., 2014)
> > > *a)* Provision of accurate and understandable information
> > > *b)* Establishment of realistic expectations regarding survivorship
> > > *c)* Provision of sensory, procedural, or medical information regarding survivorship
> > > *d)* Healthy behaviors
> > > *e)* Available resources
> > 4. Community resources
> > > *a)* Counselors and mental health professionals
> > > *b)* Support groups
> > > *c)* Organizations to assist with school reentry: Pediatric HSCT programs often have school counselors available.
> > 5. Supportive counseling
> > > *a)* Active listening
> > > *b)* Giving permission to explore and express emotions
> > > *c)* Reassurance of the normalcy of feelings
> > 6. Psychotherapy
> > > *a)* Group therapy
> > > *b)* Individual therapy

> V. QOL outcomes (Syrjala & Artherholt, 2009)
> > A. By one year post-HSCT, 75% of survivors report a return to pre-HSCT levels of physical functioning.
> > B. More than 80% of HSCT survivors return to full-time employment by three years following HSCT.
> > C. Most HSCT survivors experience good psychological health despite the intense physical and psychosocial demands of transplant.
> > D. Nevertheless, fatigue, alterations in sexual health, QOL impairments, and infertility are common among transplant survivors.
> > E. PTSD
> > > 1. PTSD incidence in adult survivors is 5%–9% and, in one report, was greater than 40% (Jacobsen et al., 2002; Lee et al., 2005; Widows, Jacobsen, & Fields, 2000).
> > > 2. In pediatric survivors, the incidence can be 10%–21% (Graf, Bergstraesser, & Landolt, 2013).
> > > 3. Risk factors or predictive variables (Jacobsen et al., 2002; Widows et al., 2000)
> > > > *a)* Pre-HSCT psychological distress

        b) Minimal social support

        c) Avoidance coping style

        d) Negative appraisal of transplant experience

    4. Signs and symptoms of PTSD in young children

        a) Bedwetting when previously potty-trained

        b) Forgetting how or being unable to talk

        c) Acting out medical events during playtime

        d) Aggressive behavior

        e) Being unusually clingy to a parent or caregiver

        f) Physical symptoms such as headaches and stomachaches

    5. Signs and symptoms of PTSD in older children, adolescents, or adults

        a) Flashbacks and nightmares

        b) Unusual behavior

        c) Losing interest in activities

        d) Feeling sad

        e) Aggressive behavior

        f) Sleep problems

  F. Facing one's mortality (McQuellon & Andrykowski, 2009)

  G. Fear of recurrence

  H. Consequences of distress

    1. Negative outcomes

    2. Nonadherence to treatment recommendations

    3. Decreased satisfaction with care

    4. Decreased QOL

    5. Difficulties with school and work

    6. Strained relationships

VI. Sexuality

  A. Sexuality is an integral component of the human experience (WHO, 1975).

    1. Sexual health is the integration of somatic, emotional, intellectual, and social aspects of sexual beings in ways that enrich personality, communication, and love (WHO, 1975).

    2. Multidimensional construct with physiologic, psychological, and social dimensions and complex interactions among these dimensions.

  B. Sexual response cycle

    1. Four linear phases: Excitement, plateau, orgasm, and resolution (Masters & Johnson, 1966)

    2. A newer model proposes a motivational incentive-based circular model with overlapping phases (Basson, 2015).

  C. Sexual dysfunctions

    1. Clinically significant disruption in an individual's ability to respond sexually or experience sexual pleasure (American Psychiatric Association, 2013)

    2. Types of sexual dysfunctions reported in HSCT survivors

        a) Hypoactive sexual desire disorder

        b) Female sexual arousal disorder

        c) Erectile dysfunction

        d) Orgasm disorders

        e) Sexual pain disorders (i.e., dyspareunia)

D. Incidence
  1. Females
      a) Eighty percent of female HSCT survivors three to five years post-HSCT report dysfunction or dissatisfaction (Syrjala, Kurland, Abrams, Sanders, & Heiman, 2008; Syrjala et al., 1998).
      b) In several studies, women report more alterations in sexual health than men (Humphreys, Tallman, Altmaier, & Barnette, 2007; Syrjala et al., 1998, 2008).
  2. Males: In men three to five years post-HSCT, the incidence of altered sexual health ranges from 29%–46% (Syrjala et al., 1998, 2008).
E. Physiologic variables contributing to altered sexual health in male HSCT survivors
  1. Damage from the preparative regimen to the hypothalamic-pituitary-gonadal axis
      a) Elevated follicle-stimulating hormone (FSH) in 47%–68%, indicating infertility (Somali et al., 2005; Tauchmanovà et al., 2002)
      b) Elevated luteinizing hormone (LH) in 52% of men (Somali et al., 2005)
      c) Testosterone levels are usually low (Somali et al., 2005; Tauchmanovà et al., 2002): A proportion of male HSCT survivors have low levels of circulating testosterone (Kauppila, Viikari, Irjala, Koskinen, & Remes, 1998).
  2. Cavernosal arterial insufficiency contributes to erectile dysfunction (Chatterjee et al., 2000): Risk of cavernosal arterial insufficiency is 79% in those treated with TBI and 30% in those receiving only chemotherapy.
F. Physiologic variables contributing to altered sexual health in female HSCT survivors
  1. Alkylating agents and radiation are associated with a dose-dependent depletion of both resting and dividing follicles, resulting in infertility and premature ovarian failure (POF).
  2. Hormonal alterations indicative of ovarian failure include elevated FSH and LH combined with low estradiol levels (Somali et al., 2005; Tauchmanovà et al., 2002).
  3. Menopausal symptoms (Beck-Peccoz & Persani, 2006; Loibl, Lintermans, Dieudonné, & Neven, 2011; Piccioni et al., 2004)
      a) Vasomotor symptoms: Hot flashes and night sweats
      b) Insomnia
      c) Mood swings, irritability, depression, and anxiety
      d) Changes in cognitive function
      e) Changes in appearance
      f) Vaginal alterations: Dryness, atrophy and fibrosis, pruritus, and urogenital symptoms
G. Risk factors for vaginal alterations
  1. POF
  2. TBI
  3. Chronic GVHD: Alterations occur in 25%–49% of women with chronic GVHD (Spinelli et al., 2003; Zantomio et al., 2006).
H. Signs and symptoms (Spinelli et al., 2003; Zantomio et al., 2006)
  1. Patient-reported symptoms
      a) Burning or burning on urination
      b) Soreness
      c) Dysuria
      d) Dyspareunia
  2. Clinical signs

        a) Vaginal redness, dryness, and ulcerations
        b) Leukokeratosis
        c) Vulvar denudation
        d) Introital stenosis
        e) Vaginal adhesions

I. Psychosocial variables contributing to altered sexual health in HSCT survivors of both genders
  1. Psychological distress (Claessens, Beerendonk, & Schattenberg, 2006; Humphreys et al., 2007; Joshi et al., 2014)
    a) Changes in body image and feeling self-conscious
    b) Fatigue
    c) Depression
    d) Decreased sexual desire
    e) Infertility
  2. Relationship factors
    a) Diminished sexual relationships
    b) Partner's uncertainty, anxiety, and issues regarding sexual health
    c) Role-shifting within the couple, in particular an increased dependence on the caregiver (usually the sexual partner) during treatment
  3. Infertility may lead to discordance in existing relationships and difficulty establishing intimate relationships.
  4. Adolescent and young adult transplant survivors struggle with complex issues regarding their developing sexuality. Adolescence is a turbulent time for any teenager, but HSCT survivors face added challenges, including the following:
    a) Delayed development of secondary sexual characteristics
    b) Poor self-image
    c) Difficulty developing a sexual identity
    d) Difficulty establishing intimate relationships

J. Barriers in assessment
  1. Silence by healthcare providers remains a significant and persistent barrier to addressing sexuality.
    a) Professional barriers include lack of education and time and personal discomfort.
    b) Thirty percent of HSCT survivors were not informed of potential alterations in sexuality, and 20% were dissatisfied with the information they received on fertility and sexual functioning (Claessens et al., 2006).
    c) Half of the survivors followed three years or more indicated they had no discussion of sexuality with their healthcare providers (Humphreys et al., 2007).
  2. Patient barriers include reluctance of patients to disclose concerns.

K. Assessing for sexual dysfunctions (Tierney, 2009)
  1. Physical examination and medical history
    a) Review medication profile.
    b) Assess lifestyle factors.
  2. Symptom assessment focusing on fatigue and physical stamina
  3. Hormonal testing (Chatterjee & Kottaridis, 2002; Shanis et al., 2012)
    a) In women: FSH, LH, estradiol and androgen levels, and thyroid function
    b) In men: Total testosterone, bioavailable testosterone, sex hormone–binding globulin, FSH, LH, prolactin, and thyroid function

4. Gynecologic examination in women
5. Female pediatric survivors are screened for ovarian failure by Tanner stages of development (van Dorp et al., 2012).
6. Urologic examination in men: Comprehensive evaluation of the functional and structural capacity of the penis (Kandeel, Koussa, & Swerdloff, 2001)
7. Male pediatric survivors are screened for testicular function by assessing Tanner stages of development, testicular volume, and sperm counts (van Dorp et al., 2012).
8. Emotional distress, particularly depression
9. Relationship factors
   a) Stress
   b) Discordance of expectations
   c) Adequacy of communication
10. Presence of other sexual dysfunctions
11. Assessment and intervention models (Krebs, 2008)
   a) PLISSIT: Give the patient permission to discuss the topic, provide limited information and specific suggestions, and refer the patient for intensive therapy.
   b) Ex-PLISSIT: Expand the PLISSIT model to have the patient give permission at each stage of the PLISSIT model (extended permission).
   c) BETTER: Bring up the topic, explain the relationship of sexual health to QOL, tell patients about available resources, time the information to patient's interest, educate patients and their partners about potential alterations in sexuality, and record key elements of the discussion.
   d) PLEASURE: Assess partner, lovemaking, emotions, attitudes, symptoms, understanding, reproduction, and energy, and intervene based on identified concerns.
   e) ALARM: Assess activity, libido, arousal, resolution, and medical history.
   f) Schover model: Evaluate past and present sexual activity, functioning and relationships, and current medical and psychological health, and identify sexual goals, desires, and knowledge.
L. Interventions
   1. Discuss sexual health with patients before transplantation.
      a) Risks of infertility
      b) POF and menopausal symptoms
      c) Possible alterations in sexual functioning
      d) Possibility of delayed development of secondary sex characteristics in pediatric HSCT survivors
      e) Safe sex
      f) Birth control
   2. Education is the first step in establishing expectations for life after HSCT and beginning the process of adaptation. Research has shown that HSCT survivors experience higher levels of psychological distress when a discrepancy exists between their expectations and experiences (Andrykowski et al., 1995).
   3. Offer reassurance that effective interventions for sexual dysfunctions are available.
   4. Include the sexual partner whenever possible.
      a) Facilitate communication.
      b) Identify the partner's anxieties.
      c) Enlist the support of the patient's partner.

5. The pre-HSCT conversation legitimatizes sexuality as a valid area of concern and identifies the healthcare provider as a resource.

6. Early interventions are critical based on a growing body of evidence that sexual dysfunctions do not appear to resolve simply with the passage of time (Syrjala et al., 1998, 2008).

7. Interventions for hypoactive sexual desire disorder
   a) In males, testosterone replacement therapy (TRT) can be effective in improving sexual desire (Somali et al., 2005).
   b) In pediatric males, TRT is reserved for those with extensive damage to the Leydig cells and those unable to progress through puberty (Cohen et al., 2008).
   c) Hormone replacement therapy (HRT) in women may improve sexual desire and functioning.
   d) Female pediatric survivors who fail to start or progress through puberty should receive HRT (Cohen et al., 2008).
   e) Testosterone therapy in women is controversial; however, some women may experience improvements in sexual desire and arousal with androgen therapy (Bancroft, 2005; Piccioni et al., 2004; Zantomio et al., 2006).
   f) Treat other sexual dysfunctions.
   g) Refer couple for counseling to address relationship issues.

8. Interventions for POF
   a) HRT is effective in relieving menopausal symptoms, including the following (Piccioni et al., 2004; Somali et al., 2005; Tichelli & Rovó, 2013):
      (1) Decreasing vasomotor symptoms
      (2) Improving sleep
      (3) Maintaining vaginal elasticity and lubrication
      (4) Decreasing changes in the appearance of the skin and breasts
   b) HRT should be offered to female HSCT survivors after assessing for contraindications such as chronic GVHD of the liver or a history of blood clotting problems (Piccioni et al., 2004; Somali et al., 2005).
   c) Initiation of HRT within the first year following HSCT may be critical to avoiding long-standing issues of sexual dysfunction (Syrjala et al., 1998).
   d) Nonhormonal strategies
      (1) Herbs
      (2) Vitamins
      (3) Yoga
      (4) Acupressure and acupuncture
      (5) Exercise
      (6) Diet modifications

9. Interventions for dyspareunia
   a) Water-soluble vaginal lubricants prior to sexual activity
   b) Vaginal estrogen
   c) Dilators to help restore vaginal patency
   d) Pelvic floor muscle exercises

10. Interventions for vaginal chronic GVHD (Zantomio et al., 2006)
    a) Prevention
       (1) Patient education

        (2) Topical estrogen

        (3) Early initiation of HRT

        (4) Vaginal dilation in the absence of sexual activity

        (5) Regular gynecologic examinations

    b) Treatment

        (1) Topical steroids

        (2) Topical cyclosporine

        (3) Vaginal dilation in women with evidence of vaginal narrowing

  11. Interventions for erectile dysfunction

    a) TRT may improve erectile function (Bancroft, 2005; Somali et al., 2005).

    b) TRT plus phosphodiesterase inhibitors has been successful in treating men with cavernosal arterial insufficiency (Chatterjee, Kottaridis, McGarrigle, & Linch, 2002).

    c) Masturbation may decrease performance anxiety (Gallo-Silver, 2000).

    d) Staying focused on sensations during sexual activity may minimize negative thoughts and performance concerns.

    e) Prolong foreplay to ensure maximum arousal.

    f) Modify contributory medications, if possible.

    g) Phosphodiesterase inhibitors may be prescribed.

VII. Infertility

A. Effects

  1. May negatively affect the QOL of HSCT survivors and their partners (Hammond et al., 2007)

  2. May negatively affect relationships (Hammond et al., 2007)

  3. May delay or prevent the onset of puberty and development of secondary sex characteristics in prepubescent HSCT survivors (Bresters et al., 2014)

B. Pathophysiology: Alkylating agents and radiation cause damage to gonadal tissue and the hypothalamic-pituitary-gonadal axis in both genders (Salooja et al., 2001).

C. Risk factors

  1. Pre-HSCT antineoplastic therapy: Diminishes gonadal reserves in both genders (Tichelli & Rovó, 2013)

  2. Exposure to alkylating agents (Tichelli & Rovó, 2013)

  3. TBI or pelvic irradiation (Anserini et al., 2002; Jadoul & Donnez, 2012)

  4. Older age (Jadoul & Donnez, 2012; Rovó et al., 2006)

D. Prevention

  1. RIC regimens: Needs to be studied prospectively

  2. Alkylating agents and TBI: Avoid when possible.

  3. Gonadotropin-releasing hormone agonists to protect gonadal tissue (Chatterjee & Kottaridis, 2002): Needs further investigation

E. Counseling

  1. Pre-HSCT counseling includes options for fertility preservation with details regarding risks, benefits, procedures, and success rates.

  2. Post-HSCT counseling on prevention of pregnancy: Recommended to avoid pregnancy for the first two years following HSCT when the risk of relapse is highest (Joshi et al., 2014; Majhail et al., 2012).

  3. Follow-up with endocrinologist to ensure transition through puberty also is recommended (Bresters et al., 2014).

F. Preservation
   1. Guidelines for fertility preservation have been published (Joshi et al., 2014; Loren et al., 2013).
   2. Remove barriers to fertility preservation (e.g., healthcare providers' lack of information and knowledge; cost and lack of insurance coverage for patients).
G. Preservation options
   1. Males (Tichelli & Rovó, 2013)
      a) Sperm banking
      b) Testicular tissue cryopreservation (experimental): Risk of tumor contamination (Nixon, 2014)
   2. Females (Tichelli & Rovó, 2013)
      a) Embryo cryopreservation
      b) Oocyte cryopreservation
      c) Ovarian tissue cryopreservation (experimental): Risk of tumor contamination (Nixon, 2014)
H. Spontaneous recovery
   1. Spermatogenesis may recover (Rovó et al., 2006; Savani, Kozanas, Shenoy, & Barrett, 2006).
   2. Among women who had received a chemotherapy-only preparative regimen, 10% had resumption of menstrual cycles. However, this is not necessarily indicative of an ability to conceive (Somali et al., 2005).
I. Pregnancy outcomes: Successful pregnancies have been reported. In one report, the conception rate was 0.6% (Salooja et al., 2001). In another report, 83 pregnancies were reported in female HSCT survivors, with 85% resulting in live births. In male HSCT survivors, 95 pregnancies were reported, with 86% leading to live births (Loren et al., 2011).
J. Pregnancy risks (Salooja et al., 2001)
   1. Increased risk of preterm birth
   2. Increased risk of low birth weight
   3. Similar rate of spontaneous abortion compared to general population
   4. Cardiac decompensation during pregnancy due to prior anthracycline exposure (Hudson, 2010)

VIII. Follow-up care
   A. Long-term care of HSCT survivors and caregivers
      1. Requires a large multidisciplinary team
      2. Coordination is essential to provide comprehensive care.
      3. Survivors play a key role in monitoring their health and health care.
   B. Pediatric survivors (Klassen et al., 2015)
      1. Education on the need for continuous follow-up with an understanding of potential late effects is necessary.
      2. A referral to an adult HSCT program with experience in dealing with late effects may be required.
      3. Pediatric survivors need to be embowered to take over their healthcare needs.
   C. Expanded healthcare team (Tierney & Robinson, 2013)
      1. Care is delivered by multiple providers, including the following:
         a) HSCT team
         b) Oncologist or hematologist

      c) Primary care provider or pediatrician
      d) Medical specialist
    2. Informed HSCT survivors play a critical role in coordinating their complex care needs (Tierney & Robison, 2013).
  D. Care coordination
    1. Frequent communication is necessary (both verbal and written).
    2. Written communications should outline required screening and preventive strategies to minimize complications.
    3. Participation in clinic trials necessitates that study calendars detailing required assessments are available to all healthcare providers and HSCT survivors.
  E. Development of HSCT survivor clinics
    1. Coordinate long-term care.
    2. A nurse coordinator or case manager can be key to the success of such clinics.
  F. Vaccinations
    1. Immunocompromised individuals may not respond to vaccinations.
    2. CD4 counts can be used as a marker of immune system recovery.
    3. Vaccination with inactive vaccines may begin at six months following HSCT, and vaccinations with live vaccines may begin at two years in the absence of ongoing immunosuppression and GVHD (Tomblyn et al., 2009).
    4. Recommended vaccinations (Centers for Disease Control and Prevention, 2016; Majhail et al., 2012; Tomblyn et al., 2009)
      a) Pneumococcal conjugate
      b) Diphtheria-tetanus
      c) Pertussis
      d) Meningococcal conjugate (in pediatric survivors aged 11 years or older)
      e) Inactivated polio
      f) Hepatitis B
      g) Recombinant hepatitis A
      h) Influenza
      i) Measles, mumps, and rubella
      j) Human papillomavirus

Key Points

- Although the majority of hematopoietic stem cell transplantation (HSCT) survivors return to a healthy and satisfying life, all HSCT survivors are at risk for long-term health problems. The HSCT team must effectively communicate with all members of the extended healthcare team regarding recommendations for screening and care.

- Educated HSCT survivors assume an integral role in their long-term health and well-being. Comprehensive and diligent monitoring ensures that problems are identified early and treatment is promptly initiated. Survivors need counseling on healthy living, preventive health maintenance, and health screening recommendations.

- Healthcare providers have an opportunity to improve the quality of life of transplant survivors by intervening to decrease physical symptoms, psychosocial distress, and alterations in sexual functioning and addressing infertility.

References

Alderfer, M.A., Long, K.A., Lown, E.A., Marsland, A.L., Ostrowski, N.L., Hock, J.M., & Ewing, L.J. (2010). Psychosocial adjustment of siblings of children with cancer: A systematic review. *Psycho-Oncology, 19,* 789–805. doi:10.1002/pon.1638

American Cancer Society. (2014). Second cancers in adults. Retrieved from http://www.cancer.org/cancer/cancercauses/othercarcinogens/medicaltreatments/secondcancerscausedbycancertreatment/index

American Psychiatric Association. (2013). *Diagnostic and statistical manual of mental disorders* (5th ed.). Arlington, VA: Author.

American Psychological Association. (n.d.). Individuals With Disabilities Education Act (IDEA). Retrieved from http://www.apa.org/about/gr/issues/disability/idea.aspx

Andorsky, D.J., Loberiza, F.R., & Lee, S.J. (2006). Pre-transplantation physical and mental functioning is strongly associated with self-reported recovery from stem cell transplantation. *Bone Marrow Transplantation, 37,* 889–895. doi:10.1038/sj.bmt.1705347

Andrykowski, M.A., Bishop, M.M., Hahn, E.A., Cella, D.F., Beaumont, J.L., Brady, M.J., ... Wingard, J.R. (2005). Long-term health-related quality of life, growth, and spiritual well-being after hematopoietic stem-cell transplantation. *Journal of Clinical Oncology, 23,* 599–608. doi:10.1200/JCO.2005.03.189

Andrykowski, M.A., Brady, M.J., Greiner, C.B., Altmaier, E.M., Burish, T.G., Antin, J.H., ... Henslee-Downey, P.J. (1995). 'Returning to normal' following bone marrow transplantation: Outcomes, expectations and informed consent. *Bone Marrow Transplantation, 15,* 573–581.

Andrykowski, M.A., Carpenter, J.S., Greiner, C.B., Altmaier, E.M., Burish, T.G., Antin, J.H., ... Henslee-Downey, P.J. (1997). Energy level and sleep quality following bone marrow transplantation. *Bone Marrow Transplantation, 20,* 669–679. doi:10.1038/sj.bmt.1700949

Andrykowski, M.A., Cordova, M.J., Hann, D.M., Jacobsen, P.B., Fields, K.K., & Phillips, G. (1999). Patients' psychosocial concerns following stem cell transplantation. *Bone Marrow Transplantation, 24,* 1121–1129. doi:10.1038/sj.bmt.1702022

Anserini, P., Chiodi, S., Spinelli, S., Costa, M., Conte, N., Copello, F., & Bacigalupo, A. (2002). Semen analysis following allogeneic bone marrow transplantation. Additional data for evidence-based counselling. *Bone Marrow Transplantation, 30,* 447–451. doi:10.1038/sj.bmt.1703651

Baileys, K.A. (2013). Neurologic complications. In S.A. Ezzone (Ed.), *Hematopoietic stem cell transplantation: A manual for nursing practice* (2nd ed., pp. 231–241). Pittsburgh, PA: Oncology Nursing Society.

Baker, K.S., DeFor, T.E., Burns, L.J., Ramsay, N.K., Neglia, J.P., & Robison, L.L. (2003). New malignancies after blood or marrow stem-cell transplantation in children and adults: Incidence and risk factors. *Journal of Clinical Oncology, 21,* 1352–1358. doi:10.1200/jco.2003.05.108

Bancroft, J. (2005). The endocrinology of sexual arousal. *Journal of Endocrinology, 186,* 411–427. doi:10.1677/joe.1.06233

Basson, R. (2015). Human sexual response. In D.B. Vodušek & F. Boller (Eds.), *Handbook of clinical neurology* (Vol. 130, pp. 11–18). doi:10.1016/B978-0-444-63247-0.00002-X

Beck-Peccoz, P., & Persani, L. (2006). Premature ovarian failure. *Orphanet Journal of Rare Diseases, 1,* 9. doi:10.1186/1750-1172-1-9

Bevans, M.F., Mitchell, S.A., Barrett, J.A., Bishop, M.R., Childs, R., Fowler, D., ... Yang, L. (2014). Symptom distress predicts long-term health and well-being in allogeneic stem cell transplantation survivors. *Biology of Blood and Marrow Transplantation, 20,* 387–395. doi:10.1016/j.bbmt.2013.12.001

Bhatia, S., & Bhatia, R. (2009). Secondary malignancies after hematopoietic cell transplantation. In S.J. Forman, F.R. Appelbaum, R.S. Negrin, & K.G. Blume (Eds.), *Thomas' hematopoietic cell transplantation* (4th ed., pp. 1638–1652). West Sussex, UK: Wiley-Blackwell.

Bhatia, S., Francisco, L., Carter, A., Sun, C.L., Baker, K.S., Gurney, J.G., ... Weisdorf, D.J. (2007). Late mortality after allogeneic hematopoietic cell transplantation and functional status of long-term survivors: Report from the Bone Marrow Transplant Survivor Study. *Blood, 110,* 3784–3792. doi:10.1182/blood-2007-03-082933

Bhatia, S., Louie, A.D., Bhatia, R., O'Donnell, M.R., Fung, H., Kashyap, A., ... Forman, S.J. (2001). Solid cancers after bone marrow transplantation. *Journal of Clinical Oncology, 19,* 464–471.

Bhatia, S., Ramsay, N.K., Steinbuch, M., Dusenbery, K.E., Shapiro, R.S., Weisdorf, D.J, ... Neglia, J.P. (1996). Malignant neoplasms following bone marrow transplantation. *Blood, 87,* 3633–3639.

Bhatia, S., Robison, L.L., Francisco, L., Carter, A., Liu, Y., Grant, M., ... Forman, S.J. (2005). Late mortality in survivors of autologous hematopoietic-cell transplantation: Report from the Bone Marrow Transplant Survivor Study. *Blood, 105,* 4215–4222. doi:10.1182/blood-2005-01-0035

Bishop, M.M., Beaumont, J.L., Hahn, E.A., Cella, D., Andrykowski, M.A., Brady, M.J., ... Wingard, J.R. (2007). Late effects of cancer and hematopoietic stem-cell transplantation on spouses or partners compared with survivors and survivor-matched controls. *Journal of Clinical Oncology, 25,* 1403–1411. doi:10.1200/JCO.2006.07.5705

Bresters, D., Emons, J.A.M., Nuri, N., Ball, L.M., Kollen, W.J.W., Hannema, S.E., … Oostdijk, W. (2014). Ovarian insufficiency and pubertal development after hematopoietic stem cell transplantation in childhood. *Pediatric Blood and Cancer, 61,* 2048–2053. doi:10.1002/pbc.25162

CancerConnect. (2014). Secondary malignancies. Retrieved from http://news.cancerconnect.com/secondary-malignancies

Carlson, C.A. (2014). Late effects of childhood cancer. In N.E. Kline (Ed.), *Essentials of pediatric hematology/oncology nursing: A core curriculum* (4th ed., pp. 391–458). Chicago, IL: Association of Pediatric Hematology/Oncology Nurses.

Carlson, L.E., Smith, D., Russell, J., Fibich, C., & Whittaker, T. (2006). Individualized exercise program for the treatment of severe fatigue in patients after allogeneic hematopoietic stem-cell transplant: A pilot study. *Bone Marrow Transplantation, 37,* 945–954. doi:10.1038/sj.bmt.1705343

Centers for Disease Control and Prevention. (2016). Birth–18 years and "catch-up" immunization schedules. Retrieved from http://www.cdc.gov/vaccines/schedules/hcp/child-adolescent.html

Chang, G., Orav, J., McNamara, T.K., Tong, M.-Y., & Antin, J.H. (2005). Psychosocial function after hematopoietic stem cell transplantation. *Psychosomatics, 46,* 34–40. doi:10.1176/appi.psy.46.1.34

Chatterjee, R., Andrews, H., McGarrigle, H.H., Kottaridis, P., Lees, W., Mackinnon, S., … Goldstone, A. (2000). Cavernosal arterial insufficiency is a major component of erectile dysfunction in some recipients of high-dose chemotherapy/chemoradiotherapy for haematological malignancies. *Bone Marrow Transplantation, 25,* 1185–1189. doi:10.1038/sj.bmt.1702391

Chatterjee, R., & Kottaridis, P.D. (2002). Treatment of gonadal damage in recipients of allogeneic or autologous transplantation for haematological malignancies. *Bone Marrow Transplantation, 30,* 629–635. doi:10.1038/sj.bmt.1703721

Chatterjee, R., Kottaridis, P.D., McGarrigle, H.H., & Linch, D.C. (2002). Management of erectile dysfunction by combination therapy with testosterone and sildenafil in recipients of high-dose therapy for haematological malignancies. *Bone Marrow Transplantation, 29,* 607–610. doi:10.1038/sj.bmt.1703421

Children's Oncology Group. (2007). *Establishing and enhancing services for childhood cancer survivors: Long-term follow-up resource guide.* Retrieved from http://www.survivorshipguidelines.org/pdf/LTFUResourceGuide.pdf

Claessens, J.J., Beerendonk, C.C.M., & Schattenberg, A.V. (2006). Quality of life, reproduction and sexuality after stem cell transplantation with partially T-cell-depleted grafts and after conditioning with a regimen including total body irradiation. *Bone Marrow Transplantation, 37,* 831–836. doi:10.1038/sj.bmt.1705350

Cohen, A., Békássy, A.N., Gaiero, A., Faraci, M., Zecca, S., Tichelli, A., & Dini, G. (2008). Endocrinological late complications after hematopoietic SCT in children. *Bone Marrow Transplantation, 41*(Suppl. 2), S43–S48. doi:10.1038/bmt.2008.54

Cooke, L., Chung, C., & Grant, M. (2011). Psychosocial care for adolescent and young adult hematopoietic cell transplant patients. *Journal of Psychosocial Oncology, 29,* 394–414. doi:10.1080/07347332.2011.582636

Curtis, R.E., Rowlings, P.A., Deeg, H.J., Shriner, D.A., Socié, G., Travis, L.B., … Boice, J.D. (1997). Solid cancers after bone marrow transplantation. *New England Journal of Medicine, 336,* 897–904. doi:10.1056/NEJM199703273361301

Curtis, R.E., Travis, L.B., Rowlings, P.A., Socié, G., Kingma, D.W., Banks, P.M., … Deeg, H.J. (1999). Risk of lymphoproliferative disorders after bone marrow transplantation: A multi-institutional study. *Blood, 94,* 2208–2216.

Duell, T., van Lint, M.T., Ljungman, P., Tichelli, A., Socié, G., Apperley, J.F., … Kolb, H.-J. (1997). Health and functional status of long-term survivors of bone marrow transplantation. *Annals of Internal Medicine, 126,* 184–192. doi:10.7326/0003-4819-126-3-199702010-00002

Felix, C.A., Walker, A.H., Lange, B.J., Williams, T.M., Winick, N.J., Cheung, N.-K., … Rebbeck, T.R. (1998). Association of CYP3A4 genotype with treatment-related leukemia. *Proceedings of the National Academy of Sciences of the United States of America, 95,* 13176–13181. doi:10.1073/pnas.95.22.13176

Ferrell, B., Grant, M., Schmidt, G.M., Rhiner, M., Whitehead, C., Fonbuena, P., & Forman, S.J. (1992). The meaning of quality of life for bone marrow transplant survivors. Part 1. The impact of bone marrow transplant on quality of life. *Cancer Nursing, 15,* 153–160. doi:10.1097/00002820-199206000-00001

Fox, C.P., Burns, D., Parker, A.N., Peggs, K.S., Harvey, C.M., Natarajan, S., … Chaganti, S. (2014). EBV-associated post-transplant lymphoproliferative disorder following in vivo T-cell-depleted allogeneic transplantation: Clinical features, viral load correlates and prognostic factors in the rituximab era. *Bone Marrow Transplantation, 49,* 280–286. doi:10.1038/bmt.2013.170

Fraser, C.J., Bhatia, S., Ness, K., Carter, A., Francisco, L., Arora, M., … Baker, K.S. (2006). Impact of chronic graft-versus-host disease on the health status of hematopoietic cell transplantation survivors: A report from the Bone Marrow Transplant Survivor Study. *Blood, 108,* 2867–2873. doi:10.1182/blood-2006-02-003954

Friedberg, J.W., Neuberg, D., Stone, R.M., Alyea, E., Jallow, H., LaCasce, A., … Freedman, A.S. (1999). Outcome in patients with myelodysplastic syndrome after autologous bone marrow transplantation for non-Hodgkin's lymphoma. *Journal of Clinical Oncology, 17,* 3128–3135.

Fromm, K., Andrykowski, M.A., & Hunt, J. (1996). Positive and negative psychosocial sequelae of bone marrow transplantation: Implications for quality of life assessment. *Journal of Behavioral Medicine, 19,* 221–240. doi:10.1007/BF01857767

Fulcher, C.D., Kim, H.-J., Smith, P.R., & Sherner, T.L. (2014). Putting evidence into practice: Evidence-based interventions for depression. *Clinical Journal of Oncology Nursing, 18*(Suppl. 1), 26–37. doi:10.1188/08.CJON.131-140

Gallagher, G., & Forrest, D.L. (2007). Second solid cancers after allogeneic hematopoietic stem cell transplantation. *Cancer, 109,* 84–92. doi:10.1002/cncr.22375

Gallo-Silver, L. (2000). The sexual rehabilitation of persons with cancer. *Cancer Practice, 8,* 10–15. doi:10.1046/j.1523-5394.2000.81005.x

Gerdemann, U., Katari, U.L., Papadopoulou, A., Keirnan, J.M., Craddock, J.A., Liu, H., … Leen, A.M. (2013). Safety and clinical efficacy of rapidly-generated trivirus-directed T cells as treatment for adenovirus, EBV, and CMV infections after allogeneic hematopoietic stem cell transplant. *Molecular Therapy, 21,* 2113–2121. doi:10.1038/mt.2013.151

Gerson, R., & Rappaport, N. (2013). Traumatic stress and posttraumatic stress disorder in youth: Recent research findings on clinical impact, assessment, and treatment. *Journal of Adolescent Health, 52,* 137–143. doi:10.1016/j.jadohealth.2012.06.018

Graf, A., Bergstraesser, E., & Landolt, M.A. (2013). Posttraumatic stress in infants and preschoolers with cancer. *Psycho-Oncology, 22,* 1543–1548. doi:10.1002/pon.3164

Hammond, C., Abrams, J.R., & Syrjala, K.L. (2007). Fertility and risk factors for elevated infertility concern in 10-year hematopoietic cell transplant survivors and case-matched controls. *Journal of Clinical Oncology, 25,* 3511–3517. doi:10.1200/JCO.2007.10.8993

Harder, H., Cornelissen, J.J., Van Gool, A.R., Duivenvoorden, H.J., Eijkenboom, W.M., & van den Bent, M.J. (2002). Cognitive functioning and quality of life in long-term adult survivors of bone marrow transplantation. *Cancer, 95,* 183–192. doi:10.1002/cncr.10627

Heinonen, H., Volin, L., Uutela, A., Zevon, M., Barrick, C., & Ruutu, T. (2001). Quality of life and factors related to perceived satisfaction with quality of life after allogeneic bone marrow transplantation. *Annals of Hematology, 80,* 137–143. doi:10.1007/s002770000249

Hjermstad, M.J., Knobel, H., Brinch, L., Fayers, P.M., Loge, J.H., Holte, H., & Kaasa, S. (2004). A prospective study of health-related quality of life, fatigue, anxiety and depression 3–5 years after stem cell transplantation. *Bone Marrow Transplantation, 34,* 257–266. doi:10.1038/sj.bmt.1704561

Horowitz, M.M. (2016). Uses and growth of hematopoietic cell transplantation. In S.J. Forman, R.S. Negrin, J.H. Antin, & F.R. Appelbaum (Eds.), *Thomas' hematopoietic cell transplantation* (5th ed., pp. 8–15). West Sussex, UK: Wiley-Blackwell.

Horton-Deutsch, S., Day, P.O., Haight, R., & Babin-Nelson, M. (2007). Enhancing mental health services to bone marrow transplant recipients through a mindfulness-based therapeutic intervention. *Complementary Therapies in Clinical Practice, 13,* 110–115. doi:10.1016/j.ctcp.2006.11.003

Hudson, M.M. (2010). Reproductive outcomes for survivors of childhood cancer. *Obstetrics and Gynecology, 116,* 1171–1183. doi:10.1097/AOG.0b013e3181f87c4b

Humphreys, C.T., Tallman, B., Altmaier, E.M., & Barnette, V. (2007). Sexual functioning in patients undergoing bone marrow transplantation: A longitudinal study. *Bone Marrow Transplantation, 39,* 491–496. doi:10.1038/sj.bmt.1705613

Jacobsen, P.B., Sadler, I.J., Booth-Jones, M., Soety, E., Weitzner, M.A., & Fields, K.K. (2002). Predictors of posttraumatic stress disorder symptomatology following bone marrow transplantation for cancer. *Journal of Consulting and Clinical Psychology, 70,* 235–240. doi:10.1037/0022-006X.70.1.235

Jadoul, P., & Donnez, J. (2012). How does bone marrow transplantation affect ovarian function and fertility? *Current Opinion in Obstetrics and Gynecology, 24,* 164–171. doi:10.1097/GCO.0b013e328353bb57

Jans, S.R., Schomerus, E., & Bygum, A. (2015). Neurofibromatosis type 1 diagnosed in a child based on multiple juvenile xanthogranulomas and juvenile myelomonocytic leukemia. *Pediatric Dermatology, 32,* e29–e32. doi:10.1111/pde.12478

Jim, H.S., Syrjala, K.L., & Rizzo, D. (2012). Supportive care of hematopoietic cell transplant patients. *Biology of Blood and Marrow Transplantation, 18*(Suppl. 1), S12–S16. doi:10.1016/j.bbmt.2011.10.029

Joshi, S., Savani, B.N., Chow, E.J., Gilleece, M.H., Halter, J., Jacobsohn, D.A., … Majhail, N.S. (2014). Clinical guide to fertility preservation in hematopoietic cell transplant recipients. *Bone Marrow Transplantation, 49,* 477–484. doi:10.1038/bmt.2013.211

Kandeel, F.R., Koussa, V.K.T., & Swerdloff, R.S. (2001). Male sexual function and its disorders: Physiology, patho-physiology, clinical investigation, and treatment. *Endocrine Reviews, 22,* 342–388. doi:10.1210/edrv.22.3.0430

Kauppila, M., Viikari, J., Irjala, K., Koskinen, P., & Remes, K. (1998). The hypothalamus–pituitary–gonad axis and testicular function in male patients after treatment for haematological malignancies. *Journal of Internal Medicine, 244,* 411–416. doi:10.1046/j.1365-2796.1998.00390.x

Kiss, T.L., Abdolell, M., Jamal, N., Minden, M.D., Lipton, J.H., & Messner, H.A. (2002). Long-term medical outcomes and quality-of-life assessment of patients with chronic myeloid leukemia followed at least 10 years after allogeneic bone marrow transplantation. *Journal of Clinical Oncology, 20,* 2334–2343. doi:10.1200/JCO.2002.06.077

Kiviat, J. (2013). Quality-of-life issues. In S.A. Ezzone (Ed.), *Hematopoietic stem cell transplantation: A manual for nursing practice* (2nd ed., pp. 283–291). Pittsburgh, PA: Oncology Nursing Society.

Klassen, A.F., Rosenberg-Yunger, Z.R.S., D'Agostino, N.M., Cano, S.J., Barr, R., Syed, I., … Nathan, P.C. (2015). The development of scales to measure childhood cancer survivors' readiness for transition to long-term follow-up care as adults. *Health Expectations, 18,* 1941–1955. doi:10.1111/hex.12241

Kolb, H.J., Socié, G., Duell, T., Van Lint, M.T., Tichelli, A., Apperley, J.F., … Prentice, H.G. (1999). Malignant neoplasms in long-term survivors of bone marrow transplantation. *Annals of Internal Medicine, 131,* 738–744. doi:10.7326/0003-4819-131-10-199911160-00004

Krebs, L.U. (2008). Sexual assessment in cancer care: Concepts, methods, and strategies for success. *Seminars in Oncology Nursing, 24,* 80–90. doi:10.1016/j.soncn.2008.02.002

Kuehnle, I., Huls, M.H., Liu, Z., Semmelmann, M., Krance, R.A., Brenner, M.K., … Heslop, H.E. (2000). CD20 monoclonal antibody (rituximab) for therapy of Epstein-Barr virus lymphoma after hematopoietic stem-cell transplantation. *Blood, 95,* 1502–1505.

Kuriyama, T., Kawano, N., Yamashita, K., & Ueda, A. (2014). Successful treatment of rituximab-resistant Epstein-Barr virus-associated post-transplant lymphoproliferative disorder using R-CHOP. *Journal of Clinical and Experimental Hematopathology, 54,* 149–153. doi:10.3960/jslrt.54.149

Kurtz, B.P., & Abrams, A.N. (2010). Psychiatric aspects of pediatric cancer. *Child and Adolescent Psychiatric Clinics of North America, 19,* 401–421. doi:10.1016/j.chc.2010.01.009

Langer, S., Abrams, J., & Syrjala, K. (2003). Caregiver and patient marital satisfaction and affect following hematopoietic stem cell transplantation: A prospective, longitudinal investigation. *Psycho-Oncology, 12,* 239–253. doi:10.1002/pon.633

Lee, S.J., Fairclough, D., Parsons, S.K., Soiffer, R.J., Fisher, D.C., Schlossman, R.L., … Weeks, J.C. (2001). Recovery after stem-cell transplantation for hematologic diseases. *Journal of Clinical Oncology, 19,* 242–252.

Lee, S.J., Kim, H.T., Ho, V.T., Cutler, C., Alyea, E.P., Soiffer, R.J., & Antin, J.H. (2006). Quality of life associated with acute and chronic graft-versus-host disease. *Bone Marrow Transplantation, 38,* 305–310. doi:10.1038/sj.bmt.1705434

Lee, S.J., Loberiza, F.R., Antin, J.H., Kirkpatrick, T., Prokop, L., Alyea, E.P., … Soiffer, R.J. (2005). Routine screening for psychosocial distress following hematopoietic stem cell transplantation. *Bone Marrow Transplantation, 35,* 77–83. doi:10.1038/sj.bmt.1704709

Loibl, S., Lintermans, A., Dieudonné, A.S., & Neven, P. (2011). Management of menopausal symptoms in breast cancer patients. *Maturitas, 68,* 148–154. doi:10.1016/j.maturitas.2010.11.013

Long, K.A., Marsland, A.L., Wright, A., & Hinds, P. (2015). Creating a tenuous balance: Siblings' experience of a brother's or sister's childhood cancer diagnosis. *Journal of Pediatric Oncology Nursing, 32,* 21–31. doi:10.1177/1043454214555194

Loren, A.W., Chow, E., Jacobsohn, D.A., Gilleece, M., Halter, J., Joshi, S., … Majhail, N.S. (2011). Pregnancy after hematopoietic cell transplantation: A report from the late effects working committee of the Center for International Blood and Marrow Transplant Research (CIBMTR). *Biology of Blood and Marrow Transplantation, 17,* 157–166. doi:10.1016/j.bbmt.2010.07.009

Loren, A.W., Mangu, P.B., Beck, L.N., Brennan, L., Magdalinski, A.J., Partridge, A.H., … Oktay, K. (2013). Fertility preservation for patients with cancer: American Society of Clinical Oncology clinical practice guideline update. *Journal of Clinical Oncology, 31,* 2500–2510. doi:10.1200/JCO.2013.49.2678

Lovett, B.D., Strumberg, D., Blair, I.A., Pang, S., Burden, D.A., Megonigal, M.D., … Felix, C.A. (2001). Etoposide metabolites enhance DNA topoisomerase II cleavage near leukemia-associated *MLL* translocation breakpoints. *Biochemistry, 40,* 1159–1170. doi:10.1021/bi002361x

Majhail, N.S. (2008). Old and new cancers after hematopoietic-cell transplantation. *ASH Education Book, 2008,* 142–149. doi:10.1182/asheducation-2008.1.142

Majhail, N.S., & Rizzo, J.D. (2013). Surviving the cure: Long term followup of hematopoietic cell transplant recipients. *Bone Marrow Transplantation, 48,* 1145–1151. doi:10.1038/bmt.2012.258

Majhail, N.S., Rizzo, J.D., Lee, S.J., Aljurf, M., Atsuta, Y., Bonfim, C., ... Tichelli, A. (2012). Recommended screening and preventive practices for long-term survivors after hematopoietic cell transplantation. *Biology of Blood and Marrow Transplantation, 18*, 348–371.

Malric, A., Defachelles, A.-S., Leblanc, T., Lescoeur, B., Lacour, B., Peuchmaur, M., ... Bourdeaut, F. (2015). Fanconi anemia and solid malignancies in childhood: A national retrospective study. *Pediatric Blood and Cancer, 62*, 463–470. doi:10.1002/pbc.25303

Masters, W.H., & Johnson, V.E. (1966). *Human sexual response.* Boston, MA: Little, Brown and Co.

McQuellon, R.P., & Andrykowski, M. (2009). Psychosocial issues in hematopoietic cell transplantation. In S.J. Forman, F.R. Appelbaum, R.S. Negrin, & K.G. Blume (Eds.), *Thomas' hematopoietic cell transplantation* (4th ed., pp. 488–501). West Sussex, UK: Wiley-Blackwell.

McQuellon, R.P., Russell, G.B., Rambo, T.D., Craven, B.L., Radford, J., Perry, J.J., ... Hurd, D.D. (1998). Quality of life and psychological distress of bone marrow transplant recipients: The 'time trajectory' to recovery over the first year. *Bone Marrow Transplantation, 21*, 477–486. doi:10.1038/sj.bmt.1701115

Megonigal, M.D., Cheung, N.K., Rappaport, E.F., Nowell, P.C., Wilson, R.B., Jones, D.H., ... Felix, C.A. (2000). Detection of leukemia-associated *MLL-GAS7* translocation early during chemotherapy with DNA topoisomerase II inhibitors. *Proceedings of the National Academy of Sciences of the United States of America, 97*, 2814–2819. doi:10.1073/pnas.050397097

Nathan, P.C., Patel, S.K., Dilley, K., Goldsby, R., Harvey, J., Jacobsen, C., ... Armstrong, F.D. (2007). Guidelines for identification of, advocacy for, and intervention in neurocognitive problems in survivors of childhood cancer: A report from the Children's Oncology Group. *Archives of Pediatric and Adolescent Medicine, 161*, 798–806. doi:10.1001/archpedi.161.8.798

National Cancer Institute. (n.d.). NCI dictionary of cancer terms. Retrieved from http://www.cancer.gov/dictionary

National Comprehensive Cancer Network. (2015). *NCCN Clinical Practice Guidelines in Oncology (NCCN Guidelines®): Distress management* [v.3.2015]. Retrieved from http://www.nccn.org/professionals/physician_gls/pdf/distress.pdf

Nixon, C. (2014). Side effects of treatment. In N.E. Kline (Ed.), *Essentials of pediatric hematology/oncology nursing: A core curriculum* (4th ed., pp. 199–262). Chicago, IL: Association of Pediatric Hematology/Oncology Nurses.

Norberg, L., Mellgren, K., Winiarski, J., & Forinder, U. (2014). Relationship between problems related to child late effects and parent burnout after pediatric hematopoietic stem cell transplantation. *Pediatric Transplantation, 18*, 302–309. doi:10.1111/petr.12228

Patel, S.K., Lo, T.T., Dennis, J.M., & Bhatia, S. (2013). Neurocognitive and behavioral outcomes in Latino childhood cancer survivors. *Pediatric Blood and Cancer, 60*, 1696–1702. doi:10.1002/pbc.24608

Piccioni, P., Scirpa, P., D'Emilio, I., Sora, F., Scarciglia, M., Laurenti, L., ... Chiusolo, P. (2004). Hormonal replacement therapy after stem cell transplantation. *Maturitas, 49*, 327–333. doi:10.1016/j.maturitas.2004.02.015

Pidala, J., Anasetti, C., & Jim, H. (2009). Quality of life after allogeneic hematopoietic cell transplantation. *Blood, 114*, 7–19. doi:10.1182/blood-2008-10-182592

Radich, J.P., Gooley, T., Sanders, J.E., Anasetti, C., Chauncey, T., & Appelbaum, F.R. (2000). Second allogeneic transplantation after failure of first autologous transplantation. *Biology of Blood and Marrow Transplantation, 6*, 272–279. doi:10.1016/S1083-8791(00)70009-7

Rizzo, J.D., Curtis, R.E., Socié, G., Sobocinski, K.A., Gilbert, E., Landgren, O., ... Deeg, H.J. (2009). Solid cancers after allogeneic hematopoietic cell transplantation. *Blood, 113*, 1175–1183. doi:10.1182/blood-2008-05-158782

Rizzo, J.D., Wingard, J.R., Tichelli, A., Lee, S.J., Van Lint, M.T., Burns, L.J., ... Socié, G. (2006). Recommended screening and preventive practices for long-term survivors after hematopoietic cell transplantation: Joint recommendations of the European Group for Blood and Marrow Transplantation, the Center for International Blood and Marrow Transplant Research, and the American Society of Blood and Marrow Transplantation. *Biology of Blood and Marrow Transplantation, 12*, 138–151. doi:10.1016/j.bbmt.2005.09.012

Rovó, A., Tichelli, A., Passweg, J.R., Heim, D., Meyer-Monard, S., Holzgreve, W., ... De Geyter, C. (2006). Spermatogenesis in long-term survivors after allogeneic hematopoietic stem cell transplantation is associated with age, time interval since transplantation, and apparently absence of chronic GvHD. *Blood, 108*, 1100–1105. doi:10.1182/blood-2006-01-0176

Salooja, N., Szydlo, R.M., Socié, G., Rio, B., Chatterjee, R., Ljungman, P., ... Apperley, J.F. (2001). Pregnancy outcomes after peripheral blood or bone marrow transplantation: A retrospective survey. *Lancet, 358*, 271–276. doi:10.1016/S0140-6736(01)05482-4

Savani, B.N., Kozanas, E., Shenoy, A., & Barrett, A.J. (2006). Recovery of spermatogenesis after total-body irradiation. *Blood, 108*, 4292–4293. doi:10.1182/blood-2006-08-044289

Shanis, D., Merideth, M., Pulanic, T.K., Savani, B.N., Battiwalla, M., & Stratton, P. (2012). Female long-term survivors after allogeneic hematopoietic stem cell transplantation: Evaluation and management. *Seminars in Hematology, 49*, 83–93. doi:10.1053/j.seminhematol.2011.10.002

Shannon, S.P. (2013). Relapse and secondary malignancies. In S.A. Ezzone (Ed.), *Hematopoietic stem cell transplantation: A manual for nursing practice* (2nd ed., pp. 245–249). Pittsburgh, PA: Oncology Nursing Society.

Shimada, K., Yokozawa, T., Atsuta, Y., Kohno, A., Maruyama, F., Yano, K., ... Morishita, Y. (2005). Solid tumors after hematopoietic stem cell transplantation in Japan: Incidence, risk factors and prognosis. *Bone Marrow Transplantation, 36,* 115–121. doi:10.1038/sj.bmt.1705020

Smith, P.R., Cope, D., Sherner, T.L., & Walker, D.K. (2014). Update on research-based interventions for anxiety in patients with cancer. *Clinical Journal of Oncology Nursing, 18*(Suppl. 1), 5–16. doi:10.1188/14.CJON.S3.5-16

Socié, G., & Rizzo, J.D. (2012). Second solid tumors: Screening and management guidelines in long-term survivors after allogeneic stem cell transplantation. *Seminars in Hematology, 49,* 4–9. doi:10.1053/j.seminhematol.2011.10.013

Somali, M., Mpatakoias, V., Avramides, A., Sakellari, I., Kaloyannidis, P., Smias, C., ... Vagenakis, A. (2005). Function of the hypothalamic-pituitary-gonadal axis in long-term survivors of hematopoietic stem cell transplantation for hematological diseases. *Gynecology and Endocrinology, 21,* 18–26. doi:10.1080/09513590500099255

Spinelli, S., Chiodi, S., Costantini, S., Van Lint, M.T., Raiola, A.M., Ravera, G.B., & Bacigalupo, A. (2003). Female genital tract graft-versus-host disease following allogeneic bone marrow transplantation. *Haematologica, 88,* 1163–1168.

Sun, C.L., Kersey, J.H., Francisco, L., Armenian, S.H., Baker, K.S., Weisdorf, D.J., ... Bhatia, S. (2013). Burden of morbidity in 10+ year survivors of hematopoietic cell transplantation: Report from the Bone Marrow Transplantation Survivor Study. *Biology of Blood and Marrow Transplantation, 19,* 1073–1080. doi:10.1016/j.bbmt.2013.04.002

Syrjala, K.L., & Artherholt, S.B. (2009). Assessment of quality of life in hematopoietic cell transplantation recipients. In S.J. Forman, F.R. Appelbaum, R.S. Negrin, & K.G. Blume (Eds.), *Thomas' hematopoietic cell transplantation* (4th ed., pp. 502–514). West Sussex, UK: Wiley-Blackwell.

Syrjala, K.L., Kurland, B.F., Abrams, J.R., Sanders, J.E., & Heiman, J.R. (2008). Sexual function changes during the 5 years after high-dose treatment and hematopoietic cell transplantation for malignancy, with case-matched controls at 5 years. *Blood, 111,* 989–996. doi:10.1182/blood-2007-06-096594

Syrjala, K.L., Langer, S.L., Abrams, J.R., Storer, B.E., & Martin, P.J. (2005). Late effects of hematopoietic cell transplantation among 10-year adult survivors compared with case-matched controls. *Journal of Clinical Oncology, 23,* 6596–6606. doi:10.1200/JCO.2005.12.674

Syrjala, K.L., Langer, S.L., Abrams, J.R., Storer, B., Sanders, J.E., Flowers, M.E., & Martin, P.J. (2004). Recovery and long-term function after hematopoietic cell transplantation for leukemia or lymphoma. *JAMA, 291,* 2335–2343. doi:10.1001/jama.291.19.2335

Syrjala, K.L., Roth-Roemer, S.L., Abrams, J.R., Scanlan, J.M., Chapko, M.K., Visser, S., & Sanders, J.E. (1998). Prevalence and predictors of sexual dysfunction in long-term survivors of marrow transplantation. *Journal of Clinical Oncology, 16,* 3148–3157.

Tauchmanovà, L., Selleri, C., Rosa, G.D., Pagano, L., Orio, F., Lombardi, G., ... Colao, A. (2002). High prevalence of endocrine dysfunction in long-term survivors after allogeneic bone marrow transplantation for hematologic diseases. *Cancer, 95,* 1076–1084. doi:10.1002/cncr.10773

Tewari, P., Franklin, A.R., Tarek, N., Askins, M.A., Mofield, S., & Kebriaei, P. (2014). Hematopoietic stem cell transplantation in adolescents and young adults. *Acta Haematologica, 132,* 313–325. doi:10.1159/000360211

Tichelli, A., & Rovó, A. (2013). Fertility issues following hematopoietic stem cell transplantation. *Expert Reviews in Hematology, 6,* 375–388. doi:10.1586/17474086.2013.816507

Tierney, D.K. (2009). Sexuality following hematopoietic cell transplantation: An important health-related quality of life issue. In S.J. Forman, F.R. Appelbaum, R.S. Negrin, & K.G. Blume (Eds.), *Thomas' hematopoietic cell transplantation* (4th ed., pp. 515–525). West Sussex, UK: Wiley-Blackwell.

Tierney, D.K., & Robinson, T. (2013). Long-term care of hematopoietic cell transplant survivors. In S.A. Ezzone (Ed.), *Hematopoietic stem cell transplantation: A manual for nursing practice* (2nd ed., pp. 251–267). Pittsburgh, PA: Oncology Nursing Society.

Tomblyn, M., Chiller, T., Einsele, H., Gress, R., Sepkowitz, K., Storek, J., ... Boeckh, M.A. (2009). Guidelines for preventing infectious complications among hematopoietic cell transplantation recipients: A global perspective. *Biology of Blood and Marrow Transplantation, 15,* 1143–1238. doi:10.1016/j.bbmt.2009.06.019

U.S. Department of Education. (2015). Protecting students with disabilities. Retrieved from http://www2.ed.gov/about/offices/list/ocr/504faq.html

U.S. Department of Labor. (2009, June 15). Americans With Disabilities Act of 1990, as amended. Retrieved from http://www.ada.gov/pubs/adastatute08.htm

van Dorp, W., van Beek, R.D., Laven, J.S., Pieters, R., de Muinck Keizer-Schrama, S.M., & van den Heuvel-Eibrink, M.M. (2012). Long-term endocrine side effects of childhood Hodgkin's lymphoma treatment: A review. *Human Reproduction Update, 18,* 12–28. doi:10.1093/humupd/dmr038

Vardiman, J.W., Harris, N.L., & Brunning, R.D. (2002). The World Health Organization (WHO) classification of the myeloid neoplasms. *Blood, 100,* 2292–2302. doi:10.1182/blood-2002-04-1199

Vaxman, I., Ram, R., Gafter-Gvili, A., Vidal, L., Yeshurun, M., Lahav, M., & Shpilberg, O. (2015). Secondary malignancies following high dose therapy and autologous hematopoietic cell transplantation-systematic review and meta-analysis. *Bone Marrow Transplantation, 50,* 706–714. doi:10.1038/bmt.2014.325

Widows, M.R., Jacobsen, P.B., Booth-Jones, M., & Fields, K.K. (2005). Predictors of posttraumatic growth following bone marrow transplantation for cancer. *Health Psychology, 24,* 266–273. doi:10.1037/0278-6133.24.3.266

Widows, M.R., Jacobsen, P.B., & Fields, K.K. (2000). Relation of psychological vulnerability factors to posttraumatic stress disorder symptomatology in bone marrow transplant recipients. *Psychosomatic Medicine, 62,* 873–882. doi:10.1097/00006842-200011000-0001

Wilson, R.W., Jacobsen, P.B., & Fields, K.K. (2005). Pilot study of a home-based aerobic exercise program for sedentary cancer survivors treated with hematopoietic stem cell transplantation. *Bone Marrow Transplantation, 35,* 721–727. doi:10.1038/sj.bmt.1704815

Wingard, J.R., Huang, I.C., Sobocinski, K.A., Andrykowski, M.A., Cella, D., Rizzo, J.D., ... Bishop, M.M. (2010). Factors associated with self-reported physical and mental health after hematopoietic cell transplantation. *Biology of Blood and Marrow Transplantation, 16,* 1682–1692. doi:10.1016/j.bbmt.2010.05.017

World Health Organization. (1946). *Preamble of the constitution of the World Health Organization* (Vol. 2). Geneva, Switzerland: Author.

World Health Organization. (1975). *Education and treatment in human sexuality: The training of health professionals* (WHO Technical Report Series, No. 572). Geneva, Switzerland: Author.

Zantomio, D., Grigg, A., MacGregor, L., Panek-Hudson, Y., Szer, J., & Ayton, R. (2006). Female genital tract graft-versus-host disease: Incidence, risk factors and recommendations for management. *Bone Marrow Transplantation, 38,* 567–572. doi:10.1038/sj.bmt.1705487

Survivorship Resources	
Topic	**Website**
Education	www.dol.gov/odep www.ed.gov www.hhs.gov/ocr/civilrights/resources/factsheets
Fertility	www.asco.org/guidelines/fertility www.livestrong.org/we-can-help/fertility-services www.myoncofertility.org www.path2parenthood.org www.reproductivefacts.org
Menopause	www.menopause.org
Preventive health maintenance and screening guidelines	www.cancer.gov/cancertopics/coping/eatinghints www.cibmtr.org/referencecenter/patient/guidelines/index.html www.health.gov/paguidelines www.livestrongcareplan.org www.survivorshipguidelines.org www.uspreventiveservicestaskforce.org
Recovery	www.bethematch.org/patient www.marrow.org/md-guidelines
Support groups and coping	www.bmtinfonet.org www.cancersupportcommunity.org www.chopra.com/ccl/guided-meditations www.lls.org www.myeloma.org www.smartpatients.com

Study Questions

1. What is a patient who received a T-cell-depleted transplant at risk for developing within the first year following transplant?
   A. Acute myeloid leukemia
   B. Breast cancer
   C. Basal cell carcinoma
   D. Post-transplant lymphoproliferative disorders

2. What is the most common secondary malignancy in pediatric patients who receive radiation as part of the transplant conditioning regimen?
   A. Esophageal cancer
   B. Thyroid cancer
   C. Nonsquamous cell carcinoma
   D. Brain stem glioma

3. Which of the following is true of human papillomavirus (HPV) infections?
   A. Exposure does not increase patients' risk of developing secondary cancers.
   B. Because patients are not at a significant risk following transplant, vaccination is not necessary.
   C. HPV can significantly increase patients' risk of developing post-transplant lymphoproliferative disorder.
   D. Patients between the ages of 9 and 26 should be revaccinated post-transplant with the HPV vaccine.

4. With which of the following are post-transplant lymphoproliferative disorders strongly associated?
   A. Donor B cells infected with the Epstein-Barr virus (EBV)
   B. Donor T cells infected with EBV
   C. They are not associated with viral infections.
   D. Sibling myeloablative transplants

5. Which of the following is NOT a risk for developing secondary solid tumors?
   A. Genetic predisposition
   B. Chronic graft-versus-host disease (GVHD)
   C. An increased incidence within the first 12 months following transplant
   D. Younger age at transplant

6. Acute myeloid leukemia without features of myelodysplastic syndrome is most often associated with patients who received which of the following?
   A. Fractionated total body irradiation
   B. Antithymocyte globulin (ATG)
   C. A topoisomerase II inhibitor
   D. An alkylating agent

7. The risk of ovarian failure, regardless of pubertal status, is associated with the use of which chemotherapy?
   A. Fludarabine and cyclophosphamide
   B. Busulfan and cyclophosphamide
   C. Etoposide and carmustine
   D. ATG and cyclophosphamide

8. Patients with vaginal chronic GVHD should consider all of the following EXCEPT:
   A. Vaginal dilation if not sexually active
   B. Early hormone replacement therapy
   C. Avoiding topical estrogen
   D. Scheduling regular gynecologic examinations

9. Which of the following is a side effect of ovarian failure in prepubescent females?
   A. Infertility alone
   B. Infertility and neurocognitive delays
   C. Infertility and impaired growth
   D. Infertility, impaired sexual development, and short stature

10. A 20-year-old patient with a history of aplastic anemia received a transplant at age eight. The conditioning regimen consisted of equine ATG (120 mg/kg) and cyclophosphamide (200 mg/kg). The patient received growth hormone therapy at age 12 but otherwise progressed through puberty without intervention. He now is about to be married and is asking about fertility. How should the nurse proceed?
    A. Explain to the patient that because he received only equine ATG and cyclophosphamide and progressed through puberty without issue, he will likely have his fertility preserved.
    B. Explain to the patient that, although it is possible to have spontaneous recovery of spermatogenesis, given the dose of cyclophosphamide, it is likely that he will be infertile.
    C. Encourage the patient to cryopreserve sperm now so that it will be available to him in the future, if he wishes to have children.
    D. Encourage the patient and endocrinology team to discuss methods to preserve his fertility.

11. A 34-year-old patient is asking about having a normal sex life following transplant. What should the nurse explain?
    A. "Most transplant survivors go on to have a normal sex life. They need to practice safe sex, even though the risk of unwanted pregnancy is low."
    B. "Testosterone levels often are low in males after transplant."
    C. "For patients who received chemotherapy alone as part of their conditions, erectile dysfunction occurs in the majority of males."
    D. "Erectile dysfunction is not affected by hypertension, hyperlipidemia, certain medications, and alcohol use."

12. In female hematopoietic stem cell transplantation (HSCT) patients, premature ovarian failure
    A. Can occur as a result of decreased levels of follicle-stimulating hormone and luteinizing hormone in combination with high estradiol levels.
    B. Is usually a subtle transition and can occur over months to years.
    C. Can be treated with hormone replacement therapy to relieve symptoms.
    D. Cannot be treated with hormone replacement therapy for patients with chronic GVHD.

13. Which of the following is a barrier to treating sexual dysfunction?
    A. Consistent follow-up with an endocrinologist to evaluate hormone levels
    B. Lack of discussion regarding sexuality by healthcare providers
    C. Lack of questions from patients regarding sexuality following HSCT
    D. Lack of relevancy or age barrier (e.g., adolescent survivors who are not yet sexually interested)

14. If a patient has moderate cutaneous chronic GVHD, which dimensions of the patient's quality of life may be affected?
    A. Physical, emotional, and social
    B. Physical, social, emotional, and functional
    C. Functional, physical, emotional, social, and functional
    D. Social, emotional, and functional

15. Neurocognitive changes can affect survivors in all of the following areas of EXCEPT:
    A. Memory
    B. Processing speed
    C. Gross motor skills
    D. Executive function

16. In what way does post-traumatic stress disorder (PTSD) affect patients?
    A. Patients may experience aggressive behavior, loss of interest in activities, and flashbacks and nightmares about the traumatic event.
    B. Patients may experience aggressive behavior, increased interest in activities, and may push parents and caretakers away in an attempt to gain independence.
    C. Patients may feel sad and may regress from previous milestones of development but are only affected immediately following transplant and resolve once engrafted.
    D. PTSD can affect young children, but because they experience no outward signs and symptoms, no intervention is necessary.

17. Children who received radiation as part of the conditioning regimen are at risk for neurocognitive delays. What should families of pediatric patients be made aware of by the nurse?
    A. Laws mandate that schools must provide children with specialized programs and services to help them achieve.
    B. Older children treated with radiation have less cognitive delays.
    C. If pediatric patients do not have issues early on in school, most will not have delays in the future.
    D. All of the above

18. Prior to reimmunizing patients, some centers may use which marker to show immune recovery?
    A. CD19
    B. CD4
    C. CD3
    D. CD34

19. Which of the following immunizations cannot be restarted once the patient's immune system has recovered, they show no clinical signs of GVHD, and they are off immuno-suppressive medications?
    A. Diphtheria, tetanus, pertussis
    B. Measles, mumps, and rubella
    C. Inactivated polio
    D. *Haemophilus influenzae* type B

20. Which of the following is a nursing intervention for long-term survivors?
    A. Instruct female patients to perform monthly breast self-examinations and male patients to perform testicular self-examinations.
    B. Provide information to patients and families on school reentry programs.
    C. Encourage patients to understand their disease and their past treatments so that they can have an active role in their future health and well-being.
    D. All of the above

21. Which of the following is true of late effects clinics?
    A. It is just as important that patients be seen regularly by a primary physician.
    B. Patients should have a primary physician for general healthcare needs, and the late effects team should provide the doctor with written and verbal communications on required screenings.
    C. Long-term follow-up clinics can be combined with oncology late effects clinics (but only for patients who received HSCT for oncologic diseases).
    D. Patients do not require a primary physician. All of their healthcare needs should be managed by a late effects clinic.

CHAPTER 8

Professional Practice

Kelli Thoele, MSN, RN, ACNS-BC, BMTCN®, OCN®

I. Introduction: All nurses caring for hematopoietic stem cell transplant (HSCT) recipients must be knowledgeable about professional practice. Nursing practice is influenced by professional organizations, state boards of nursing, accreditation agencies, and ethical and legal issues. In order to advance the nursing profession, research, evidence-based practice (EBP), and continuous quality improvement are essential. As knowledge advances over time, evidence-based practice and continuous quality improvement serve to improve the quality of care provided to HSCT recipients.

A. Professional organizations, such as the American Nurses Association (ANA) and Oncology Nursing Society (ONS), have published scopes and standards of nursing practice that inform thinking, describe the role of nursing, guide practice, and identify competencies of standard nursing care.

B. Professional nursing practice also is influenced by standards that are set by accreditation agencies, including the Joint Commission (TJC) and the Foundation for the Accreditation of Cellular Therapy.

C. To advocate for patients and remain within the scope of nursing practice, nurses must be familiar with ethical and legal issues, including delegation, confidentiality, advance directives, informed consent, and professional boundaries.

D. Self-care also is important; nurses must be aware of the signs and symptoms of compassion fatigue and moral distress to intervene when needed.

II. Nursing professional practice

A. Definition: ANA (2015b) defined nursing as "the protection, promotion, and optimization of health and abilities, prevention of illness and injury, facilitation of healing, alleviation of suffering through the diagnosis and treatment of human response, and advocacy in the care of individuals, families, groups, communities, and populations" (p. 1).

B. Characteristics of a profession

1. A profession is characterized by specialized knowledge, altruism, autonomy, and ethical practice (Chitty & Black, 2011).

2. Houle's (1980) characteristics of a profession
   a) Clarification of the function and openness to change
   b) Mastery of theoretical knowledge
   c) Ability to solve problems
   d) Use of practical knowledge

   e) Self-enhancement

   f) Formal training or education

   g) Credentialing

   h) Creation of subculture

   i) Legal reinforcement of standards

   j) Ethical practice

   k) Public acceptance

   l) Autonomous practice and role distinction

   m) Penalties for failure to comply with standards

   n) Altruism

 C. Model of professional practice regulation (Styles, Schumann, Bickford, & White, 2008)

  1. Contributors to professional practice regulation

   a) Scope and standards of practice developed by nursing professional organizations; certification; and code of ethics

   b) Rules, regulations, and nurse practice acts

   c) Institutional policies and procedures

   d) The nurse's self-determination

  2. The outcome is nursing practice that is safe, high quality, and evidence based.

III. Scope and standards of practice

 A. Definition

  1. *Scope* is defined as "the 'who,' 'what,' 'where,' 'when,' 'why,' and 'how' of nursing practice that addresses the range of nursing practice activities common to all registered nurses" (ANA, 2015b, p. 89).

  2. *Standards* are "authoritative statements defined and promoted by the profession by which the quality of practice, service, or education can be evaluated" (ANA, 2015b, p. 89).

 B. Timeline of oncology nursing scope and standards

  1. 1979: ONS and ANA published *ONS-ANA Outcome Standards for Cancer Nursing Practice: Models for Implementation.*

  2. 1987: ONS and ANA published *Standards of Oncology Nursing Practice.*

  3. 1990: ONS published *Standards of Advanced Practice in Oncology Nursing.*

  4. 1996: ONS and ANA published *Statement on the Scope and Standards of Oncology Nursing Practice.*

  5. 1997: ONS published *Statement on the Scope and Standards of Advanced Practice in Oncology Nursing.*

  6. 2003: ONS published *Statement on the Scope and Standards of Advanced Practice Nursing in Oncology.*

  7. 2004: ONS published *Statement on the Scope and Standards of Oncology Nursing Practice.*

  8. 2013: ONS published *Statement on the Scope and Standards of Oncology Nursing Practice: Generalist and Advanced Practice.*

 C. Scope of oncology nursing practice (Brant & Wickham, 2013)

  1. Generalist

   a) RNs are in a variety of roles, including researcher, educator, direct care nurse, and leader.

   b) Nursing care occurs in a variety of settings, including acute care, outpatient clinics or infusion centers, home care, and hospice.

        c) The goals of oncology nursing practice are cancer prevention, early detection, and supporting patients with cancer and their families.

        d) Patient-centered nursing care involves the diagnosis and treatment of patients' response to disease.

    2. Advanced nursing

        a) Oncology advanced practice registered nurses (APRNs) are nurse practitioners or clinical nurse specialists; advanced practice nurses have a master's or doctoral degree and must demonstrate competency.

        b) APRNs take on a variety of roles, including researcher, educator, direct caregiver, mentor, and change agent.

        c) APRNs must possess knowledge about theory, research, and the analysis of clinical and nonclinical problems.

        d) Oncology APRNs care for patients with cancer or a potential diagnosis of cancer.

  D. Standards of nursing practice

    1. Components of each standard

        a) ANA (2015b)

           (1) Standard

           (2) Competencies (RN and graduate-level prepared RN)

        b) ONS (Brant & Wickham, 2013)

           (1) Standard

           (2) Rationale

           (3) Measurement criteria (RN and APRN)

    2. Standards of practice (ANA, 2015b)

        a) Assessment

        b) Diagnosis

        c) Outcomes identification

        d) Planning

        e) Implementation

           (1) Coordination of care

           (2) Health teaching and health promotion

         f) Evaluation

    3. Standards of professional performance (ANA, 2015b)

        a) Ethics

        b) Education

        c) EBP and research

        d) Quality of practice

        e) Communication

        f) Leadership

        g) Collaboration

        h) Professional practice evaluation

        i) Resource utilization

        j) Environmental health

        k) Culturally congruent practice

IV. State nurse practice acts

  A. State nurse practice acts are statutory laws passed by state legislature and include the following (Russell, 2012):

1. Definition of terms used in statutes
2. Establishment of a board of nursing with authority to develop administrative laws
3. Standards for education programs
4. Scope and standards of nursing practice
5. Establishment of titles, licensure requirements, and protection of titles
6. Process to address incompetent care or unacceptable behavior
   B. Nurse practice acts vary by state; additional information can be found at the National Council of State Boards of Nursing (NCSBN) website (www.ncsbn.org).

V. Accreditation
   A. Definition: This process recognizes that an institution maintains standards set by the accrediting agency. Accreditation involves continuous improvement and monitoring of outcomes within an organization.
   B. TJC
   1. History
      a) TJC was founded in 1951, and the goal of the organization is to improve health care.
      b) TJC develops standards to improve the safety, efficiency, quality, and value of health care and evaluates organizations based on compliance with standards.
   2. Accreditation services
      a) Ambulatory care
      b) Behavioral health care
      c) Home care
      d) Hospitals
      e) Nursing care centers
      f) Laboratories
      g) Office-based surgery centers
   3. Standards
      a) TJC standards are developed based on information from experts, consumers, scientific literature, and government agencies. Each standard must improve patient outcomes and the quality or safety of care. In addition, the standards must be measurable. The Board of Commissioners approves each standard.
      b) Categories of standards for hospital accreditation
         (1) Accreditation participation requirements
         (2) Environment of care
         (3) Emergency management
         (4) Human resources
         (5) Infection prevention and control
         (6) Information management
         (7) Leadership
         (8) Life safety
         (9) Medication management
         (10) Medical staff
         (11) National Patient Safety Goals
         (12) Nursing
         (13) Provision of care, treatment, and services
         (14) Performance improvement

(15) Record of care, treatment, and services
(16) Rights and responsibilities of individuals
(17) Transplant safety
(18) Waived testing
C. HSCT accreditation
  1. Foundation for the Accreditation of Cellular Therapy (FACT)
    a) FACT was founded in 1996 by the International Society for Cellular Therapy (ISCT) and the American Society for Blood and Marrow Transplantation (ASBMT).
    b) FACT is a nonprofit corporation; its standards promote quality practice in cellular therapy from donation to administration.
  2. Joint Accreditation Committee (JACIE) (www.jacie.org)
    a) JACIE was founded in 1998 by ISCT and the European Society for Blood and Marrow Transplantation (EBMT).
    b) The goal of JACIE, a nonprofit entity, is to promote quality practice in cellular therapy.
  3. FACT-JACIE standards (FACT-JACIE, 2012)
    a) FACT and JACIE collaborate to develop and maintain standards regarding the minimum guidelines for quality practice in cellular therapy.
    b) Four major categories of standards currently exist.
      (1) Clinical program standards
      (2) Marrow collection facility standards
      (3) Apheresis collection facility standards
      (4) Processing facility standards
    c) Each category has multiple standards related to topics such as personnel, quality management, policies and procedures, process controls, data management, research, storage and transportation, and documentation.
    d) Examples of FACT-JACIE standards significant to HSCT nursing practice (FACT-JACIE, 2012)
      (1) Nurses should have formal training in the care of HSCT recipients. This training must include care of hematology/oncology patients, administration of chemotherapy and blood products, management of transplant complications, and provision of end-of-life care.
      (2) Written policies regarding the care of HSCT recipients, including central venous access device care, care of immunocompromised patients, and administration of chemotherapy, blood products, and cellular therapy products, need to be established.
      (3) The number of trained staff and the nurse–patient ratio should be satisfactory.
      (4) Prior to chemotherapy administration, two people who are qualified to administer chemotherapy must verify the drug, dose, route, and patient.
      (5) Cellular therapy products should be labeled before being removed from the proximity of the patient.
      (6) Aseptic technique should be used in the collection of cellular therapy products to prevent contamination.
      (7) A quality management plan and documentation of staff training, competency, and continuing education should be established.
      (8) Staff members must follow applicable standard operating procedures.

D. Ethical and legal issues in standards and accreditation
  1. ONS's *Statement on the Scope and Standards of Oncology Nursing Practice: Generalist and Advanced Practice* (Brant & Wickham, 2013)
     a) Decision making and patient advocacy in nursing practice are based on ethical principles.
     b) Rationale: Ethical dilemmas occur in cancer care and may lead to moral distress. Potential ethical dilemmas may include end-of-life decisions, misunderstanding or disagreement among the healthcare team, or complementary and alternative medicine.
  2. ANA's *Nursing's Social Policy Statement: The Essence of the Profession* (ANA, 2010): The foundation of nursing professional practice includes adherence to professional standards, including the professional code of ethics.
  3. FACT-JACIE standards (FACT-JACIE, 2012)
     a) Training for staff members should include ethical, legal, and regulatory issues relevant to practice.
     b) HSCT programs must comply with local, national, and international laws and regulations.

VI. Ethics
  A. Nurses caring for HSCT recipients will face ethical situations and must be aware of ethical principles and decision making in order to advocate for patients.
  B. Ethical challenges may arise when nurses are "in the middle" of the patient and another party, such as the physician, the organization, a family member, or even the nurse's own personal values and beliefs (Hamric, 2001).
  C. Ethical principles (Beauchamp & Childress, 2013)
     1. Respect for autonomy: Respect for the decision-making capabilities of autonomous people
     2. Nonmaleficence: Avoidance of causing harm
     3. Beneficence: Balance of benefits and risks, providing benefits to the patient
     4. Justice: Fair distribution of resources, benefits, and risks
  D. Professional–patient relationships (Beauchamp & Childress, 2013)
     1. Privacy: The patient has a right to space and time alone.
     2. Veracity: Healthcare providers should provide information that is honest, truthful, and accurate.
     3. Confidentiality: Patient information should not be disclosed without permission.
     4. Fidelity: Healthcare providers should honor commitments.
  E. Framework for ethical decision making (Purtilo & Doherty, 2011)
     1. Assess the situation and gather information.
     2. Identify the ethical problem.
     3. Analyze the problem.
     4. Explore alternative options.
     5. Implement an alternative option.
     6. Evaluate the outcome.
  F. Codes of ethics
     1. ANA's *Code of Ethics for Nurses With Interpretive Statements* (ANA, 2015a)
        a) Describes the ethical duties of nurses, provides a standard, and delineates commitment to society

b) Contains nine provisions

    (1) The nurse practices with respect and compassion in all professional relationships.

    (2) The nurse maintains a primary commitment to the patient, which may be an individual, family, group, or community.

    (3) The nurse promotes and protects the rights, health, and safety of the patient.

    (4) The nurse is accountable for own practice and delegation of tasks.

    (5) The nurse is responsible for individual growth, integrity, and competence.

    (6) The nurse influences and improves the healthcare environment.

    (7) The nurse advances the nursing profession.

    (8) The nurse collaborates with other healthcare professionals to meet healthcare needs and maintains the integrity of the nursing profession.

    (9) The nurse influences social policy and maintains integrity of the nursing profession.

2. The International Council of Nurses' (ICN's) *ICN Code of Ethics for Nurses* (ICN, 2012)

    a) Responsibilities of nurses

        (1) Prevent illness.

        (2) Promote health.

        (3) Restore health.

        (4) Alleviate suffering.

    b) Principal elements of ethical conduct: Nurses' responsibilities to people, practice, the profession, and coworkers

VII. Legal issues

  A. A law is "the formalization of a body of rules of action or conduct prescribed that is enforced by binding legal authority or as the sum total of rules and regulations by which society is governed" (Westrick & Dempski, 2009, p. 2).

  B. The preamble to the U.S. Constitution states that the purpose of law is to ensure order, promote general welfare, protect individuals, and establish fairness.

  C. Types of laws (Black, 2011; Westrick & Dempski, 2009)

    1. Statutory law: Written laws created through the legislative process

    2. Administrative law

      a) Laws delegated by the legislative body to governmental agencies in order to meet statutes

      b) In the United States, federal and state administrative laws are established.

    3. Common law

      a) Laws that result from judicial decisions during the resolution of disputes

      b) Common laws guide decisions in future similar circumstances.

  D. Regulation of nursing practice (Black, 2011; Westrick & Dempski, 2009)

    1. Licensure: A license granted by a governmental agency confirms that the person has met minimum requirements to practice. RNs are licensed through state boards of nursing.

    2. Accreditation: Evaluation of compliance with standards

      a) Healthcare accreditation agencies

        (1) FACT

        (2) TJC

        (3) American College of Surgeons Commission on Cancer

    b) Nursing education accreditation agencies

        (1) National League for Nursing Commission for Nursing Education Accreditation

        (2) Commission on Collegiate Nursing Education

  3. Certification: Endorsement of advanced knowledge in a specific area

  4. Education: Formal process of receiving instruction

    a) RNs must have a diploma or associate or bachelor's degree in nursing.

    b) Advanced practice nurses must have a master's or doctorate degree.

E. Ethical and legal issues in HSCT nursing

  1. Professional boundaries (ANA, 2015a; ICN, 2012; NCSBN, 2011)

    a) The purpose of the nurse–patient relationship is to alleviate suffering, prevent illness, and protect and promote health. This relationship is based on the needs of the patient and not on the needs of the nurse.

    b) In this working relationship, a power differential exists between the nurse's power and the patient's vulnerability.

        (1) The nurse has specialized knowledge and skills, influence, and access to information.

        (2) The patient is in an unfamiliar environment and potentially stressful situation.

    c) Professional behavior is on a continuum from too little provider involvement (neglect, disinterest) to too much provider involvement (boundary violations).

    d) A therapeutic nurse–patient relationship is in the center of the behavior continuum and requires acting in the patient's best interest and within the intended purpose of the relationship.

    e) Every nurse is responsible for maintaining appropriate professional boundaries and seeking assistance when boundaries are breached.

    f) Potential boundary violations in the nurse–patient relationship

        (1) The nurse believes and behaves as though he or she is the only nurse who understands the patient and can meet the patient's needs.

        (2) The nurse discusses intimate details of his or her life or personal problems.

        (3) The nurse spends an inappropriate amount of time with the patient or gives the patient special treatment.

        (4) The nurse has selective communication and does not explain all aspects of care to the patient or report all aspects of patient behavior.

        (5) The nurse's communication with the patient is inappropriate (e.g., flirtatious, offensive).

  2. Informed consent

    a) Process of communication between patient and clinician that allows the patient to make a decision about his or her own health care. Elements of informed consent include the following (Wilkinson, 2012):

        (1) Information

            (a) Treatment and alternatives

            (b) Potential benefits and risks of the treatment and alternatives

        (2) Comprehension

            (a) The clinician should explain the informed consent in terms that the patient can understand. The patient should have time to review the consent.

            (b) The clinician must address the patient's concerns and questions.

    (3) Voluntary consent: The patient must voluntarily consent (without coercion).

  b) Ethical considerations

    (1) Autonomy: The informed consent process allows the patient to make informed decisions (Jacoby et al., 1999).

    (2) Vulnerability: HSCT may be the only option available to the patient. The patient's vulnerability should be considered (Jacoby et al., 1999).

    (3) During the informed consent process, providers must balance beneficence and autonomy (D'Souza, Pasquini, & Spellecy, 2014; Jacoby et al., 1999).

    (4) Because the patient's expectation of HSCT often is different from the actual experience, the informed consent process should continue throughout the transplant continuum (D'Souza et al., 2014).

    (5) The donor also should go through the informed consent process. During the process, the donor should not feel pressured or coerced to donate stem cells (Chen, Wang, & Yang, 2013).

  c) Legal considerations (U.S. Department of Health and Human Services [DHHS], 2009b)

    (1) For patients who participate as subjects in research, federal regulations specify basic requirements of informed consent.

    (2) Some studies may require additional information in the informed consent; the basic requirements have some exceptions (e.g., no risk to participation in the study).

    (3) Basic requirements of an informed consent form for patients in research

      (a) Information about the research

        i. Purpose

        ii. Expected duration of participation

        iii. Identification and explanation of experimental procedures

      (b) Potential risks and benefits

      (c) Alternatives to participation in the study

      (d) Information about the extent of confidentiality of patient data

      (e) Resources for medical treatment or compensation if research has more than minimal risk

      (f) Contact information in case of injury or research-related questions

      (g) A statement about the participant's rights

        i. At any point in the study, the participant can stop participating in the study without penalty.

        ii. Participation is voluntary.

        iii. If the participant chooses not to participate in the study, there will be no penalty or loss of benefit.

        iv. State laws regarding informed consent vary; it also is necessary to consider institutional and regulatory requirements.

  d) Potential barriers to informed consent (D'Souza et al., 2014; Wilkinson, 2012)

    (1) Patient related: Age extremes, limited health literacy, language barrier, stress or anxiety, misunderstanding of the information discussed, lack of time to process the information, discomfort asking questions to ensure comprehension

    (2) Provider related: Lack of time to present information and answer questions, misperception that patient comprehended the information

     (3) Process related: Consent forms or educational information that are inaccurate, confusing, or inconsistent

  3. Malpractice: When a person deviates from the normal standard of care or acts in a way that differs from how a reasonably prudent provider would act in similar circumstances (Black, 2011)

    a) Malpractice can be through omission (failure to act) or commission (inappropriate action).

    b) Negligence is malpractice (failure to act).

    c) Required elements of malpractice

      (1) Duty

      (2) Breach of duty

      (3) Injury

      (4) Causation

  4. Delegation: When a nurse transfers the responsibility of completing a task or activity to another person (ANA & NCSBN, 2006)

    a) Nurses cannot delegate the nursing process of assessment, diagnosis, planning, implementation, and evaluation.

    b) Nurses can delegate components of care if the other professional has the knowledge and skills necessary to perform the task.

    c) The nurse remains responsible and accountable for tasks that are delegated to nursing assistive personnel.

    d) The Five Rights of Delegation (ANA & NCSBN, 2006)

      (1) The right task

      (2) Under the right circumstance

      (3) To the right person

      (4) With the right directions and communication

      (5) Under the right supervision and evaluation

  5. Confidentiality

    a) Maintaining patient confidentiality has legal and ethical implications (Black, 2011).

    b) The Health Insurance Portability and Accountability Act of 1996 is a federal law that protects patients' private health information (U.S. DHHS, 2003).

      (1) This law applies to healthcare providers, health plans (e.g., insurers, Medicare), and healthcare clearinghouses (e.g., billing services, health management systems).

      (2) Data about mental or physical health, care provided, and payment for health care are considered protected health information.

      (3) Protected health information can be disclosed only with written permission of the patient or as the law permits.

      (4) Protected health information must be disclosed to the individual or representative when requested and to the DHHS during a review or investigation.

      (5) Healthcare entities must provide patients with written information explaining their rights regarding protected health information.

    c) ANA and ICN both address confidentiality in their codes of ethics.

      (1) *Code of Ethics for Nurses With Interpretive Statements* (ANA, 2015a)

        (a) The third provision states that nurses must promote patient rights of privacy and confidentiality.

   (b) Confidentiality is a patient right that must be maintained by nurses to establish a trusting relationship and protect the patient's well-being.

   (c) Any decision regarding disclosure of confidential information must first and foremost consider patient rights, including the right to confidentiality.

   (d) Disclosure of patient information may be required to protect the patient or another person or for public health purposes.

  (2) *ICN Code of Ethics for Nurses* (ICN, 2012)

   (a) The nurse's responsibility to other people is one of the principal elements of ethical conduct.

   (b) Part of the responsibility to patients includes the need to keep personal information confidential.

6. Advance directives

 a) Advance directives are legal documents that provide guidance regarding medical care decisions in the case that the patient is unable to communicate his or her wishes (National Cancer Institute [NCI], 2013).

  (1) Advance directives should be completed before the patient is seriously ill.

  (2) Medical care preferences should be communicated with loved ones.

  (3) Legal requirements vary from state to state. The National Hospice and Palliative Care Organization provides information about advance directives; state-specific legal forms can be downloaded from its website (www.caringinfo.org).

  (4) The patient can update advance directives if circumstances change.

  (5) If a patient does not have written advance directives, state law determines who is able to make healthcare decisions for the patient.

 b) In 1990, U.S. Congress passed the Patient Self-Determination Act, which took effect December 1, 1991 (La Puma, Orentlicher, & Moss, 1991).

  (1) The purpose of the act is to encourage completion of advance directives and ensure that healthcare institutions inform patients about their rights regarding medical care.

  (2) Hospitals, nursing homes, home health agencies, hospices, and other healthcare institutions must abide by the following:

   (a) Inform the patient of his or her rights to complete an advance directive and accept or refuse medical treatment.

   (b) Determine if the patient has an advance directive and document appropriately.

   (c) Implement policies regarding patient rights and advance directives.

   (d) Provide education for the community and healthcare staff regarding advance directives.

  (3) Healthcare institutions cannot discriminate against patients based on advance directive status.

 c) Types of advance directives

  (1) Living will (NCI, 2013): A living will addresses preferences regarding the refusal or acceptance of life-sustaining medical interventions: dialysis, intubation, parenteral nutrition and hydration, organ and tissue donation, and CPR.

  (2) Medical power of attorney (National Hospice and Palliative Care Organization, 2008)

       (a) This is a person, designated by the patient, who can make health-care decisions if the patient is temporarily or permanently unable to make his or her own decisions.

       (b) State documents for power of attorney have different terms, including durable power of attorney, healthcare proxy, and healthcare representative.

   d) Advance directives in HSCT

      (1) ASBMT states that physicians caring for HSCT recipients should be competent in effective communication about advance directives (Khan, Juckett, Komanduri, Krishnan, & Burns, 2012).

      (2) Advance care planning with HSCT recipients has several potential barriers (Joffe, Mello, Cook, & Lee, 2007; Loggers et al., 2014; Snyder, 2009).

        (a) Younger patients

        (b) Possibility of cure with HSCT for potentially fatal diseases

        (c) Provider discomfort discussing end-of-life issues

        (d) Patient or provider desire to focus on the positive

      (3) A study of 155 HSCT recipients found that the majority of recipients (63%) reportedly discussed advance care planning with family and friends, but written advance directives were present in only 39% of medical charts (Joffe et al., 2007).

      (4) Loggers et al. (2014) found that the majority of HSCT recipients would like to discuss advance care planning with their physicians prior to transplantation.

VIII. Compassion fatigue and moral distress

  A. Compassion fatigue: When a person indirectly experiences trauma through helping someone who is experiencing trauma (Figley, 2002a, 2002b)

    1. The caregiver may relive the traumatic event through recurring thoughts or recollections, dreams about the trauma or the patient, distress when helping others, or feelings that the event is recurring.

    2. The caregiver may avoid situations associated with trauma such as thoughts, feelings, places, or people associated with the trauma. The caregiver may also exhibit a decreased interest in activities.

    3. Potential manifestations of compassion fatigue (Coetzee & Klopper, 2010; Figley, 2002b)

      a) Physical (e.g., changes in sleep patterns, becoming accident prone)

      b) Emotional (e.g., apathy, sense of helplessness, difficulty coping with stress)

      c) Intellectual (e.g., disorderliness, confusion or decreased concentration)

      d) Social (e.g., indifference, unresponsiveness)

    4. Potential contributing factors (Coetzee & Klopper, 2010; Figley, 2002a)

      a) Stress

      b) Prolonged contact with patients

      c) Lack of professional boundaries

      d) Life disruption

      e) Recollection of a traumatic event

    5. Compassion fatigue in nursing (Coetzee & Klopper, 2010)

      a) Compassion fatigue is a cumulative process that begins with compassion discomfort and then progresses to compassion stress and, finally, compassion fatigue.

b) Strategies for compassion fatigue (Cooke, Gemmill, Kravits, & Grant, 2009; Figley, 2002a)

(1) Enhance social support and support a caring environment.

(2) Maintain professional boundaries.

(3) Promote a balance between work life and personal life.

(4) Practice stress management techniques.

B. Moral distress

1. Definition (Jameton, 1984)

a) Moral uncertainty: A potential ethical dilemma with uncertainty around the need to take action

b) Moral dilemma: The need to choose between multiple conflicting principles or values

c) Moral distress: The inability to take the right course of action due to institutional constraints

2. Sources (Hamric, Borchers, & Epstein, 2012)

a) Clinical situations (e.g., futile treatment, inappropriate use of resources, incompetent care, treatment that is against the patient's wishes)

b) Internal constraints (e.g., self-doubt, lack of knowledge regarding ethical issues, passiveness)

c) External constraints (e.g., inadequate administrative support, lack of the appropriate number of staff or appropriately trained staff, care compromised by cost-reduction efforts)

3. Symptoms (Gutierrez, 2005)

a) Physical (e.g., pain, changes in sleep pattern)

b) Emotional (e.g., sadness, frustration, discouragement, guilt, anger)

c) Social (e.g., withdrawal from loved ones, verbalization of concerns with family or friends)

d) Professional (e.g., desire to miss work, withdrawal from colleagues)

4. Interventions

a) The American Association of Critical-Care Nurses (AACN) developed a framework, the 4 A's to Rise Above Moral Distress, for addressing moral distress in nurses to create a healthy work environment (AACN, n.d.).

(1) Ask: Engage in self-reflection to determine if manifestations of distress are present and if distress is work related. The goal of this step is to identify moral distress.

(2) Affirm: Affirm commitment to self-care and responsibility to support a healthy work environment. The goal of this step is to commit to addressing moral distress.

(3) Assess: Assess the circumstances that result in distress and your readiness to act. The goal of this step is to prepare to develop an action plan.

(4) Act: Prepare a plan and implement change strategies. The goal of this step is to "preserve integrity and authenticity" (AACN, n.d., p. 2).

(5) This ongoing process is cyclic and requires continuous evaluation to sustain change.

b) AACN (2008) also recommended organizational interventions to prevent or address moral distress in nurses.

(1) Develop and implement strategies to recognize moral distress and situations that may lead to moral distress.

        (2) Recognize and analyze organizational issues that may contribute to moral distress.

        (3) Provide opportunities for staff support, including tools to manage moral distress, ethics committees with nurse representation, grief counseling, and stress debriefings.

IX. Education and chemotherapy/biotherapy competence
- A. Standards and accreditation
    1. ONS's *Statement on the Scope and Standards of Oncology Nursing Practice: Generalist and Advanced Practice* (Brant & Wickham, 2013)
        - a) Oncology nurses must be aware of the current evidence in cancer care and contribute to the professional development of themselves and colleagues.
        - b) Rationale: As the evidence of cancer care evolves, nurses must continue to acquire new knowledge to provide evidence-based care.
    2. ANA's *Nursing's Social Policy Statement: The Essence of the Profession* (ANA, 2010)
        - a) Continuing education is necessary to maintain current knowledge, and certification is one way to demonstrate competence.
        - b) Nurses are responsible for self-regulation and accountability regarding their knowledge base.
    3. FACT-JACIE standards (FACT-JACIE, 2012)
        - a) Mid-level practitioners, including advanced practice nurses, must regularly participate in educational programs about HSCT.
        - b) Nurses caring for HSCT patients must have initial training and, at least, annual education and evaluation of nurse competency.
- B. ONS position on lifelong learning (ONS, 2014)
    1. ONS states that lifelong learning is required for nurses to advance health and lead change in health care.
    2. Lifelong learning opportunities
        - a) Ongoing assessment of learning needs and the pursuit of learning opportunities throughout the nurse's career
        - b) Development and use of a variety of approaches to learning
        - c) Acquisition of certification
        - d) Sharing of knowledge and skills with other nurses
        - e) Participation in research, quality improvement, and EBP
        - f) Interdisciplinary collaboration to improve cancer care
        - g) Advocacy in health policy
- C. Chemotherapy and biotherapy competence
    1. ONS position on chemotherapy and biotherapy education (ONS, 2015)
        - a) RNs who administer chemotherapy and biotherapy should receive initial and annual competency assessment.
        - b) Educational content should include current evidence regarding the following:
            - (1) Information about chemotherapy and biotherapy, including pharmacology, routes of administration, indications, drug classifications, and pertinent molecular biomarkers
            - (2) Safe handling and disposal practices, including the use of personal protective equipment
            - (3) Administration procedures

        (4) Patient and family considerations, including patient assessment and management, patient safety, patient and family education, symptom management, and survivorship

     c) A clinical practicum should occur after completion of the didactic component of chemotherapy education. A chemotherapy-competent nurse should evaluate and document competency during the clinical practicum (see Figure 8-1).

  2. American Society of Clinical Oncology/ONS Chemotherapy Administration Safety Standards (Neuss et al., 2013)

     a) Each institution should develop an educational program or use an established program for the administration of chemotherapy.

     b) In addition to education, initial competency should be assessed.

     c) Competency should be reassessed on a regular basis (annual competency assessment is recommended).

X. EBP and clinical trials

  A. Standards and accreditation

    1. ONS's *Statement on the Scope and Standards of Oncology Nursing Practice: Generalist and Advanced Practice* (Brant & Wickham, 2013)

     a) Oncology nurses improve patient outcomes by incorporating current knowledge into practice. Oncology nurses also contribute through research, quality improvement, education, and management.

     b) Rationale: Oncology nurses' research involvement may be direct or indirect.

    2. ANA's *Nursing's Social Policy Statement: The Essence of the Profession* (ANA, 2010)

     a) The foundation of quality care is EBP.

     b) Nurses use theoretical and evidence-based knowledge in the nursing process.

    3. FACT-JACIE standards (FACT-JACIE, 2012)

     a) Clinical trials should be reviewed and approved by an institutional review board (IRB) or ethics committee.

     b) Informed consent for participation in clinical trials is required.

     c) Mid-level practitioners must participate in regular educational activities to maintain current knowledge regarding evidence in HSCT care.

  B. EBP

    1. EBP is the use of current evidence to guide patient care.

    2. EBP should result in improved patient outcomes, high-quality care, and reduction in healthcare costs.

    3. Several factors should be considered when making an evidence-based clinical decision (Melnyk & Fineout-Overholt, 2015).

     a) External evidence: Theory, research, and expert panels

     b) Clinical expertise: Resource availability and internal evidence

     c) Patient values and preference

    4. Barriers to EBP may be personal, professional, or organizational (Schmidt & Brown, 2015).

     a) Perceived lack of time

     b) Lack of knowledge about EBP, research, or the value of EBP

     c) Lack of resources or technological skills to search for evidence

     d) Resistance to change

     e) Organizational resistance to EBP

Figure 8-1. Clinical Practicum Evaluation

Chemotherapy Administration Competency Record

Employee Name _____

Chemotherapy-competent RN evaluators must observe practice and validate that the nurse meets all of the following criteria. Administer at least one vesicant under supervision.

RN Evaluators	Date	Drugs Administered

PRIOR TO ADMINISTRATION — Initials

1. Coordinates time of administration with pharmacy and others as needed.

2. Verifies signed consent for treatment.

3. Verifies laboratory values are within acceptable parameters and reports results to provider as needed.

4. Performs independent double check of original orders with a second RN for accuracy of
   - Protocol or regimen
   - Agents
   - Recalculated body surface area
   - Patient dose
   - Schedule
   - Route

5. Verifies that patient education, premedication, prehydration, and other preparations are completed.

ADMINISTRATION

1. Compares original order to dispensed drug label at the bedside or chairside with another RN.

2. Verifies patient identification.

3. Applies gloves and gown and uses safe handling precautions.

4. Verifies adequacy of venous access and appropriate IV site selection.

5. Checks IV patency and flushes line with 5–10 ml normal saline.

6. Demonstrates safe administration:
   - Pushes through side arm or at hub closest to patient; checks patency every 2–5 ml (every 2–3 ml for pediatric patients).
   - Verifies appropriate rate of administration.

7. Demonstrates appropriate monitoring/observation for specific acute drug effects.

8. Verbalizes appropriate action in the event of extravasation.

9. Verbalizes appropriate action in the event of hypersensitivity reaction.

AFTER ADMINISTRATION

1. Flushes line with enough fluid to clear IV tubing of drug.

2. Removes peripheral IV device or flushes/maintains vascular access device.

3. Disposes of chemotherapy waste according to policy.

4. Documents medications, education, and patient response.

5. Communicates post-treatment considerations to the patient, caregivers, and appropriate personnel.

(Continued on next page)

Figure 8-1. Clinical Practicum Evaluation *(Continued)*

Check the appropriate column to indicate whether the nurse performs the listed activities satisfactorily. If the nurse has not had the opportunity to perform an activity, check the N/A (not applicable) column. Under Comments, provide examples of how the nurse met each objective or performed each activity. Include plans for remediation for all activities for which "No" is indicated.

	Yes	No	N/A
1. Participates in interdisciplinary care planning with physicians, nurses, and other healthcare professionals (e.g., home care or dietary workers). Comments:			
2. Anticipates complications of chemotherapy and takes action to prevent or minimize the complications. Comments:			
3. Involves patients and caregivers in care planning and provides interventions specific to individual patient needs. Comments:			
4. Instructs patients about hair, scalp, and skin care and takes measures to preserve body image. Comments:			
5. Reviews laboratory values and provides patients with information about myelosuppression, prevention of infection, fatigue, and prevention of bleeding according to ONS Putting Evidence Into Practice (PEP) evidence. Comments:			
6. Identifies patients at risk for oral mucositis and provides education regarding oral hygiene according to ONS PEP evidence. Comments:			
7. Demonstrates knowledge of interventions (drug therapy and nonpharmacologic) for prevention and management of nausea and vomiting according to ONS PEP evidence. Comments:			
8. Instructs patients about the prevention and management of gastrointestinal complications (e.g., constipation, diarrhea, anorexia) according to ONS PEP evidence. Comments:			
9. Identifies and takes nursing action to prevent or manage potential or actual hypersensitivity and anaphylactic reactions. Comments:			
10. Uses appropriate safe handling precautions in the preparation, handling, and disposal of hazardous drugs. Comments:			
11. Demonstrates knowledge and skill in the assessment, management, and follow-up care of extravasations. Comments:			
12. Assesses patients for the most appropriate type of venous access device (peripheral or central) based on type and duration of intended therapy. Comments:			
13. Demonstrates knowledge of research trials by participating in data collection, drug administration, patient education, and follow-up. Comments:			

Note. From *Chemotherapy and Biotherapy Guidelines and Recommendations for Practice* (4th ed., pp. 469–470), by M. Polovich, M. Olsen, and K.B. LeFebvre (Eds.), 2014, Pittsburgh, PA: Oncology Nursing Society. Copyright 2014 by Oncology Nursing Society. Reprinted with permission.

f) Communication gap between clinicians and researchers

g) Inability to read and appraise research

C. Seven steps of EBP described by Melnyk and Fineout-Overholt (2015)

   1. Encourage inquiry in the clinical environment.

      a) A culture of inquiry allows clinicians to question current practice and look for ways to improve practice.

      b) The organization should include EBP within the organizational philosophy and mission and provide EBP tools, mentors, and support for clinicians.

      c) The organization should recognize successful implementation of EBP.

   2. Ask a clinical question.

      a) The clinical question helps effectively guide the search for evidence.

      b) The PICOT format is an example of a clinical question.

         (1) **P**opulation to be studied: Age, disease, gender, and ethnicity are characteristics that may define patient populations.

         (2) **I**ssue or intervention: This is an issue of interest to the clinician or an intervention such as a treatment, an action, or a diagnostic test.

         (3) **C**omparison group: This group will be compared to the issue of interest or intervention. The comparison group may have a different intervention, a placebo, or no intervention.

         (4) **O**utcome: The outcome of interest may include the rate of adverse outcomes, risk of disease, or other outcome related to the intervention.

         (5) **T**ime frame: This could be either the time the population will be observed or the time required to observe an outcome related to the intervention.

      c) An example of a PICOT question in HSCT: In adult HSCT recipients, does chlorhexidine bathing decrease central line infections during hospitalization?

         (1) P: Adult HSCT recipients

         (2) I: Chlorhexidine bathing

         (3) C: Bathing without chlorhexidine

         (4) O: Central line infections

         (5) T: During hospitalization

   3. Collect the evidence. Sources of evidence include the following (see Table 8-1):

      a) External evidence

         (1) Systematic reviews: Summarize current evidence of a given topic

         (2) Meta-analyses: Use statistical methods to combine results from multiple studies

         (3) Research-based evidence

            (a) Randomized controlled trials

            (b) Controlled trials

            (c) Cohort studies

            (d) Case-control studies

            (e) Descriptive studies

            (f) Correlational studies

         (4) Evidence-based theories

         (5) Expert panels

      b) Internal evidence

         (1) Quality improvement projects

         (2) Available resources

      c) Patient values and preferences

Table 8-1. Selected Sources of Data for Evidence-Based Practice

Source	Website
Organizations	
American Society for Blood and Marrow Transplantation	www.asbmt.org
American Society for Pain Management Nursing	www.aspmn.org
American Society of Clinical Oncology	www.asco.org
Association of Pediatric Hematology/Oncology Nurses	www.aphon.org
Centers for Disease Control and Prevention	www.cdc.gov
Hospice and Palliative Nurses Association	www.hpna.org
Infectious Diseases Society of America	www.idsociety.org
Infusion Nurses Society	www.ins1.org
National Cancer Institute	www.cancer.gov
National Comprehensive Cancer Network®	www.nccn.org
Oncology Nursing Society	www.ons.org
World Health Organization	www.who.int
Databases	
Cochrane Database of Systematic Reviews	www.cochranelibrary.com
Cumulative Index to Nursing and Allied Health Literature	www.ebscohost.com/nursing/products/cinahl-databases/cinahl-complete
PsycINFO®	www.apa.org/pubs/databases/psycinfo
PubMed	www.ncbi.nlm.nih.gov/pubmed
Publications	
Biology of Blood and Marrow Transplantation	www.bbmt.org
Bone Marrow Transplantation	www.nature.com/bmt/index.html
Cancer Nursing	www.lww.com/product/0162-220X
Clinical Journal of Oncology Nursing	https://cjon.ons.org
Journal of Clinical Oncology	www.jco.ascopubs.org
Journal of Infusion Nursing	www.ins1.org/journalofinfusionnursing.aspx

(Continued on next page)

Table 8-1. Selected Sources of Data for Evidence-Based Practice *(Continued)*	
Source	**Website**
Journal of Palliative Medicine	www.liebertpub.com/overview/journal-of-palliative-medicine/41
Journal of Pediatric Oncology Nursing	http://jpo.sagepub.com
Oncology Nursing Forum	https://onf.ons.org
Pain Management Nursing	www.painmanagementnursing.org
Seminars in Oncology Nursing	www.seminarsoncologynursing.com
Additional Resources	
Agency for Healthcare Research and Quality	www.ahrq.gov/index.html
National Database of Nursing Quality Indicators	www.pressganey.com/solutions/clinical-quality/nursing-quality
National Guideline Clearinghouse	www.guideline.gov
Oncology Nursing Society Putting Evidence Into Practice	www.ons.org/practice-resources/pep
Internal Evidence	
Data from internal quality improvement projects	–
Internal clinical experts (e.g., clinical nurse specialists, infection control practitioners, expert nurses)	–

4. Appraise the evidence.
   a) Critical appraisal of evidence (Fineout-Overholt, Melnyk, Stillwell, & Williamson, 2010)
      (1) Hierarchy of evidence (Melnyk & Fineout-Overholt, 2015)
         (a) Level 1: Systematic reviews, meta-analyses of randomized controlled trials
         (b) Level 2: Randomized controlled trials
         (c) Level 3: Controlled trials without randomization
         (d) Level 4: Cohort studies, case-control studies
         (e) Level 5: Systematic reviews of qualitative or descriptive studies
         (f) Level 6: Descriptive or qualitative studies
         (g) Level 7: Opinions of experts or authorities
      (2) Scientific rigor (i.e., was the study conducted following strict scientific methods?)
      (3) Applicability to practice (i.e., does the evidence apply to the patient population of interest?)
   b) Critical appraisal of studies (Fineout-Overholt et al., 2010)
      (1) Significance of the problem

          (a) Is relevant literature summarized?

          (b) Is there a gap in literature that specifies a need for the study?

          (c) Is the problem stated with evidence that the problem is important?

  (2) Aim of the study

          (a) Is the purpose of the study stated?

          (b) Does the purpose of the study address the problem?

          (c) What is the research question or hypothesis?

  (3) Theoretical or conceptual framework

          (a) Is the study based on a theory or conceptual framework?

          (b) Is the theory congruent with the problem and purpose?

  (4) Study design

          (a) Is the study design stated?

          (b) Is the design appropriate for the study?

  (5) Subjects

          (a) How were the subjects chosen?

          (b) Is there an adequate number of subjects?

  (6) Variables

          (a) How were the data collected?

          (b) Are there independent and dependent variables?

          (c) How will the variables be measured?

          (d) Are the tools used reliable and valid?

  (7) Analysis

          (a) How were the data analyzed?

          (b) If statistical tests were used, were they the appropriate tests?

  (8) Findings

          (a) Are the findings of the study stated?

          (b) Do the findings address the problem and purpose of the study?

          (c) Are the findings applicable to practice?

          (d) What are the limitations to this study?

5. Integrate the evidence into clinical practice.

  a) Form a team for EBP implementation.

  b) Discuss the need for a change.

  c) Review the evidence with stakeholders.

  d) Review documentation and workflow processes that will be affected by a change.

  e) Implement a series of smaller changes.

  f) Celebrate the successes of the team.

  g) Several models exist for the implementation of EBP.

    (1) The Advancing Research and Clinical Practice Through Close Collaboration Model (Melnyk & Fineout-Overholt, 2005)

    (2) The Iowa Model of Evidence-Based Practice to Promote Quality Care (Titler et al., 2001)

    (3) The Johns Hopkins Nursing Evidence-Based Practice Model (Newhouse, Dearholt, Poe, Pugh, & White, 2007)

6. Evaluate the outcomes.

  a) Did outcomes change when the evidence was integrated into practice?

  b) Are the tools used to measure outcomes reliable and valid?

  c) Was the change an improvement?

    d) Were there any unintended consequences?

  7. Disseminate the outcomes.

    a) Staff meetings

    b) EBP or research committees

    c) Local, regional, or national conferences

    d) Publication in peer-reviewed journals or newsletters

D. Clinical trials

  1. Definition: A clinical trial is a scientific process in which researchers test the efficacy and safety of an intervention in voluntary human participants (National Institutes of Health [NIH], 2012).

  2. Potential interventions in clinical trials (World Health Organization, n.d.)

    a) Medication

    b) Surgical or radiologic procedure

    c) Medical device

    d) Cellular or biologic product

    e) Change in process

    f) Change in behavior

  3. For clinical trials involving medications, the U.S. Food and Drug Administration (FDA) has described four phases (U.S. FDA, 2013a).

    a) Phase I

      (1) Determine safety, frequent side effects, metabolism, and excretion of the drug.

      (2) Clinical trial usually includes 20–80 healthy volunteers.

    b) Phase II

      (1) Study the effectiveness of the drug (compared to patients receiving a different drug or placebo) and continue to evaluate safety and side effects.

      (2) Clinical trial includes approximately 100–300 volunteers with the condition that the drug intends to treat.

    c) Phase III

      (1) Study different dosages and the drug in combination with other drugs, compare drug to current standard treatment, and continue to evaluate safety and effectiveness.

      (2) Clinical trial includes approximately 1,000–3,000 volunteers with the condition that the drug intends to treat.

    d) Phase IV

      (1) This phase occurs after the drug has been approved by FDA and is on the market.

      (2) Goals are to examine long-term effects, test the drug in different populations, and determine optimal use of the drug.

  4. Protecting patients in clinical trials (U.S. DHHS, 2009a; U.S. FDA, 2013b)

    a) Informed consent: The informed consent process is required in clinical trials.

    b) Ethical guidelines

      (1) Ethical guidelines are established to protect patients. Many guidelines were developed in response to unethical practices in research.

      (2) Nurses have a duty to protect patients involved in research and report research that is morally objectionable (ANA, 2010).

    c) IRBs

(1) IRBs are required in each institution that will conduct or support clinical trials.

(2) This committee evaluates clinical trials and determines if each trial follows ethical, legal, and institutional guidelines.

    (a) Based on the review, the IRB can approve or disapprove the trial.

    (b) The IRB also can require modifications to the trial for the protection of patients.

(3) The IRB monitors and oversees trials to ensure that risks are minimized.

  d) FDA

(1) FDA has developed regulations that address good clinical practices and human subjects protection in clinical trials.

(2) For clinical trials regulated by FDA, the Office of Good Clinical Practice addresses the protection of human subjects.

  e) Office for Human Research Protections

(1) This office protects patients who participate in trials conducted or supported by U.S. DHHS.

(2) Leadership on the protection of patient rights and welfare is provided through education, compliance oversight, policy development, and expert opinion.

5. Clinical trials in HSCT

  a) Blood and Marrow Transplant Clinical Trials Network (BMT CTN)

(1) BMT CTN was established in 2001 and works to improve outcomes in BMT patients by conducting multi-institutional clinical trials.

    (a) Supports the development of well-designed trials with timely initiation and completion of the trial

    (b) Protects donors and recipients who participate in clinical trials

    (c) Ensures that the trials meet regulatory requirements

    (d) Promotes dissemination of clinical trial results

    (e) Provides statistical support and quality data

(2) Funded by NIH and is a collaboration of the Center for International Blood and Marrow Transplant Research, the National Marrow Donor Program, the EMMES Corporation, and transplant centers.

  b) ASBMT (2011) has identified research priorities in HSCT.

(1) Stem cell biology

(2) Tumor relapse

(3) Graft-versus-host disease

(4) Applying new technology to HSCT

(5) Expanded indications for HSCT

(6) Survivorship

(7) Transplants in older adult patients

(8) Improving current use of HSCT

6. Potential barriers to clinical trials in HSCT recipients (BMT CTN, 2015)

  a) Limited number of eligible patients

  b) Variety of indications for HSCT

  c) Post-transplant complications

  d) Complexity of transplants

  e) Potential delays related to consenting and randomizing the donor and the recipient

7. The nurse's role in clinical trials
   a) NIH Clinical Center: Clinical Research Nursing 2010 Domain of Practice Committee (2009) identified two nursing roles in clinical trials.
      (1) Clinical research nurse
         (a) Cares for patients who are participating in clinical trials
         (b) Works in the clinical staff nurse role
      (2) Research nurse coordinator
         (a) Involved in data management and coordination of a study
         (b) Supports adherence to regulatory requirements
         (c) Involved in recruitment of participants
   b) Five domains of practice were identified.
      (1) Clinical practice
         (a) Provide patient education and direct nursing care.
         (b) Identify and report potential adverse events.
         (c) Document pertinent data.
      (2) Human subjects protection
         (a) Facilitate the informed consent process.
         (b) Address ethical concerns.
         (c) Minimize risk to participants of the study.
      (3) Contribution to the science
         (a) Mentor new investigators and students.
         (b) Disseminate the results of clinical trials.
         (c) Identify areas of future research and clinical nursing research.
      (4) Care coordination and continuity
         (a) Coordinate referrals and study activities and meetings.
         (b) Educate healthcare providers on study requirements.
         (c) Communicate with research participants regarding the effect of procedures involved in the study and address inquiries from participants.
      (5) Study management
         (a) Participate in development of the study, recruitment of participants, and site visits.
         (b) Communicate within the research team and among research sites.
         (c) Collect and record data, identify trends, and participate in reporting outcomes.
         (d) Identify clinical implications of the study and provide nursing expertise.
   c) *Oncology Clinical Trials Nurse Competencies* (ONS, 2010)
      (1) Protocol compliance: Assist with compliance of the research protocol requirements (including regulations, institutional policies, IRB policies, and clinical trial objectives).
      (2) Clinical trials–related communication
         (a) Communicate with team members, research participants, clinicians, and referring physicians regarding the clinical trial.
         (b) Educate others about clinical trials and promote safe care for participants.
      (3) Informed consent process
         (a) Ensure that the informed consent process occurs and is documented appropriately.

(b) Assess for potential barriers to informed consent and assist in the removal of barriers.

(c) Ensure comprehension of information and continue to educate the patient throughout the clinical trial.

(4) Management of clinical trial patients

(a) Assess patients and assist in symptom management, report adverse events as required, and communicate with the principal investigator.

(b) Assist with adherence to clinical trial requirements.

(5) Documentation

(a) Document patient information as required by protocol.

(b) Ensure that reports and regulatory documents are completed and accurate.

(6) Patient recruitment

(a) Identify and recruit potential clinical trial participants.

(b) Assess for barriers to recruitment and use available resources to enhance the recruitment process.

(7) Ethical issues

(a) Ensure that the clinical trial is conducted ethically.

(b) Advocate for clinical trial participants and promote ethical care.

(8) Financial implications: Consider financial implications of patient participation in the study and identify patients who may benefit from financial counseling.

(9) Professional development: Continue to participate in activities that contribute to professional growth.

XI. Quality and quality improvement

A. Standards and accreditation

1. ONS's *Statement on the Scope and Standards of Oncology Nursing Practice: Generalist and Advanced Practice* (Brant & Wickham, 2013)

a) Oncology nurses evaluate nursing practice related to quality, safety, and effectiveness.

b) Rationale: Patient safety is dependent on minimizing risks and responding to errors. As new evidence emerges, nurses must appraise the evidence and incorporate best evidence to promote a culture of safety.

2. ANA's *Nursing's Social Policy Statement: The Essence of the Profession* (ANA, 2010)

a) Nurses are responsible and accountable for providing quality care.

b) Nurses partner with other healthcare colleagues, patients, families, and the community to promote quality care.

3. FACT-JACIE standards (FACT-JACIE, 2012)

a) The HSCT program must have a quality management program and a written quality management plan.

b) The quality management plan must include an organizational chart and requirements for members of the program (e.g., education, training, experience, competency).

c) Quality performance must be reported annually.

d) Relevant policies and procedures should be included in the quality management plan.

B. Quality
1. Quality has been defined as "conformance of a product or process with pre-established specifications or standards" (FACT-JACIE, 2012, p. 11).
2. The structure and processes of nursing care can influence patient and organizational outcomes; outcomes influenced by nursing practice may be referred to as *nursing-sensitive indicators*.
    a) In 2004, the National Quality Forum identified nursing-sensitive indicators, and TJC developed an implementation guide (TJC, 2009).
    b) Nursing-sensitive indicators
        (1) Mortality due to treatable complications in postoperative patients
        (2) Hospital-acquired pressures ulcers
        (3) Patient falls and falls with injury
        (4) Catheter-associated urinary tract infections and central line–associated bloodstream infections in intensive care patients
        (5) Ventilator-associated pneumonia
        (6) Nursing skill mix and hours per patient per day
        (7) Nurse turnover
        (8) Nursing practice environment
3. The National Database of Nursing Quality Indicators® allows for comparison of unit-level quality data in acute care hospitals (www.pressganey.com/solutions/clinical-quality/nursing-quality).
C. Quality improvement
1. The DHHS Health Resources and Services Administration (2011) defined quality improvement as "systematic and continuous actions that lead to measurable improvement in health care services and the health status of targeted patient groups" (p. 1).
2. JACIE was founded in 1998 to improve quality in HSCT care. Gratwohl et al. (2014) found that overall mortality in HSCT decreased from 1999 to 2006. HSCT programs accredited by JACIE had earlier reductions in mortality and significantly longer relapse-free survival and overall survival in allogeneic stem cell recipients than programs that were not accredited by JACIE.
3. Health and Medicine Division of the National Academies of Sciences, Engineering, and Medicine, formerly the Institute of Medicine (IOM)
    a) *Crossing the Quality Chasm: A New Health System for the 21st Century,* a 2001 report by IOM, states that high-quality consistent care is not currently available to all people in the United States and calls for improvement in the delivery of health care.
    b) Six aims for improvement
        (1) Safe
        (2) Effective
        (3) Patient-centered
        (4) Timely
        (5) Efficient
        (6) Equitable
    c) Health system redesign rules
        (1) Relationship-based care
        (2) Individualized patient care based on needs and values
        (3) Patient as source of control

(4) Shared knowledge and information

(5) Evidence-based decision making

(6) System focus on safety

(7) Transparency regarding system performance

(8) Anticipation of patient needs

(9) Reduction of waste

(10) Cooperation among clinicians

D. Principles of quality improvement (Massoud, 2013; U.S. DHHS, 2011)

  1. Understand the system and processes

    a) Quality improvement requires an understanding of the processes and systems within an organization.

    b) Effective quality improvement is individualized to the needs of the organization.

    c) Quality improvement in healthcare systems (Donabedian, 1980)

      (1) Structure: Resources and the attributes of the system

        (a) Organizational structure

        (b) People

        (c) Facilities

        (d) Financial resources

      (2) Process: Delivery of health care

        (a) What is done in providing and receiving care

        (b) How it is done

      (3) Outcomes: Result of health care

        (a) Patient behavior

        (b) Patient knowledge

        (c) Patient satisfaction

        (d) Health status of the patient or population

  2. Focus on teamwork

    a) Different members of the team provide expertise and insight to quality improvement.

      (1) Data entry and analysis

      (2) Operations

      (3) Clinical expertise

      (4) Leadership

    b) Team member involvement in quality improvement increases ownership.

  3. Use data

    a) Data should be used to establish current outcomes, identify areas of potential improvement, and monitor outcomes to determine if the change is an improvement.

    b) Data can be quantitative or qualitative.

  4. Focus on the patient: Improvements should aim to meet the needs and expectations of patients.

E. Quality improvement models

  1. Lean Model (Womack & Jones, 2003)

    a) Identifies value, as specified by the customer, and the steps necessary to provide value

    b) Creates continuous flow through the value-added steps

    c) Decreases steps that do not add value

  2. Model for Improvement (Langley et al., 2009)

a) Asks three questions to determine the aim or goal, identify measures of success, and select a change for improvement

b) Incorporates a Plan-Do-Study-Act cycle to test series of incremental changes

c) Functions as a continuous process in which lessons learned in each cycle contribute to subsequent cycles

d) Establishes a relationship between changes in process and outcome

3. FADE (U.S. DHHS, 2011)

    a) Four steps: Focus, analyze, develop, and execute

    b) Focuses on the process

4. Six Sigma (Munro, Maio, Nawaz, Ramu, & Zrymiak, 2008)

    a) Uses data and statistical analysis to improve processes and reduce variation

    b) Five steps: Define, measure, analyze, improve, and control

    c) By controlling aspects of a process, nurses can control the outcome.

Key Points

- Since Florence Nightingale founded modern nursing in the 1800s, the profession has continued to evolve in response to cultural, societal, and political changes, as well as advancements in technology, scientific knowledge, and theoretical basis for practice.

- As the number of hematopoietic stem cell transplantations (HSCTs) worldwide and indications for transplantation increase, it is especially vital for HSCT nurses to maintain specialized knowledge and ethical practice regarding this unique patient population.

- Autonomous nursing practice and collaboration with members of the healthcare team are required to lead change and advance health for HSCT donors and recipients. The American Nurses Association and Oncology Nursing Society have developed the scope of practice in general and advanced practice oncology nursing; these documents describe the activities performed by nurses caring for patients with cancer.

- Standards of nursing practice and professional performance are minimum competencies required by nurses and provide a framework for evaluation.

- For the evaluation of quality within a healthcare organization, accrediting agencies such as the Joint Commission develop practice standards and assess organizations based on the standards.

- The European Society for Blood and Marrow Transplantation (EBMT) and International Society for Cellular Therapy (ISCT) have founded the Joint Accreditation Committee-ISCT & EBMT (JACIE). The Foundation for the Accreditation of Cellular Therapy collaborates with JACIE to evaluate the quality of care provided by healthcare organizations to HSCT donors and recipients. Potential ethical and legal issues are common in HSCT nursing.

- Because of the severity of illness, risks associated with transplantation, and relatively younger patient population, nurses caring for these patients must be familiar with the ethical principles of autonomy, beneficence, nonmaleficence, and justice.

- In the case of conflicting ethical principles or moral distress, nurses are advocates for patients, families, and healthcare providers. Legal requirements vary at the local, state, national, and international levels, and each nurse has a professional responsibility to practice according to applicable laws.

- Scientific knowledge advances through clinical trials by testing an intervention to determine the safety and efficacy. Nurses may be involved in the development or coordination of trials or provide care to patients who participate in clinical trials.
- The domains of clinical trial nursing include clinical practice, human subjects protection, contribution to science, care coordination, and study management.
- Evidence from clinical trials, research, internal experts, and patient preferences must be incorporated into nursing practice to provide high-quality care to patients.
- Evidence-based practice requires a culture that promotes clinical inquiry.
- Continuous quality improvement must occur to ensure best practice in HSCT nursing.

Recommended Resources

The following websites provide extensive resources for nurses and patients.
- American Society for Blood and Marrow Transplantation: www.asbmt.org
- Blood and Marrow Transplant InfoNet: www.bmtinfonet.org/resources
- Center for International Blood and Marrow Transplant Research: www.cibmtr.org/pages/index.aspx
- Cleveland Clinic: http://my.clevelandclinic.org/health/treatments_and_procedures
- Leukemia and Lymphoma Society: www.lls.org
- Miceli, T., Lilleby, K., Noonan, K., Kurtin, S., Faiman, B., & Mangan, P.A. (2013). Hematopoietic stem cell transplantation and multiple myeloma: From the International Myeloma Foundation Nurse Leadership Board supplement. *Clinical Journal of Oncology Nursing, 17*(Suppl. 6), 7–11. Available at https://cjon.ons.org/cjon/17/6/supplement/autologous-hematopoietic-stem-cell-transplantation-patients-multiple-myeloma/html/full
- National Marrow Donor Program: https://bethematch.org/for-patients-and-families and www.marrow.org/md-guidelines

---

References

American Association of Critical-Care Nurses. (n.d.). The 4A's to rise above moral distress. Retrieved from http://www.aacn.org/WD/Practice/Docs/4As_to_Rise_Above_Moral_Distress.pdf

American Association of Critical-Care Nurses. (2008). AACN position statement: Moral distress. Retrieved from http://www.aacn.org/wd/practice/docs/moral_distress.pdf

American Nurses Association. (2010). *Nursing's social policy statement: The essence of the profession.* Silver Spring, MD: Author.

American Nurses Association. (2015a). *Code of ethics for nurses with interpretive statements.* Silver Spring, MD: Author.

American Nurses Association. (2015b). *Nursing: Scope and standards of practice.* Silver Spring, MD: Author.

American Nurses Association & National Council of State Boards of Nursing. (2006). Joint statement on delegation. Retrieved from https://www.ncsbn.org/Delegation_joint_statement_NCSBN-ANA.pdf

American Society for Blood and Marrow Transplantation. (2011). ASBMT research priorities. Retrieved from http://www.asbmt.org

Beauchamp, T.L., & Childress, J.F. (2013). *Principles of biomedical ethics* (7th ed.). New York, NY: Oxford University Press.

Black, B.P. (2011). Legal aspects of nursing. In K.K. Chitty & B.P. Black (Eds.), *Professional nursing: Concepts and challenges* (6th ed., pp. 77–98). Maryland Heights, MO: Elsevier Saunders.

Blood and Marrow Transplant Clinical Trials Network. (2015). *Blood and Marrow Transplant Clinical Trials Network progress report 2015.* Retrieved from https://web.emmes.com/study/bmt2/public/Progress%20report/BMT%20CTN%20Progress%20Report%202015.pdf

Brant, J.M., & Wickham, R. (Eds.). (2013). *Statement on the scope and standards of oncology nursing practice: Generalist and advanced practice.* Pittsburgh, PA: Oncology Nursing Society.

Chen, S.-H., Wang, T.-F., & Yang, K.-L. (2013). Hematopoietic stem cell donation. *International Journal of Hematology, 97,* 446–455. doi:10.1007/s12185-013-1298-8

Chitty, K.K., & Black, B.P. (Eds.). (2011). *Professional nursing: Concepts and challenges* (6th ed.). Maryland Heights, MO: Elsevier Saunders.

Clinical Research Nursing 2010 Domain of Practice Committee. (2009). *Building the foundation for clinical research nursing: Domain of practice for the specialty of clinical research nursing.* Retrieved from http://www.cc.nih.gov/nursing/crn/DOP_document.pdf

Coetzee, S.K., & Klopper, H.C. (2010). Compassion fatigue within nursing practice: A concept analysis. *Nursing and Health Sciences, 12,* 235–243. doi:10.1111/j.1442-2018.2010.00526.x

Cooke, L., Gemmill, R., Kravits, K., & Grant, M. (2009). Psychological issues of stem cell transplant. *Seminars in Oncology Nursing, 259,* 139–150. doi:10.1016/j.soncn.2009.03.008

Donabedian, A. (1980). *Explorations in Quality Assessment and Monitoring: Vol. 1. The definition of quality and approaches to its assessment.* Ann Arbor, MI: Health Administration Press.

D'Souza, A., Pasquini, M., & Spellecy, R. (2015). Is 'informed consent' an 'understood consent' in hematopoietic cell transplantation? *Bone Marrow Transplantation, 50,* 10–40. doi:10.1038/bmt.2014.207

Figley, C.R. (2002a). Compassion fatigue: Psychotherapists' chronic lack of self-care. *Journal of Clinical Psychology, 58,* 1433–1441. doi:10.1002/jclp.10090

Figley, C.R. (2002b). Introduction. In C.R. Figley (Ed.), *Treating compassion fatigue* (pp. 1–16). New York, NY: Brunner-Routledge.

Fineout-Overholt, E., Melnyk, B.M., Stillwell, S.B., & Williamson, K.M. (2010). Evidence-based practice step by step: Critical appraisal of the evidence: Part I. *American Journal of Nursing, 110*(7), 47–52. doi:10.1097/01.NAJ.0000383935.22721.9c

Foundation for the Accreditation of Cellular Therapy & Joint Accreditation Committee-ISCT & EBMT. (2012). *International standards for cellular therapy product collection, processing, and administration: Accreditation manual* [v.5.3]. Retrieved from https://www.factweb.org/forms/store/ProductFormPublic/search?action=1&Product_productNumber=621

Gratwohl, A., Brand, R., McGrath, E., van Biezen, A., Sureda, A., Ljungman, P., … Apperley, J. (2014). Use of the quality management system "JACIE" and outcome after hematopoietic stem cell transplantation. *Haematologica, 99,* 908–915. doi:10.3324/haematol.2013.096461

Gutierrez, K.M. (2005). Critical care nurses' perceptions of and responses to moral distress. *Dimensions of Critical Care Nursing, 24,* 229–241. doi:10.1097/00003465-200509000-00011

Hamric, A.B. (2001). Reflections on being in the middle. *Nursing Outlook, 49,* 254–257. doi:10.1067/mno.2001.120247

Hamric, A.B., Borchers, C.T., & Epstein, E.G. (2012). Development and testing of an instrument to measure moral distress in healthcare professionals. *American Journal of Bioethics Primary Research, 3*(2), 1–9. doi:10.1080/21507716.2011.652337

Houle, C.O. (1980). *Continuing learning in the professions.* San Francisco, CA: Jossey-Bass.

Institute of Medicine. (2001). *Crossing the quality chasm: A new health system for the 21st century.* Washington, DC: National Academies Press.

International Council of Nurses. (2012). *The ICN code of ethics for nurses.* Retrieved from http://www.icn.ch/images/stories/documents/about/icncode_english.pdf

Jacoby, L.H., Maloy, B., Cirenza, E., Shelton, W., Goggins, T., & Balint, J. (1999). The basis of informed consent for BMT patients. *Bone Marrow Transplantation, 23,* 711–717. doi:10.1038/sj.bmt.1701631

Jameton, A. (1984). *Nursing practice: The ethical issues.* Englewood Cliffs, NJ: Prentice-Hall.

Joffe, S., Mello, M.M., Cook, E.F., & Lee, S.J. (2007). Advance care planning in patients undergoing hematopoietic cell transplantation. *Biology of Blood and Marrow Transplantation, 13,* 65–73. doi:10.1016/j.bbmt.2006.08.042

Joint Commission. (2009). *Implementation guide for the NQF endorsed nursing-sensitive care measure set.* Retrieved from http://www.jointcommission.org/assets/1/6/NSC%20Manual.pdf

Khan, S., Juckett, M.B., Komanduri, K.V., Krishnan, A., & Burns, L.J. (2012). American Society of Blood and Marrow Transplantation guidelines for training in hematopoietic progenitor cell transplantation. *Biology of Blood and Marrow Transplantation, 18,* 1322–1328. doi:10.1016/j.bbmt.2012.04.007

Langley, G.L., Moen, R.D., Nolan, K.M., Nolan, T.W., Norman, C.L., & Provost, L.P. (2009). *The improvement guide: A practical approach to enhancing organizational performance* (2nd ed.). San Francisco, CA: Jossey-Bass.

La Puma, J., Orentlicher, D., & Moss, R.J. (1991). Advance directives on admission: Clinical implications and analysis of the Patient Self-Determination Act of 1990. *JAMA, 266,* 402–405. doi:10.1001/jama.1991.03470030102032

Loggers, E.T., Lee, S., Chilson, K., Back, A.L., Block, S., & Loberiza, F.R. (2014). Advance care planning among hematopoietic cell transplant patients and bereaved caregivers. *Bone Marrow Transplantation, 49,* 1317–1322. doi:10.1038/bmt.2014.152

Massoud, M.R.F. (2013). *Advances in quality improvement: Principles and framework.* Retrieved from http://www .smbs.buffalo.edu/GME/pdf/Advances_in_Quality_Improvement.pdf

Melnyk, B.M., & Fineout-Overholt, E. (2005). *ARCC: Advancing research and clinical practice through close collaboration.* Gilbert, AZ: ARCC Publishing.

Melnyk, B.M., & Fineout-Overholt, E. (2015). *Evidence-based practice in nursing and healthcare: A guide to best practice* (3rd ed.). Philadelphia, PA: Wolters Kluwer Health/Lippincott Williams & Wilkins.

Munro, R.A., Maio, M.J., Nawaz, M.B., Ramu, G., & Zrymiak, D.J. (Eds.). (2008). *The certified Six Sigma green belt handbook.* Milwaukee, WI: ASQ Quality Press.

National Cancer Institute. (2013). Advance directives. Retrieved from http://www.cancer.gov/about-cancer/managing -care/advance-directives

National Council of State Boards of Nursing. (2011). *A nurse's guide to professional boundaries.* Retrieved from https:// www.ncsbn.org/ProfessionalBoundaries_Complete.pdf

National Hospice and Palliative Care Organization. (2008). *Understanding advance directives.* Retrieved from http:// www.caringinfo.org/files/public/brochures/Understanding_Advance_Directives.pdf

National Institutes of Health. (2012). Learn about clinical studies. Retrieved from https://clinicaltrials.gov/ct2/ about-studies/learn

Neuss, M.N., Polovich, M., McNiff, K., Esper, P., Gilmore, T.R., LeFebvre, K.B., ... Jacobson, J.O. (2013). 2013 updated American Society of Clinical Oncology/Oncology Nursing Society chemotherapy administration safety standards including standards for the safe administration and management of oral chemotherapy. *Oncology Nursing Forum, 40,* 225–233. doi:10.1188/13.ONF.40-03AP2

Newhouse, R.P., Dearholt, S.L., Poe, S.S., Pugh, L.C., & White, K.M. (2007). *Johns Hopkins nursing evidence-based practice model and guidelines.* Indianapolis, IN: Sigma Theta Tau International.

Oncology Nursing Society. (2010). *Oncology clinical trials nurse competencies.* Retrieved from http://www.ons.org/sites/ default/files/ctncompetencies.pdf

Oncology Nursing Society. (2014). Lifelong learning for professional oncology nurses [Position statement]. Retrieved from https://www.ons.org/advocacy-policy/positions/education/lifelong

Oncology Nursing Society. (2015). Education of the nurse who administers and cares for the individual receiving chemotherapy and biotherapy [Position statement]. Retrieved from https://www.ons.org/advocacy-policy/positions/ education/chemotherapy-biotherapy

Purtilo, R., & Doherty, R. (2011). *Ethical dimensions in the health professions* (5th ed.). St. Louis, MO: Elsevier Saunders.

Russell, K.A. (2012). Nurse practice acts guide and govern nursing practice. *Journal of Nursing Regulation, 3*(3), 36–42. doi:10.1016/S2155-8256(15)30197-6

Schmidt, N.A., & Brown, J.M. (2015). What is evidence-based practice? In N.A. Schmidt & J.M. Brown (Eds.), *Evidence-based practice for nurses: Appraisal and application of research* (3rd ed., pp. 3–42). Burlington, MA: Jones & Bartlett Learning.

Snyder, D.S. (2009). Ethical issues in hematopoietic cell transplantation. In F.R. Appelbaum, S.J. Forman, R.S. Negrin, & K.G. Blume (Eds.), *Thomas' hematopoietic cell transplantation: Stem cell transplantation* (4th ed., pp. 478–487). Oxford, UK: Wiley-Blackwell.

Styles, M.M., Schumann, M.J., Bickford, C., & White, K.M. (2008). *Specialization and credentialing in nursing revisited: Understanding the issues, advancing the profession.* Silver Spring, MD: Nursesbooks.org.

Titler, M.G., Kleiber, C., Steelman, V.J., Rakel, B.A., Budreau, G., Everett, L.Q., ... Goode, C.J. (2001). The Iowa model of evidence-based practice to promote quality care. *Critical Care Nursing Clinics of North America, 13,* 497–509.

U.S. Department of Health and Human Services. (2003). Summary of the HIPAA privacy rule. Retrieved from http://www.hhs.gov/hipaa/for-professionals/privacy/laws-regulations

U.S. Department of Health and Human Services. (2009a). Office for Human Research Protections. Retrieved from http://www.hhs.gov/ohrp/about/facts/ohrpfactsheetdec09.pdf.pdf

U.S. Department of Health and Human Services. (2009b). Protection of human subjects (45 C.F.R. pt. 46). Retrieved from http://www.hhs.gov/ohrp/humansubjects/guidance/45cfr46.html

U.S. Department of Health and Human Services Health Resources and Services Administration. (2011). *Quality improvement.* Retrieved from http://www.hrsa.gov/quality/toolbox/508pdfs/qualityimprovement.pdf

U.S. Food and Drug Administration. (2013a). Inside clinical trials: Testing medical products in people. Retrieved from http://www.fda.gov/Drugs/ResourcesForYou/Consumers/ucm143531.htm

U.S. Food and Drug Administration. (2013b). Office of Good Clinical Practice. Retrieved from http://www.fda .gov/AboutFDA/CentersOffices/OfficeofMedicalProductsandTobacco/OfficeofScienceandHealthCoordination/ ucm2018191.htm

Westrick, S.J., & Dempski, K. (2009). *Essentials of nursing law and ethics.* Burlington, MA: Jones & Bartlett Learning.

Wilkinson, K. (2012). Informed consent and patients with cancer: Role of the nurse as advocate. *Clinical Journal of Oncology Nursing, 16,* 348–350. doi:10.1188/12.CJON.348-350

Womack, J., & Jones, D. (2003). *Lean thinking: Banish waste and create wealth in your corporation, revised and updated.* New York, NY: Simon & Schuster.

World Health Organization. (n.d.). International Clinical Trials Registry Platform: Glossary. Retrieved from http:// www.who.int/ictrp/glossary/en

Study Questions

1. A patient with multiple myeloma is receiving high-dose melphalan. The nurse has the patient chew on ice during the infusion to reduce the risk of mucositis. This is an example of which of the following?
   A. A clinical trial
   B. Evidence-based practice
   C. Outcome identification
   D. Research

2. In *Statement on the Scope and Standards of Oncology Nursing Practice: Generalist and Advanced Practice*, Standard XII states that nurses should display leadership in the nursing profession and healthcare setting. Which of the following measurement criteria supports this standard?
   A. The nurse evaluates how his or her personal beliefs and values influence practice.
   B. The nurse incorporates research findings into practice.
   C. The nurse sets professional goals and evaluates progress and completion of goals.
   D. The nurse participates in a professional organization and mentors colleagues interested in obtaining a specialty certification.

3. A patient is participating in a phase II clinical trial and states, "I don't think I can do this anymore." What would be the nurse's best response?
   A. "You have already agreed to participate and signed the informed consent."
   B. "OK. I will tell the physician that you are dropping out of the trial."
   C. "Can you tell me more about your concerns?"
   D. "You will feel better soon."

4. A patient with grade IV gastrointestinal graft-versus-host disease states that he does not want to receive parenteral nutrition, but his wife disagrees with his decision. The wife states, "You can't let my husband starve to death." What ethical principle applies in this situation?
   A. Respect for autonomy
   B. Nonmaleficence
   C. Confidentiality
   D. Privacy

5. An advanced practice hematopoietic stem cell transplantation (HSCT) nurse is going to move from Texas to Indiana and would like to determine the requirements for licensure in Indiana. What would be the best resource?
   A. The policies and procedures at the hiring hospital
   B. The state's nurse practice act
   C. A national professional nursing organization
   D. The Foundation for the Accreditation of Cellular Therapy

6. Because of an increase in central line–associated bloodstream infections in HSCT patients, an advanced practice nurse formed an interdisciplinary team. The team established a goal and analyzed current data, practice, research, and guidelines. What would be the next step?
   A. Continue to collect data.
   B. Apply for a grant to study central line–associated bloodstream infections in HSCT recipients.
   C. Select a change in practice or process.
   D. Define central line–associated bloodstream infections.

7. Which of the following is a violation of professional boundaries?
   A. The nurse stays after his or her scheduled shift to assist with a bone marrow biopsy.
   B. The nurse discusses his or her children with patients.
   C. The nurse is grieving a recent loss and asks a patient for advice about coping.
   D. The patient requests to be assigned to a particular nurse.

8. A nurse is caring for a patient with severe thrombocytopenia. While the nurse and patient were walking in the hallway, the patient fell and developed intracranial hemorrhaging as a result of the fall. Over the next few weeks, the nurse had difficulty sleeping, missed work, and avoided walking in the hallway with patients. The nurse's actions are an example of what?
   A. Compassion fatigue
   B. Moral distress
   C. Violation in professional boundaries
   D. Malpractice

Answer Key

Chapter 1. Basic Concepts and Indications for Transplantation

1. C	3. A	5. D	7. D
2. B	4. C	6. C	

Chapter 2. Types of Transplants and Sources of Stem Cells

1. D	2. A	3. A

Chapter 3. Pretransplant Issues

1. B	2. C	3. D

Chapter 4. Transplant Preparative Regimens, Cellular Infusion, Acute Complications, and Engraftment

1. C	4. A	7. C	10. D
2. D	5. C	8. A	11. B
3. D	6. B	9. A	12. C

Chapter 5. Graft-Versus-Host Disease

1. D. The patient's immunosuppressive drugs need to be at a therapeutic level. Try to use as little additional immunosuppression as is necessary to control GVHD so as to maintain allo-effect of the transplant against any residual leukemia. Often, grade 1 or 2 skin GVHD responds to topical steroids.
2. C. Infectious etiology must always be ruled out (e.g., *Clostridium difficile* [*C. difficile*], rotavirus). Medications should be changed from PO to IV to ensure absorption. GI consult to follow and assess need for colonoscopy. GI GVHD grading is based on volume of stool, so an accurate assessment of amount of diarrhea is important. Once *C. difficile* is ruled out, antidiarrheal agents may be started.
3. A
4. B. No preferred second-line therapy with acute GVHD currently exists. It often is physician or institution preference. Any of the drugs in B are acceptable. No data show that increasing steroids above 2 mg/kg per day is effective.
5. D
6. D. The Rule of Nines determines that her chest is 9% and her bilateral arms are 9% anteriorly and 9% posteriorly. It would need to be known whether the patient's front or back of arms are involved. If only C.W.'s anterior arms are involved, the total surface area is 18%. If both front and back of arms are involved, the total surface area is 36%.
7. C. Skin: Using the Rule of Nines, the body surface area (BSA) is 9% on C.W.'s chest and 9% on her back. Her face is 4.5%, and arms are 9% anteriorly and 9% posteriorly. Total BSA is 40.5%, which is stage 2. GI: She has 1–2 L of diarrhea/24 hours, which is stage 2–3. The Eastern Cooperative Oncology Group performance status is 2 at best (i.e., out of bed to chair only once a day). Therefore, C.W. is stage 2 skin and stage 3 GI. Overall grading of GVHD is grade 3.
8. D
9. D

10. C. The drug–drug interaction is related to cytochrome P450, and the patient will not require as much CNI to maintain therapeutic levels.
11. A
12. D
13. C
14. C
15. D
16. A
17. A
18. D
19. D
20. A
21. C
22. A
23. D. The exact pathophysiology of chronic GVHD is not understood, but hypotheses include cytokine dysregulation, T-lymphocyte imbalances, and high levels of cytokines—including IL-2, IL-6, and TNF-α. Research also is focusing now on the role of B cells in chronic GVHD.
24. B. Infections and long-term immunosuppression places patients at high risk for developing infectious complications such as pneumonia (PCP or viral), CMV, and fungal and encapsulated organisms.
25. D. Most cases of chronic GVHD are diagnosed within the first year, with median of four to six months after transplant. Traditionally, chronic GVHD has been defined as occurring after day 100 post-HSCT; however, recent recommendations are to base diagnosis on clinical features rather than time of occurrence.
26. A. Prior acute GVHD is the strongest risk factor, and the risk of developing chronic GVHD increases with increasing severity of acute GVHD. Even patients with mild grade 1 acute GVHD have significantly increased risk of chronic GVHD. However, chronic GVHD may develop in patients who have not had acute GVHD.
27. B
28. D
29. D
30. A
31. D
32. B
33. D
34. D
35. E
36. D
37. F
38. D
39. B
40. E

Chapter 6. Post-Transplant Issues

1. D
2. B
3. C
4. A
5. B
6. A
7. B
8. D
9. D
10. C
11. B
12. E
13. A
14. B
15. A
16. E
17. E
18. D
19. A
20. E
21. E
22. A
23. D
24. A
25. B
26. D
27. C
28. A
29. C
30. B
31. A
32. C
33. B
34. C
35. A
36. C
37. A
38. D
39. D
40. A. Polys (22%) + bands (4%) × white blood cells (2,100) = 546
41. C
42. A
43. A
44. D
45. C
46. A. According to National Cancer Institute Common Terminology Criteria for Adverse Events grading for diarrhea, grade 2 is an increase of 4–6 stools per day over baseline.
47. B
48. D
49. A
50. B
51. C
52. B
53. C
54. C
55. C
56. E
57. A
58. D

Chapter 7. Survivorship Issues

1. D	7. B	13. B	19. B
2. C	8. C	14. C	20. D
3. D	9. D	15. C	21. B
4. A	10. B	16. A	
5. C	11. A	17. A	
6. C	12. C	18. B	

Chapter 8. Professional Practice

1. B	3. C	5. B	7. C
2. D	4. A	6. C	8. A

Index

The letter *f* after a page number indicates that relevant content appears in a figure; the letter *t,* in a table.